Mental Health Nursing

Reviews & Rationales

Mary Ann Hogan, RN, CS, MSN

Clinical Assistant Professor
University of Massachusetts, Amherst

George Byron Smith, ARNP, MSN, PhD(c)

Instructor of Nursing
Hillsborough Community College
Tampa, Florida

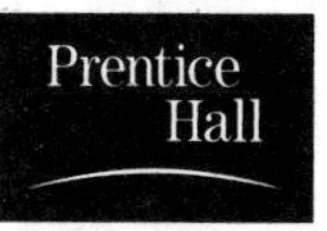

Upper Saddle River, New Jersey 07458

Library of Congress Cataloging-in-Publication Data

Mental health nursing: reviews & rationales / [edited by] Mary Ann Hogan, George Byron Smith
p.; cm.
Includes bibliographical references and index.
ISBN: 0-13-0300458-1
1. Psychiatric nursing.
[DNLM: 1. Mental Disorders–nursing. 2. Psychiatric Nursing–methods. WY 160 M5487 2003] I. Hogan, Mary Ann, MSN. II. Smith, George Byron.
RC440.M3545 2003
610.73'68–dc21

2002002266

Publisher: Julie Levin Alexander
Assistant to Publisher: Regina Bruno
Executive Editor: Maura Connor
Managing Development Editor: Marilyn Meserve
Development Editor: Jeanne Allison
Director of Production and Manufacturing: Bruce Johnson
Managing Production Editor: Patrick Walsh
Production Liaison: Danielle Newhouse
Production Editor: Jessica Balch, Pine Tree Composition
Manufacturing Buyer: Pat Brown
Design Director: Cheryl Asherman
Design Coordinator: Maria Guglielmo
Interior Designer: Jill Little
Cover Designer: Joseph DePinho
Electronic Art Creation: Precision Graphics
Marketing Manager: Nicole Benson
Assistant Editor: Yesenia Kopperman
Editorial Assistant: Sladjana Repic
Production Information Manager: Rachele Triano
Media Editor: Sarah Hayday
New Media Production Manager: Amy Peltier
New Media Project Manager: Stephen Hartner
Composition: Pine Tree Composition, Inc.
Printer/Binder: Courier/Westford

Pearson Education Ltd., *London*
Pearson Education Australia Pty. Limited, *Sydney*
Pearson Education Singapore, Pte. Ltd.
Pearson Education North Asia Ltd., *Hong Kong*
Pearson Education Canada, Ltd., *Toronto*
Pearson Educaión de Mexico, S.A. de C.V.
Pearson Education—Japan, *Tokyo*
Pearson Education Malaysia, Pte. Ltd.
Pearson Education, Upper Saddle River, New Jersey

Notice: Care has been taken to confirm the accuracy of the information presented in this book. The authors, editors, and the publisher, however, cannot accept any responsibility for errors or omissions or for the consequences for application of the information in this book and make no warranty, express or implied, with respect to its contents.

The authors and the publisher have exerted every effort to ensure that drug selections and dosages set forth in this text are in accord with current recommendations and practice at time of publication. However, in view of ongoing research, changes in government regulations, and the constant flow of information relating to drug therapy and drug reactions, the reader is urged to check the pakage inserts of all drugs for any change in indications of dosage and for added warnings and precautions. This is particularly important when the recommended agent is a new and/or infrequently employed drug.

The authors and publisher disclaim all responsibility for any liability, loss, injury, or damage incorred as a consequence, directly or indirectly, of the use and application of any of the contents of this volume.

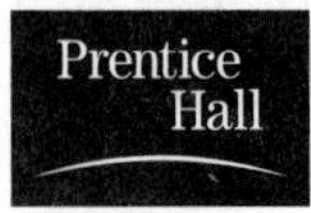

10 9 8 7 6 5
ISBN 0-13-030458-1

Contents

Preface

INTRODUCTION

Welcome to the new Prentice Hall Reviews and Rationales Series! This 9-book series has been specifically designed to provide a clear and concentrated review of important nursing knowledge in the following content areas:

- Child Health Nursing
- Maternal-Newborn Nursing
- Mental Health Nursing
- Medical-Surgical Nursing
- Pathophysiology
- Pharmacology
- Fundamentals and Skills
- Nutrition and Diet Therapy
- Fluid, Electrolyte, & Acid-Base Balance

The books in this series have been designed for use either by current nursing students as a study aid for nursing course work or NCLEX-RN licensing exam preparation, or by practicing nurses seeking a comprehensive yet concise review of a nursing specialty or subject area.

This series is truly unique. One of its most special features is that it has been authored by a large team of nurse educators from across the United States and Canada to ensure that each chapter is written by a nurse expert in the content area under study. Prentice Hall Health representatives from across North America submitted names of nurse educators and/or clinicians who excel in their respective fields, and these authors were then invited to write a chapter in one or more books. The consulting editor for each book, who is also an expert in that specialty area, then reviewed all chapters submitted for comprehensiveness and accuracy. The series editor designed the overall series in collaboration with a core Prentice Hall team to take full advantage of Prentice Hall's cutting edge technology, and also reviewed the chapters in each book.

All books in the series are identical in their overall design for your convenience (further details follow at the end of this section). As an added value, each book comes with a comprehensive support package, including free CD-ROM, free companion website access, and a Nursing Notes card for quick clinical reference.

Study Tips

Use of this review book should help simplify your study. To make the most of your valuable study time, also follow these simple but important suggestions:

- Use a weekly calendar to schedule study sessions.
  - Outline the timeframes for all of your activities (home, school, appointments, etc.) on a weekly calendar.
  - Find the "holes" in your calendar—the times in which you can plan to study. Add study sessions to the calendar at times when you can expect to be mentally alert and follow it!
- Create the optimal study environment.
  - Eliminate external sources of distraction, such as television, telephone, etc.
  - Eliminate internal sources of distraction, such as hunger, thirst, or dwelling on items or problems that cannot be worked on at the moment.
  - Take a break for 10 minutes or so after each hour of concentrated study both as a reward and an incentive to keep studying.
- Use pre-reading strategies to increase comprehension of chapter material.
  - Skim the headings in the chapter (because they identify chapter content).
  - Read the definitions of key terms, which will help you learn new words to comprehend chapter information.
  - Review all graphic aids (figures, tables, boxes) because they are often used to explain important points in the chapter.
- Read the chapter thoroughly but at a reasonable speed.
  - Comprehension and retention are actually enhanced by not reading too slowly.
  - Do take the time to reread any section that is unclear to you.
- Summarize what you have learned.
  - Use questions supplied with this book, CD-ROM, and companion website to test your recall of chapter content.
  - Review again any sections that correspond to questions you answered incorrectly or incompletely.

Test Taking Strategies

Use the following strategies to increase your success on multiple-choice nursing tests or examinations:

- Get sufficient sleep and have something to eat before taking a test. Take deep breaths during the test as needed. Remember, the brain requires oxygen and glucose as fuel. Avoid concentrated sweets before a test, however, to avoid rapid upward and then downward surges in blood glucose levels.
- Read each question carefully, identifying the stem, the four options, and any key words or phrases in either the stem or options.
  - Key words in the stem such as "most important" indicate the need to set priorities, since more than one option is likely to contain a statement that is technically correct.
  - Remember that the presence of absolute words such as "never" or "only" in an option is more likely to make that option incorrect.

- Determine who is the client in the question; often this is the person with the health problem, but it may also be a significant other, relative, friend, or another nurse.
- Decide whether the stem is a true response stem or a false response stem. With a true response stem, the correct answer will be a true statement, and vice-versa.
- Determine what the question is really asking, sometimes referred to as the issue of the question. Evaluate all answer options in relation to this issue, and not strictly to the "correctness" of the statement in each individual option.
- Eliminate options that are obviously incorrect, then go back and reread the stem. Evaluate the remaining options against the stem once more.
- If two answers seem similar and correct, try to decide whether one of them is more global or comprehensive. If the global option includes the alternative option within it, it is likely that the more global response is the correct answer.

THE NCLEX-RN LICENSING EXAMINATION

The NCLEX-RN licensing examination is a Computer Adaptive Test (CAT) that ranges in length from 75 to 265 individual (stand-alone) test items, depending on individual performance during the examination. Upon graduation from a nursing program, successful completion of this exam is the gateway to your professional nursing practice. The blueprint for the exam is reviewed and revised every three years by the National Council of State Boards of Nursing according to the results of a job analysis study of new graduate nurses (practicing within the first six months after graduation). Each question on the exam is coded to one *Client Need Category* and one or more *Integrated Concepts and Processes.*

Client Need Categories

There are 4 categories of client needs, and each exam will contain a minimum and maximum percent of questions from each category. Each major category has subcategories within it. The *Client Need* categories according to the NCLEX-RN Test Plan effective April 2001 are as follows:

- Safe, Effective Care Environment
  - Management of Care (7–13%)
  - Safety and Infection Control (5–11%)
- Health Promotion and Maintenance
  - Growth and Development Throughout the Lifespan (7–13%)
  - Prevention and Early Detection of Disease (5–11%)
- Psychosocial Integrity
  - Coping and Adaptation (5–11%)
  - Psychosocial Adaptation (5–11%)
- Physiological Integrity
  - Basic Care and Comfort (7–13%)
  - Pharmacological and Parenteral Therapies (5–11%)
  - Reduction of Risk Potential (12–18%)
  - Physiological Adaptation (12–18%)

Integrated Concepts and Processes

The integrated concepts and processes identified on the NCLEX-RN Test Plan effective April 2001, with condensed definitions, are as follows:

- Nursing Process: a scientific problem-solving approach used in nursing practice; consisting of assessment, analysis, planning, implementation, and evaluation.

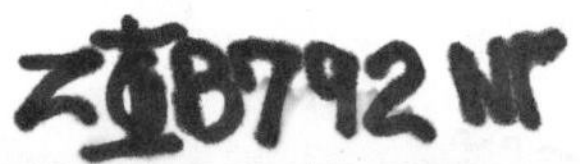

- Caring: client-nurse interaction(s) characterized by mutual respect and trust and directed toward achieving desired client outcomes.
- Communication and Documentation: verbal and/or nonverbal interactions between nurse and others (client, family, health care team); a written or electronic recording of activities or events that occur during client care.
- Cultural Awareness: knowledge and sensitivity to the client's beliefs/values and how these might impact on the client's healthcare experience.
- Self-Care: assisting clients to meet their health care needs, which may include maintaining health or restoring function.
- Teaching/Learning: facilitating client's acquisition of knowledge, skills, and attitudes that lead to behavior change.

More detailed information about this examination may be obtained by visiting the National Council of State Boards of Nursing website at http://www.ncsbn.org and viewing the *NCLEX-RN Examination Test Plan for the National Council Licensure Examination for Registered Nurses.* *

How to Get the Most Out of This Book

Chapter Organization

Each chapter has the following elements to guide you during review and study:

- Chapter Objectives: describe what you will be able to know or do after learning the material covered in the chapter.

Objectives

- Review basic principles of growth and development.
- Describe major physical expectations for each developmental age group.
- Identify developmental milestones for various age groups.
- Discuss the reactions to illness and hospitalization for children at various stages of development.

- Review at a Glance: contains a glossary of key terms used in the chapter, with definitions provided up-front and available at your fingertips, to help you stay focused and make the best use of your study time.

Review at a Glance

anticipatory guidance *the process of understanding upcoming developmental needs and then teaching caregivers to meet those needs*

cephalocaudal development *the process by which development proceeds from the head downward through the body and towards the feet*

chronological age *age in years*

critical periods *times when an individual is especially responsive to certain environmental effects, sometimes called sensitive periods*

development *an increase in capability or function; a more complex concept that is a continuous, orderly series of conditions that lead to activities, new motives for activities; and eventual patterns of behavior*

developmental age *age based on functional behavior and ability to adapt to the environment; does not necessarily correspond to chronological age*

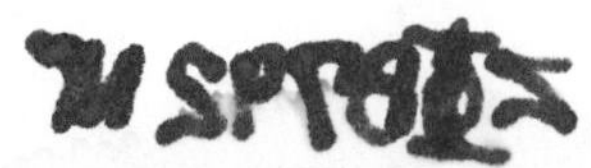

- Pretest: this 10-question multiple choice test provides a sample overview of content covered in the chapter and helps you decide what areas need the most—or the least—review.

Pretest

1 The nurse discusses dental care with the parents of a 3-year-old. The nurse explains that by the age of 3, their child should have:

(1) 5 "temporary" teeth.
(2) 10 "temporary" teeth.
(3) 15 "temporary" teeth.
(4) 20 "temporary" teeth.

2 The mother of a 6-month-old infant is concerned that the infant's anterior fontanel is still open. The nurse would inform the mother that further evaluation is needed if the anterior fontanel is open after:

(1) 6 months.
(2) 10 months.
(3) 18 months.
(4) 24 months.

- Practice to Pass questions: these are open-ended questions that stimulate critical thinking and reinforce mastery of the chapter content.

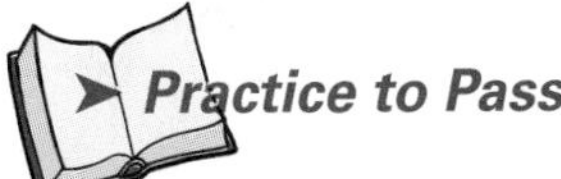

What would you explain as normal motor development for a 10-month old infant?

- NCLEX Alerts: the NCLEX icon identifies information or concepts that are likely to be tested on the NCLEX licensing examination. Be sure to learn the information flagged by this type of icon.

NCLEX!

- Case Study: found at the end of the chapter, it provides an opportunity for you to use your critical thinking and clinical reasoning skills to "put it all together;" it describes a true-to-life client case situation and asks you open-ended questions about how you would provide care for that client and/or family.

Case Study

A 6-month-old female infant is brought into the pediatric clinic for a well-baby visit. You as the pediatric nurse will be assigned to care for this family.

1. Identify the primary growth and development expectations for a 6-month-old.
2. What type common behavior is expected of this 6-month-old towards the nurse?
3. What immunization(s) are recommended at this age to maintain health and wellness?

For suggested responses, see page 406.

- Posttest: a 10-question multiple-choice test at the end of the chapter provides new questions that are representative of chapter content, and provide you with feedback about mastery of that content following review and study. All pretest and posttest questions contain rationales for the correct answer, and are coded according to the phase of the nursing process used and the NCLEX category of client need (called the Test Plan). The Test plan codes are PHYS (Physiological Integrity), PSYC (Psychosocial Integrity), SECE (Safe Effective Care Environment), and HPM (Health Promotion and Maintenance).

Posttest

1 When using the otoscope to examine the ears of a 2-year-old child, the nurse should:

(1) Pull the pinna up and back.
(2) Pull the pinna down and back.
(3) Hold the pinna gently but firmly in its normal position.
(4) Hold the pinna against the skull.

2 To assess the height of an 18-month-old child who is brought to the clinic for routine examination, the nurse should:

(1) Measure arm span to estimate adult height.
(2) Use a tape measure.
(3) Use a horizontal measuring board.
(4) Have the child stand on an upright scale and use the measuring arm.

CD-ROM

For those who want to practice taking tests on a computer, the CD-ROM that accompanies the book contains the pretest and posttest questions found in all chapters of the book. In addition, it contains 10 NEW questions for each chapter to help you further evaluate your knowledge base and hone your test-taking skills. In several chapters, one of the questions will have embedded art to use in answering the question. Some of the newly developed NCLEX test items are also designed in this way, so these items will give you valuable practice with this type of question.

Companion Website (CW)

The companion website is a "virtual" reference for virtually all your needs! The CW contains the following:

- 50 NCLEX-style questions: 10 pretest, 10 posttest, 10 CD-ROM, and 20 additional new questions
- Definitions of key terms: the glossary is also stored on the companion website for ease of reference
- In Depth With NCLEX: features drawings or photos that are each accompanied by a one- to two-paragraph explanation. These are especially useful when describing something that is complex, technical (such as equipment), or difficult to mentally visualize.
- Suggested Answers to Practice to Pass and Case Study Questions: easily located on the website, these allow for timely feedback for those who answer chapter questions on the web.

Nursing Notes Clinical Reference Card

This laminated card provides a reference for frequently used facts and information related to the subject matter of the book. These are designed to be useful in the clinical setting, when quick and easy access to information is so important!

About the Mental Health Nursing Book

Chapters in this book cover "need-to-know" information about mental health nursing, including major diagnostic categories. Additional chapters focus on special topics such as crisis intervention and suicide; victims of abuse; loss and grief; and the psychological adaptation to medical illness. Since mental health questions are unique and cause many students distress, Chapter 1 discusses effective test-taking techniques and strategies that will be specifically helpful when answering mental health questions. Mastery of the information in this book and effective use of the test-taking strategies described will help the student be confident and successful when answering psychosocial integrity questions on the NCLEX-RN.

Acknowledgments

This book is a monumental effort of collaboration. Without the contributions of many individuals, this first edition of *Mental Health Nursing: Reviews and Rationales* would not have been possible. We gratefully acknowledge all the contributors who devoted their time and talents to this book. Their chapters will surely assist both students and practicing nurses alike to extend their knowledge in the area of mental health.

We owe a special debt of gratitude to the wonderful team at Prentice Hall Health for their enthusiasm for this project, as well as their good humor, expertise, and encouragement as the series developed. Maura Connor, Executive Editor for Nursing, was unending in her creativity, support, encouragement, and belief in the need for this series. Marilyn Meserve, Senior Managing Editor for Nursing, devoted many long hours to coordinating different facets of this project, and tirelessly and cheerfully encouraged our efforts as well. Her high standards and attention to detail contributed greatly to the final "look" of this series. Jeanne Allison, Developmental Editor, actively kept in communication with the different writers in this book and also facilitated getting the book itself into production. Editorial assistants, including Beth Ann Romph, Sladjana Repic, and others, helped to keep the project moving forward on a day-to-day basis, and we are grateful for their efforts as well. A very special thank you goes to the designers of the book and the production team, led by Danielle Newhouse, who brought our ideas and manuscript into final form.

Thank you to the team at Pine Tree Composition, led by Project Coordinator Jessica Balch, for the detail-oriented work of creating this book. We greatly appreciate their hard work, attention to detail, and spirit of collaboration. A special thanks also goes to Yesenia Kopperman, Assistant Editor for Nursing at Prentice Hall, and to Carlos Cooper, Lisa Donovan, and staff at the Pearson Education Development Group for designing and producing the *Nursing Notes* clinical reference card that accompanies this book.

Mary Ann Hogan acknowledges and gratefully thanks husband Michael, and children Mike Jr., Katie, Kristen, and Billy, who sacrificed hours of time that would have been spent with them, to bring this book to publication. Your love and support kept me energized, motivated, and at times, even sane. I love you all!

George Byron Smith acknowledges and sends a special thank you to my family, who- have always believed in me and never faltered in their love and support. My family is surely "the wind beneath my wings." I particularly dedicate my work in this book to my mother, Patricia Ruth Smith, who has always been my role model in promoting mental health and in caring for others. I love you!

---

*Reference: National Council of State Boards of Nursing, Inc. *NCLEX Examination Test Plan for National Council Licensure Examination for Registered Nurses.* Effective April, 2001. Retrieved from the World Wide Web September 5, 2001 at http://www.ncsbn.org/public/resources/res/NCSBNRNTestPlan Booklet.pdf.

Contributors

Susan Bobek, RN, PhD
Associate Professor, Nursing
University of North Alabama
Florence, Alabama
Chapter 5

Jane E. Bostick, Doctoral Candidate, MSN, RN
Instructor of Clinical Nursing
Sinclair School of Nursing
University of Missouri – Columbia
Columbia, Missouri
Chapter 10

Sara L. Campbell, DNS, RN
Assistant Professor
Mennonite College of Nursing
at Illinois State University
Normal, Illinois
Chapter 14

Karma Castleberry, PhD, RN, APRN, BC
Professor, School of Nursing
Radford University
Radford, Virginia
Chapters 6 and 7

Pamela Gaurkee, RN, BSN
Residence Director
Alterra Wynwood
Bayside, Wisconsin
Chapter 3

David S. Hodson, RN, MS, ARNP
Instructor of Nursing
St. Petersburg Junior College
St. Petersburg, Florida
Chapter 1

Ann Koranda, RN, CNS, LADC, CGP
Clinical Nurse Specialist in Addiction Services
Mayo Foundation
Rochester, Minnesota
Chapter 11

Linda Manfrin-Ledet, APRN, MN, CS
Assistant Professor of Nursing
Nicholls State University
Thibodaux, Louisiana
Chapter 9

Lee Murray, MSN, RN, CS, CADAC
Assistant Professor of Nursing
Holyoke Community College
Holyoke, Massachusetts
Chapter 4

Marybeth O'Neil, RN, MSN, CS
Clinical Nurse Specialist
Mayo Foundation
Rochester, Minnesota
Chapter 12

Mark D. Soucy, MS, RN, CS
Assistant Professor
The University of Texas
Health Science Center
at San Antonio School of Nursing
San Antonio, Texas
Chapter 2

Carol Stubblefield, RN, PhD
Associate Professor of Nursing
Jewish Hospital College of Nursing and Allied Health
St. Louis, Missouri
Chapter 8

George Byron Smith, ARNP, MSN, PhD(C)
Instructor of Nursing
Hillsborough Community College
Tampa, Florida
Chapters 1 and 13

Reviewers

Diana M. Crowell, PhD, RN, CS, CNAA
Assistant Professor
University of New Hampshire
Durham, New Hampshire

Susan B. Del Bene, PhD, RN
Associate Professor
Pace University
Pleasantville, New York

Marilyn S. Fetter, PhD, RN, CS
Assistant Professor
Villanova University
Villanova, Pennsylvania

Carol Holdcraft, DNS, RN
Assistant Dean
Wright State University-Miami Valley
Dayton, Ohio

Jaya Jambunathan, PhD, RN
Professor, College of Nursing
University of Wisconsin-Oshkosh
Oshkosh, Wisconsin

Michael Landry, RN, BS, BSN, MN, DNS
Nursing Instructor
University of Louisiana-Lafayette
Lafayette, Louisiana

Melissa Lickteig, RN, MSN
Instructor
Georgia Southern University
Statesboro, Georgia

Ruby J. Martinez, RN, PhD, CS
Assistant Professor
University of Colorado
Denver, Colorado

Jean Rubino, EdD, PN, APN, C
Assistant Professor
Seton Hall University
South Orange, New Jersey

Judi Sateren, RN, MSN
Associate Professor of Nursing
St. Olaf College
Northfield, Minnesota

Beatrice Crofts Yorker, JD, RN, MS, CS, FAAN
Professor and Director
San Francisco State University
San Francisco, California

Student Consultants

Alisa Beaulieu
Santa Fe Community College
Gainesville, Florida

Alison Cody
Germanna Community College
Locust Grove, Virginia

Daniel Dale
Valdosta State University
Valdosta, Georgia

Stephanie Hornby
George Mason University
Fairfax, Virgina

Amy Jeter
Ohio University-Chillicothe
Chillicothe, Ohio

Joan Lawrence
Auburn University
Auburn, Alabama

Lisa Marie Mays
Boise State University
Boise, Idaho

Shawn Shaughnessy
Santa Fe Community College
Gainesville, Florida

Phyllis Thieken
Ohio University-Chillicothe
Chillicothe, Ohio

Jenefer Thomas
Boise State University
Boise, Idaho

Gyleen Vickerman
Boise State University
Boise, Idaho

Carolyn Wilkinson
Auburn University
Auburn, Alabama

A Guide To

Prentice Hall's Reviews and Rationales Series

Each chapter has the following **feature elements** to guide you during review and study.

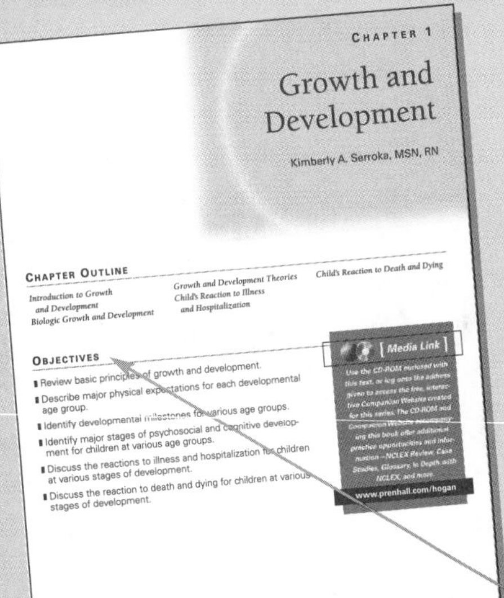

CHAPTER 1

Growth and Development

Kimberly A. Serroka, MSN, RN

CHAPTER OUTLINE

Introduction to Growth and Development
Biologic Growth and Development
Growth and Development Theories
Child's Reaction to Illness and Hospitalization
Child's Reaction to Death and Dying

OBJECTIVES

- Review basic principles of growth and development.
- Describe major physical expectations for each developmental age group.
- Identify developmental milestones for various age groups.
- Identify major stages of psychosocial and cognitive development for children at various age groups.
- Discuss the reactions to illness and hospitalization for children at various stages of development.
- Discuss the reaction to death and dying for children at various stages of development.

[Media Link]
Use the CD-ROM enclosed with this text, or log onto the address given to access the free, interactive Companion Website created for this series. The CD-ROM and Companion Website accompanying this book offer additional practice opportunities and information – NCLEX Review, Case Studies, Glossary, In Depth with NCLEX, and more.
www.prenhall.com/hogan

1

Chapter **Objectives** describe what you will be able to know or do after learning the material covered in the chapter.

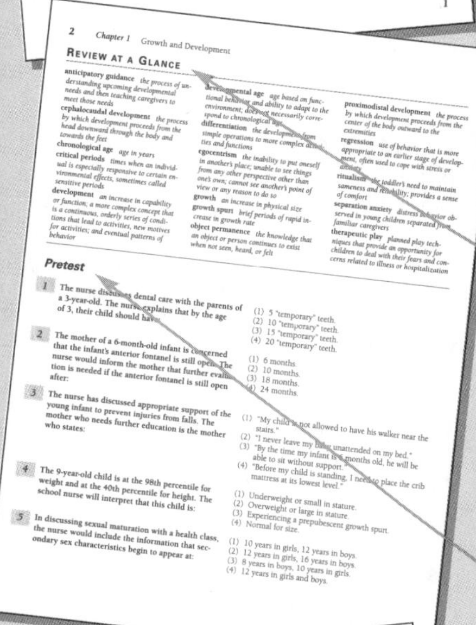

2 *Chapter 1* Growth and Development

REVIEW AT A GLANCE

anticipatory guidance *the process of understanding upcoming developmental needs and then teaching caregivers to meet those needs*
cephalocaudal development *the process by which development proceeds from the head downward through the body and towards the feet*
chronological age *age in years*
critical periods *times when an individual is especially responsive to certain environmental effects, sometimes called sensitive periods*
development *an increase in capability or function; a more complex concept that is a continuous, orderly series of conditions that lead to activities, new motives for activities, and eventual patterns of behavior*
developmental age *age based on functional behavior and ability to adapt to the environment; does not necessarily correspond to chronological age*
differentiation *the development from simple operations to more complex activities and functions*
egocentrism *the inability to put oneself in another's place; unable to see things from any other perspective other than one's own; cannot see another's point of view or any reason to do so*
growth *an increase in physical size*
growth spurt *brief periods of rapid increase in growth rate*
object permanence *the knowledge that an object or person continues to exist when not seen, heard, or felt*
proximodistal development *the process by which development proceeds from the center of the body outward to the extremities*
regression *use of behavior that is more appropriate to an earlier stage of development, often used to cope with stress or anxiety*
ritualism *the toddler's need to maintain sameness and reliability; provides a sense of comfort*
separation anxiety *distress behavior observed in young children separated from familiar caregivers*
therapeutic play *planned play techniques that provide an opportunity for children to deal with their fears and concerns related to illness or hospitalization*

Pretest

1 The nurse discusses dental care with the parents of a 3-year-old. The nurse explains that by the age of 3, their child should have:

(1) 5 "temporary" teeth.
(2) 10 "temporary" teeth.
(3) 15 "temporary" teeth.
(4) 20 "temporary" teeth.

2 The mother of a 6-month-old infant is concerned that the infant's anterior fontanel is still open. The nurse would inform the mother that further evaluation is needed if the anterior fontanel is still open after:

(1) 6 months.
(2) 10 months.
(3) 18 months.
(4) 24 months.

3 The nurse has discussed appropriate support of the young infant to prevent injuries from falls. The mother who needs further education is the mother who states:

(1) "My child is not allowed to have his walker near the stairs."
(2) "I never leave my baby unattended on my bed."
(3) "By the time my infant is 6 months old, he will be able to sit without support."
(4) "Before my child is standing, I need to place the crib mattress at its lowest level."

4 The 9-year-old child is at the 98th percentile for weight and at the 40th percentile for height. The school nurse will interpret that this child is:

(1) Underweight or small in stature.
(2) Overweight or large in stature.
(3) Experiencing a prepubescent growth spurt.
(4) Normal for size.

5 In discussing sexual maturation with a health class, the nurse would include the information that secondary sex characteristics begin to appear at:

(1) 10 years in girls, 12 years in boys.
(2) 12 years in girls, 16 years in boys.
(3) 8 years in boys, 10 years in girls.
(4) 12 years in girls and boys.

Review at a Glance contains a glossary of key terms used in the chapter, with definitions provided up-front and available at your fingertips, to help you stay focused and make the best use of your study time.

The **Pretest** is a 10-question multiple choice test providing a sample overview of content covered in the chapter and helps you decide what areas need the most – or the least – review.

Chapter 6 Neurologic Health Problems 133

7. Child and family education
   a. Teach parents use of physical therapy strategies such as range-of-motion exercises to use at home
   b. Child will need to learn self-care skills such as how to feed and dress self and perform hygiene activities
   c. Teach parents special feeding techniques and use of adaptive devices such as special silverware and dishes; parents may need to be taught how to do gastrostomy tube feedings if indicated
8. Evaluation
   a. Child establishes optimal physical mobility and self-care skills
   b. Child demonstrates adequate nutrition, as evidenced by age-appropriate maintenance or increase in height and weight
   c. Child is free from injury
   d. All individuals interacting with the child are able to comprehend the child's communication
   e. Child demonstrates adequate energy level, as evidenced by ability to participate in daily routine
   f. Family copes with the management of the child's health problems

B. Neural tube defects

1. Description: neural tube defects (also known as spina bifida or myelodysplasia) develop during the first trimester of fetal development; the defect can occur at any place along the spinal canal (see Figure 6-2)
2. Etiology and pathophysiology
   a. Etiology is unknown but thought to be associated with folic acid deficiency in mother's diet; the degree of disability is determined by the location of

Practice to Pass

Describe the multidisplinary team that will be needed in the rehabilitation of the child with cerebral palsy.

NCLEX!

Figure 6-2

Infant with lumbarsacral myelomeningocele.
Source: Ball, J. & Bindler, R. (1999). *Pediatric nursing: Caring for children.* (2nd ed.), Stamford, CT: Appleton & Lange, p. 787.

The **Practice to Pass** questions are open-ended questions that stimulate critical thinking and reinforce mastery of the chapter content.

NCLEX The NCLEX icon identifies information or concepts that are likely to be tested on the NCLEX licensing examination.

A detailed **Outline Review** of core content is given to provide both a comprehensive overview and review.

The **Case Study**, found at the end of the chapter, provides an opportunity for you to use your critical thinking and clinical reasoning skills to "put it all together." It describes a true-to-life client case situation and asks you open-ended questions about how you would provide care for that client and/or family.

The **Posttest** is a 10-question multiple-choice test at the end of the chapter providing new questions that are representative of chapter content. This posttest provides you with feedback about mastery of that content following review and study.

Answers and Rationales For all questions, answers and rationales for each correct answer are provided.

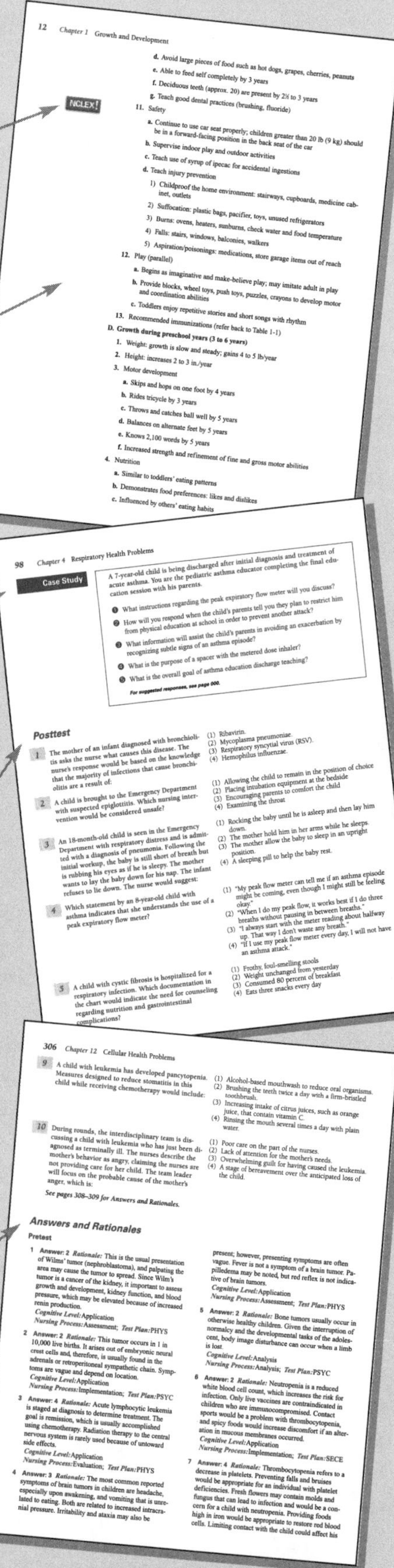

CHAPTER 1

Overview of Psychiatric–Mental Health Nursing

David S. Hodson RN, MS, ARNP

George Byron Smith, ARNP, PhD(c)

CHAPTER OUTLINE

OBJECTIVES

- Describe mental health and mental illness.
- Discuss psychiatric–mental health nursing from a historical perspective.
- Discuss basic theoretical assumptions of at least two theoretical approaches to mental illness.
- Differentiate the use of the nursing process as applied to psychiatric–mental health nursing.
- Identify the roles of neuroanatomy and neurophysiology in brain dysfunction.
- Describe effective communication techniques.
- Differentiate between normal age-related changes and mental health disorders in older populations.
- Explain the importance of understanding cultural diversity in mental illness.
- Identify key elements of legal/ethical issues in mental health nursing.

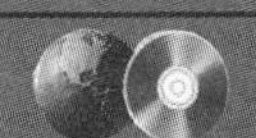

[Media Link]

Use the CD-ROM enclosed with this text, or log onto the address given to access the free, interactive Companion Website created for this series. The CD-ROM and Companion Website accompanying this book offer additional practice opportunities and information—NCLEX Review, Case Studies, Glossary, In Depth with NCLEX, and more.

www.prenhall.com/hogan

Review at a Glance

ageism *a process of systematic stereotyping and discrimination against older people simply on the basis of their age*

competency *a legal determination that a client can make reasonable judgments and decisions about treatment and other significant areas of personal life*

countertransference *the nurse's emotional reaction to clients based on feelings for significant people in the past*

culture *a pattern of learned behavior based on values, beliefs, and perceptions of the world taught and shared by members of a group or society*

Diagnostic and Statistical Manual of Mental Disorders (DSM-IV) *a classification of medical diagnoses of mental illness*

discrimination *prejudice that is expressed behaviorally*

ethnocentrism *the belief that one's own culture is more important than, and preferable to, any other*

ethnicity *ethnic affiliation and a sense of belonging to a particular cultural group*

mental health *the ability to see oneself as others do and to fit into the culture and society where one lives*

mental illness *the inability to see oneself as others do and not having the ability to conform to the norms of the culture and society*

negative bias *a refusal to recognize that there are other points of view*

neurotransmitters *chemical messengers of the nervous system; manufactured in one neuron, released from the axon into the synapse, and received by the dendrite of the next neuron*

prejudice *a negative feeling about people who are different from oneself*

stereotypes *a way of organizing information; arising out of negative biases, they are images frozen in time that cause us to see what we expect to see, even when the facts differ from our expectations*

subculture *a smaller group within a large cultural group that shares values, beliefs, behaviors, and language*

therapeutic communication *the process of influencing the behavior of others by sending, receiving, and interpreting messages*

therapeutic relationship *a nurse–client interaction that focuses on client needs and is goal-specific, theory-based, and open to supervision*

transference *the unconscious process of displaying feelings for significant people in the past onto the nurse in the present relationship*

values *a set of personal beliefs about what is meaningful and significant in life*

Pretest

1 **Which of the following responses by the nurse is the best example of clarifying?**

(1) "Tell me about what you were thinking before you went to talk to him."
(2) "When did you first notice these feelings?"
(3) "Instead of talking about your mother, I want to know how you feel."
(4) "I'm having difficulty understanding. Could you explain that to me?"

2 **During the initial interview with a client, the nurse begins to feel uncomfortable and realizes the client's behaviors and mannerisms remind the nurse of her abusive mother. The nurse realizes this phenomena is known as:**

(1) Transference.
(2) Countertransference.
(3) Denial.
(4) Reaction formation.

3 **A female client has asked the nurse what she should do about leaving her husband. The nurse replies, "I think you should divorce your husband because it is just too stressful." This is an ineffective communication technique for which reason?**

(1) It demands an explanation from the client.
(2) It disagrees with the client's actions.
(3) It belittles the client's feelings.
(4) It tells the client how to solve her problem.

4 **The nurse who is communicating with a client provides feedback about the client's statement for which of the following primary purposes?**

(1) To give advice
(2) To explore feelings
(3) To offer information
(4) To explain behavior

5 The nurse assesses a client as being on the mental health end of the continuum. Which of the following statements by the client *best* supports this assessment?

(1) The client enjoys growth opportunities and is satisfied with life.
(2) The client has no evidence of an organic brain disease.
(3) The client is dissatisfied with her marriage.
(4) The client says her life is boring, and she experiences little stress.

6 The nurse strives to accomplish which of the following while engaged in a nurse–client relationship in supportive therapy?

(1) The nurse is accepted as a beneficent authority, and a congenial atmosphere is maintained.
(2) Confidence is inspired in a nonblaming atmosphere.
(3) Negative feelings are encouraged as soon as they start to develop.
(4) The nurse helps the client look at the client's inferiority feelings.

7 A client presents at the physician's office with profound feelings of depression and indicates that since the death of her father she has been experiencing crying spells. During a conversation, the nurse notes that the client is highly verbal and intellectual. She talked at great length about her father's illness and subsequent death. The client's ability to talk meaningfully about her feelings and circumstances indicates that:

(1) Irreversible psychological damage has occurred.
(2) She is a candidate for long-term psychotherapy.
(3) She is highly anxious as well as depressed.
(4) She is a good candidate for short-term, focused psychotherapy.

8 When a client purposefully attempts to embarrass a nurse by making a sexually explicit comment, the *best* response by the nurse is to:

(1) Clarify the intention of the client.
(2) Leave the situation altogether.
(3) Refuse to talk with the client any further.
(4) Continue to interact as if the comments did not cause embarrassment.

9 An emergency psychiatric client presents with hyperthermia and unexplained loss of appetite. The nurse concludes that these symptoms are consistent with trauma to which area of the brain?

(1) Thalamus
(2) Hypothalamus
(3) Cerebrum
(4) Cerebellum

10 In evaluating the effectiveness of teaching a client with depression, the client demonstrates understanding of depressive symptoms if the client states the symptoms are a result of:

(1) Excessive serotonin activity in the central nervous system (CNS).
(2) Insufficient serotonin activity in the CNS.
(3) Excessive dopamine activity in the CNS.
(4) Insufficient dopamine activity in the CNS.

See pages 26–27 for Answers and Rationales.

I. Overview of Psychiatric Mental-Health Nursing

NCLEX!

A. *Mental health:* is related to the ability to see oneself as others do and fit into the culture and society where one lives; indicators of mental health include positive attitudes toward self, growth, development, self-actualization, integration, autonomy, reality perception, and environmental mastery

NCLEX!

B. ***Mental illness:*** the inability to see oneself as others do and not having the ability to conform to the norms of the culture and society

1. Medical diagnoses of mental illness are classified according to the ***Diagnostic and Statistical Manual of Mental Disorders,*** fourth edition (***DSM-IV***), of the American Psychiatric Association

2. The DSM-IV uses a multi-axial system that gives attention to various mental disorders, general medical conditions, aspects of the environment, and areas of functioning that might be overlooked if the focus were exclusively on assessing a single mental illness problem (see Box 1-1)

C. **Mental health and mental illness** can be viewed as end points on a continuum, with movement back and forth throughout life

D. **The mental health–mental illness continuum** cuts across physical, personal, interpersonal, and societal levels

1. Physical level: in the structure and function of the brain

2. Personal level: in caring for and about the self

3. Interpersonal level: in interactions with others

4. Societal level: in social conditions and the cultural context

E. **On the mental health–mental illness continuum,** each level is so intertwined with the others that it is often difficult to pinpoint the original source of the distress; see Figure 1-1 to see how personal, interpersonal, and cultural factors interact in ways that produce movement toward mental health or mental illness

F. **Mental health is not a concrete goal to be achieved;** rather, it is a lifelong process and includes a sense of harmony and balance for the individual, family, friends, and community; it is more than the mere absence of a mental disorder, in that it also entails a continuous process of growing toward one's potential

G. **Mental disorders**

1. In the United States, approximately one in four Americans will suffer a serious mental disorder during their lifetime (25 percent lifetime chance)

2. One in five children or adolescents may have a diagnosable mental disorder

3. Nearly one-third of the homeless population suffers from a psychiatric disability

4. More than 51 million Americans have a mental disorder in any single year

5. The majority of the 29,000 Americans who commit suicide each year have a mental disorder

Practice to Pass

You are conducting a class on mental health and mental illness with a group of well adults in the community. How would you use the mental health–mental illness continuum?

Box 1-1

DSM-IV Axes

Axis I: Adult and child clinical disorders; conditions not attributable to a mental disorder that are a focus of clinical attention
Axis II: Personality disorders; mental retardation
Axis III: General medical conditions
Axis IV: Psychosocial and environmental problems
Axis V: Global assessment of functioning (0–100)

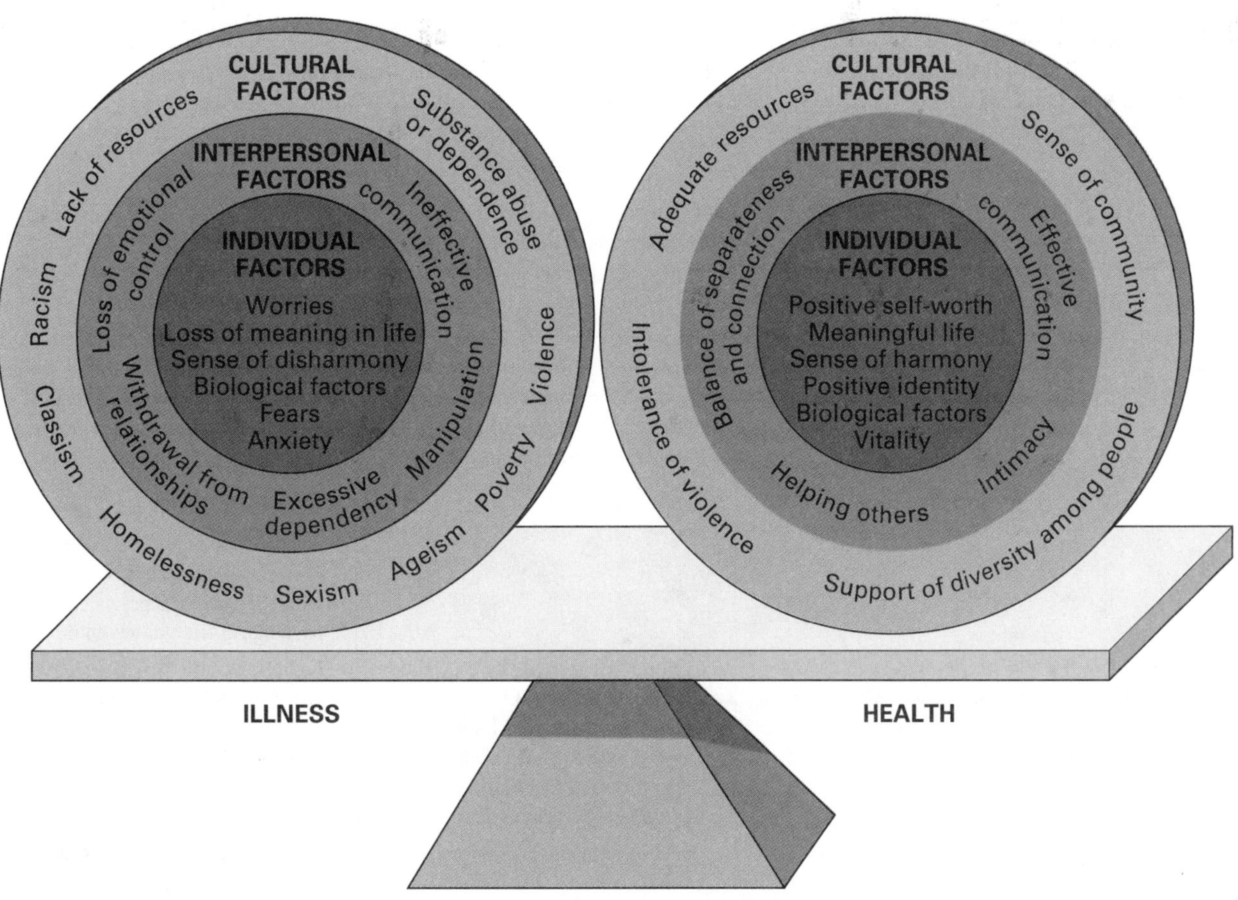

Figure 1-1 **Factors contributing to the mental health–mental illness continuum.**

II. Historical Perspective (see Table 1-1 for historical timeline)

A. Mental illness

1. Historically the care of the mentally ill in western society has been marred with cruelty and ignorance
2. Prior to the enactment of the Community Mental Health Act (1963), mental health treatment was provided in state or private hospitals for the mentally ill that were usually isolated and located away from well-populated areas
3. NCLEX! The Community Mental Health Act (1963) shifted the focus of funding and treatment away from these large hospitals to newly established community mental health centers, which provided emergency services, in-patient hospitalization, outpatient services, community support, and education
4. Currently treatment for mental illness is focused on managing a client with a mental disorder(s) across the continuum of care and services
   a. Managed behavioral health care: utilizes case management, utilization management, and interdisciplinary treatment planning to ensure the coordination and resource management of services

Table 1-1 Mental Health/Mental Illness and Psychiatric–Mental Health Nursing Historical Developments

Time Period	Significant Change in Thinking	Mental Health/ Mental Illness	Psychiatric–Mental Health Nursing
1800s	• The mentally ill were no longer treated as less than human. • Human dignity was upheld. • Scientific studies held promise for treating and curing mental health problems.	• Treatment of the mentally ill was provided in asylums. • The study of the mind and the effectiveness of treatment approaches to psychiatric conditions flourished.	• Linda Richards, the first psychiatric nurse, directed a school of psychiatric nursing at the McLean Psychiatric Asylum (1880).
1950–1960	• Least restrictive environment evolved. • Patient rights for the mentally ill begin to be discussed and evolve.	• Discovery of significant psychotropic medications, including lithium, chlorpromazine, monoamine oxidase inhibitors (MAOIs), haloperidol, tricyclic antidepressants (TCAs), and benzodiazepines.	• Hildegarde Peplau developed a framework for psychiatric nursing with an emphasis on the nurse–client relationship and theoretical constructs to explain patient problems and provided the foundation for psychiatric nursing practice. • ANA established the Conference Group on Psychiatric Nursing, which defined the practice of psychiatric–mental health nursing.
1960–1980	• The Deinstitutionalization Movement began. • People with mental illness have a right to be treated in their own communities.	• Community Mental Health Centers Act is passed (1963). • Treatment shifts from long-term hospital care to shorter inpatient stays, followed by community-based treatment after discharge.	• Founding of the American Psychiatric Nurses Association. • ANA first published standards of mental health and psychiatric nursing practice (1973).
1980–Present	• Significant changes in mental health treatment and delivery across the continuum. • Population-based community care focuses on mental illness prevention and mental health promotion.	• Behavioral managed health care evolved. • Delivery of care focuses on case management and critical pathways or inter-disciplinary planning. • "Decade of the Brain" (1990) focused on mental illness as a brain disease.	• Coalition of Psychiatric Nursing Organizations and the ANA jointly published a description of two levels of practice, the generalist and the specialist (1994).

NCLEX!

b. The least restrictive care setting is the goal for placement of clients; the aim of treatment is to manage the severity of mental illness and assist the client to live at the highest, most independent level of functioning within the community

c. The Americans with Disabilities Act (ADA) of 1990 was enacted to ensure that people with disabilities, including mental illnesses, were able to fully participate in the economic and social mainstream of society; the ADA has been able to ensure these rights for the medical disabled but has had less success with ensuring the rights of the mentally ill

d. Consumer organizations have worked to remove the stigma of mental illness in American society and have promoted a legislative agenda to protect rights of the mentally ill and to ensure parity for mental illness coverage

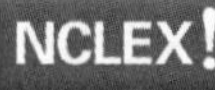

e. The decade of the 1990s was titled the "Decade of the Brain," which produced great promise in the treatment and recovery of mental disorders;

more medications and treatments have been discovered, which have offered individuals with mental illness more options and opportunities for treatment and recovery

B. Psychiatric–mental health nursing (refer again to Table 1-1 for historical timeline)

1. Psychiatric–mental health nursing can be traced as far back as the late 17th century
2. Linda Richards (1880) was credited with being the first American psychiatric nurse; she spent much of her professional career developing nursing care in psychiatric hospitals and directed one of the first schools of psychiatric nursing at the McLean Psychiatric Asylum in Massachusetts
3. Harriet Baily (1920) wrote the first psychiatric nursing textbook, *Nursing in Mental Diseases*
4. Hildegarde Peplau (1952) wrote *Interpersonal Relations in Nursing,* the first nursing framework for psychiatric nursing practice, in which she defined nursing as "a significant, therapeutic, interpersonal process . . . an educative instrument, a maturing force, that aims to promote forward movement of personality in the direction of creative, constructive, productive, personal, and community living"

III. Psychiatric–Mental Health Nursing Practice

A. Generalist: requires a baccalaureate degree in nursing with validation of clinical competencies

1. Works with individuals, families, groups, and the community to assess mental health needs, develop diagnoses, plan, implement, and evaluate nursing care
2. The psychiatric–mental health generalist uses interventions that include:
   - **a.** Health promotion and maintenance
   - **b.** Assessment and evaluation
   - **c.** Case management
   - **d.** Provision of a therapeutic milieu
   - **e.** Education of clients about factors that influence mental health and mental illness
   - **f.** Promotion of self-care and independence
   - **g.** Administration and monitoring of psychobiological treatment regimens
   - **h.** Crisis intervention and counseling
   - **i.** Engaging in social and community mental health efforts
3. Practice settings include:
   - **a.** Psychiatric hospitals
   - **b.** Community mental health centers
   - **c.** General hospitals
   - **d.** Community health agencies (i.e., home health, primary-care centers, homeless clinics, etc.)

e. Outpatient services

f. Senior centers and daycare centers

g. Schools

h. Prisons

i. Health maintenance organizations (HMOs)

j. Emergency and crisis centers

B. **Specialist:** requires a masters degree in psychiatric–mental health nursing with validation of clinical competencies

1. Psychiatric nurse practitioners (APN or APRN) provide primary care including both medical and mental health services

2. Clinical nurse specialists (CNS) provide direct care as therapists or indirect care as consultants, educators, or researchers

C. **Standards of care and practice:** ANA (1994) devised standards of clinical practice for psychiatric–mental health nursing

1. Standards of care

a. Identify the function of the psychiatric–mental health nurse

b. Outline the activities and accountability for both the psychiatric–mental health generalist and specialist nurses

2. Standards of professional performance

a. Identify the role of the psychiatric–mental health nurse

b. Include such things as quality of care, performance appraisals, education, collegiality, ethics, research, and resource utilization

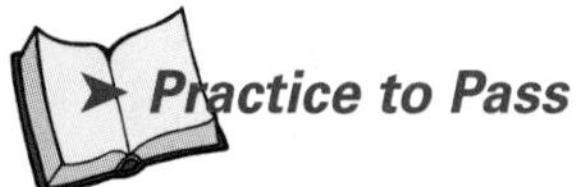

A client experiencing depression, who has been hospitalized after taking an overdose of narcotics, states, "I really wasn't trying to kill myself, I had just had a very stressful day and drank a few too many beers. I am fine. I should be going home now." You suspect the client is using which defense mechanism?

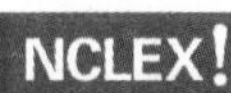

IV. Theoretical Contributions Significant to Psychiatric–Mental Health Nursing

A. Intrapersonal theory

1. Intrapersonal theory focuses on the behaviors, feelings, thoughts, and experiences of each individual

2. Sigmund Freud divided all aspects of consciousness into three categories: conscious, preconscious, and unconscious; he theorized that there were three components of the personality: the id, ego, and superego

a. Freud defined anxiety as a feeling of tension, distress, and discomfort produced by a perceived or threatened loss of inner control

b. He identified processes called defense mechanisms, which alleviate anxiety by denying, misinterpreting, or distorting reality; for the most part, defense mechanisms operate at an unconscious level

c. See Table 1-2 for definitions and examples of defense mechanisms

3. Erik Erikson saw personality as developing throughout the entire life span rather than stopping at adolescence; he felt personality was shaped by conflict between needs and culture; Erikson identified eight development stages: sensory, muscular, locomotor, latency, adolescence, young adult,

Table 1-2 **Defense Mechanisms**

Defense Mechanism	Example
Compensation. Covering up weaknesses by emphasizing a more desirable trait or by overachievement in a more comfortable area.	A high school student too small to play football becomes the star long-distance runner for the track team.
Denial. An attempt to screen or ignore unacceptable realities by refusing to acknowledge them.	A woman, though told her father has metastatic cancer, continues to plan a family reunion 18 months in advance.
Displacement. The transferring or discharging of emotional reactions from one object or person to another object or person.	A husband and wife are fighting, and the husband becomes so angry he hits a wall instead of his wife.
Identification. An attempt to manage anxiety by imitating the behavior of someone feared or respected.	A student nurse imitates the nurturing behavior she observes one of her instructors using with clients.
Intellectualization. A mechanism by which an emotional response that normally would accompany an uncomfortable or painful incident is evaded by the use of rational explanations that remove from the incident any personal significance and feelings.	The pain over a parent's sudden death is reduced by saying, "He wouldn't have wanted to live disabled."
Introjection. A form of identification that allows for the acceptance of others' norms and values into oneself, even when contrary to one's previous assumptions.	A 7-year-old tells his sister, "Don't talk to strangers." He has introjected this value from the instructions of parents and teachers.
Minimization. Not acknowledging the significance of one's behavior.	A person says, "Don't believe everything my wife tells you. I wasn't so drunk I couldn't drive."
Projection. A process in which blame is attached to others or the environment for unacceptable desires, thoughts, shortcomings, and mistakes.	A mother is told her child must repeat a grade in school, and she blames this on the teacher's poor instruction.
Rationalization. Justification of certain behaviors by faulty logic and ascription or motives that are socially acceptable but did not in fact inspire the behavior.	A mother spanks her toddler too hard and says it was all right because he couldn't feel it through the diaper anyway.
Reaction Formation. A mechanism that causes people to act exactly opposite to the way they feel.	An executive resents his bosses for calling in a consulting firm to make recommendations for change in his department but verbalizes complete support for the idea and is exceedingly polite and cooperative.
Regression. Resorting to an earlier, more comfortable level of functioning that is characteristically less demanding and responsible.	An adult throws a temper tantrum when he does not get his own way.
Repression. An unconscious mechanism by which threatening thoughts, feelings, and desires are kept from becoming conscious; the repressed material is denied entry into consciousness.	A teenager, seeing his best friend killed in a car accident, becomes amnesic about the circumstances surrounding the accident.
Sublimation. Displacement of energy associated with more primitive sexual or aggressive drives into socially acceptable activities.	A person with excessive, primitive sexual drives invests psychic energy into a well-defined religious value system.
Substitution. The replacement of a highly valued, unacceptable, or unavailable object by a less valuable, acceptable, or available object.	A woman wants to marry a man exactly like her dead father and settles for someone who looks a little bit like him.
Undoing. An action or words designed to cancel some disapproved thoughts, impulses, or acts in which the person relieves guilt by making reparation.	A father spanks his child and the next evening brings home a present for the child.

Source: Fontaine, K. L. (1999). Introduction to mental health nursing. In K. L. Fontaine & J. S. Fletcher (Eds.), *Mental health nursing* (4th ed.). Menlo Park, CA: Addison-Wesley, pp. 9–10.

Table 1-3

Erik Erikson's Stages of Social Growth and Development

Stage of Development	Period	Developmental Task	Defining Characteristics
Sensory	Birth–18 months	Trust vs. mistrust	Child learns to develop trusting relationships
Muscular	1–3 years	Autonomy vs. shame and doubt	Child starts the process of separation; starts learning to live autonomously
Locomotor	3–6 years	Initiative vs. guilt	Learns about environmental influences; becomes more aware of own identity
Latency	6–12 years	Industry vs. inferiority	Energy is directed at accomplishments, creative activities, and learning
Adolescent	12–20 years	Identity vs. role confusion	Transitional period; movement toward adulthood; starts incorporating beliefs and value systems that have been acquired previously
Young Adult	18–25 years	Intimacy vs. isolation	Learns the ability to have intimate relationships
Adulthood	24–45 years	Generativity vs. stagnation	Emphasis on maintaining intimate relationships; movement toward developing a family
Maturity	45 years—death	Integrity vs. despair	Acceptance of life as it has been; acceptance of both good and bad aspects of past life; maintaining a positive self-concept

Source: Fontaine, K. L. (1999). Introduction to mental health nursing. In K. L. Fontaine & J. S. Fletcher (Eds.), *Mental health nursing* (4th ed.). Menlo Park, CA: Addison-Wesley, p. 11.

A 72-year-old retired and recently widowed man is hospitalized on a geropsychiatric unit for major depression. He says, "My life is meaninglessness now that my wife is gone. What do I have to live for? There is no hope for the future now, and I do not have any family around who cares enough to help me. I would be better off dead." Using Erikson's stages of growth and development, describe the stage this client is currently experiencing and how you would assist him.

adulthood, and maturity; see Table 1-3 for Erikson's stages of growth and development

4. Intrapersonal models provide a way of looking at how individuals develop, how they are still trying to achieve developmental tasks, and how they have learned to cope with anxiety

B. Social-interpersonal theory

1. The focus of social-interpersonal theory is on relationships and events in the social context
2. Harry Stack Sullivan believed that personality could not be observed apart from interpersonal relationships; he identified three principal components of the interpersonal sphere: dynamisms, personifications, and cognitive processes

NCLEX!

3. Abraham Maslow identified basic physiological needs and growth-related metaneeds; his humanistic theory emphasized health rather than illness
   a. Maslow conceptualized these needs on a hierarchy, often symbolized by a pyramid
   b. There are five levels of needs in the hierarchy, and are identified (from bottom to top of the pyramid) as physiological needs, safety needs, love and

belonging needs, esteem and recognition needs, and self-actualization needs

1) Physiological needs include the needs for oxygen, food, water, sleep, shelter, and sexual expression
2) Safety needs include physical safety, avoiding harm, and attaining security and order
3) Love and belonging needs include companionship, the giving and receiving of affection, and identification with a group
4) Esteem and recognition needs include self esteem, the respect of others, prestige, and success at work
5) Self-actualization is the fulfillment of one's unique potential

NCLEX!

4. Hildegarde Peplau saw nursing as an interpersonal process, with the therapeutic nurse–client relationship at its core; the major components of her theory are growth, development, communication, and roles

5. Feminist theory is an androgynous model of mental health; theorists examine how gender roles limit the psychological development of all people and inhibit the development of mutually satisfying and non-coercive intimacy

6. Social-interpersonal models enable the nurse to assess the influences of culture, social interaction, gender stereotypes, and support systems on the behavior of clients

C. Behavioral theory

1. The focus of behavioral theory is on a person's actions, not on thoughts and feelings

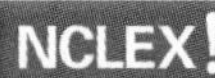

2. The major emphasis of B. F. Skinner's theory is the functional analysis of behavior

a. Reinforcements are consequences that lead to an increase in a behavior; punishments are consequences that lead to a decrease in the behavior

b. The principle of reinforcement states that a response is strengthened when reinforcement is given

3. Behavioral models are helpful in planning client education and designing programs for a variety of mental health clients and families

D. Cognitive theory

1. Cognitive theory explains how we interpret our daily lives, adapt and make changes, and develop the insights to make those changes

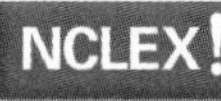

2. Jean Piaget thought that children learn by the changing stimuli that challenge their experiences and perceptions; he identified four major stages of cognitive development: sensorimotor, preoperational, concrete operational, and formal operational

3. Aaron Beck's cognitive theory focuses on how people view themselves and their world; he identified cognitive schemas as personal controlling beliefs that influence the way people process data about themselves and others; cognitive distortions result from the cognitive triad of an inadequate view of self, a negative misinterpretation of the present, and a negative view of the future

4. Albert Ellis's work with cognitive restructuring is often used as part of treatment today

5. Cognitive models help the nurse assess clients' learning capabilities; they also help the nurse analyze cognitive distortions that are symptoms of a number of mental disorders

E. Biogenic theory

1. In studying genetic factors in mental disorders, researchers must first establish that there is a higher-than-expected rate of incidence within the family and then must identify what parts are caused by genetic factors and what parts are caused by environmental factors

2. Biogenic theory looks at how genetic factors, neuroanatomy, neurophysiology, and biological rhythms relate to the cause, course, and prognosis of mental disorders

   a. The cerebrum compromises the majority (60 percent) of the brain and is composed of two cerebral hemispheres with each hemisphere being divided into four lobes

      1) Frontal lobe: primary functions—higher-order thinking, abstract reasoning, decision making, speech, and voluntary muscle movement

      2) Parietal lobe: primary functions—sensory function and proprioception (body position information)

      3) Occipital lobe: primary function—visual function

      4) Temporal lobe: primary functions—judgment, memory, smell, sensory interpretation, and understanding sound

   b. Diencephalon: extends from the cerebrum and sits above the brain stem; the diencephalon has three primary structures

      1) Thalamus: receives and relays sensory information and plays a role in memory and in regulating mood

      2) Hypothalamus: control's the body homeostasis; it regulates the autonomic nervous system, body temperature, appetite, water balance, biologic rhythms and drives, and hormonal output of the anterior pituitary gland

      3) Limbic system: comprised of the limbic lobe and the numerous structures functioning with it, including the frontal cortex, hypothalamus, amygdala, hippocampus, brain stem, and autonomic nervous system; the limbic system is primarily responsible for regulating emotional responses

You are conducting a medication education group for a group of clients who are experiencing major depression. How would you explain this disease as a chemical imbalance in the brain?

NCLEX!

NCLEX!

3. Mental disorders are often related to dysfunctional neuronal receptors or a deficiency, excess, or imbalance of **neurotransmitters** (chemical messengers of the nervous system, manufactured in one neuron and released from the axon into the synapse and received by the dendrite of the next neuron); a synapse is the gap between one membrane of one neuron and the membrane of another and is the point at which nerve impulse transmission occurs

NCLEX!

   a. Serotonin (5-HT) is involved primarily in depressive and anxiety disorders, and possibly eating disorders; many antidepressants target the synapses to increase serotonin levels

NCLEX!

b. Norepinephrine (NE) is a catecholamine neurotransmitter of the sympathetic nervous system, which mediates fight or flight response; depressive disorders, including bipolar disorder, are involved with changes in norepinephrine levels

NCLEX!

c. Dopamine (DA) is involved with schizophrenic disorders; many antipsychotic medications block dopamine from binding to its receptors

d. Acetylcholine (ACH) is a major neurotransmitter of the parasympathetic nervous system, which controls muscles, memory, and coordination; changes in acetylcholine levels are involved with Alzheimer's disease

e. Gamma-aminobutyric acid (GABA) is an inhibitory neurotransmitter; antianxiety medications increase the effects of GABA

4. Biological rhythms: circadian rhythms are regular fluctuations of a variety of physiological factors over a period of 24 hours

a. Temperature, energy, sleep, arousal, motor activity, appetite, hormones, and mood all demonstrate circadian rhythms

NCLEX!

b. The "biological clock" is located in the hypothalamus and may be desynchronized by external or internal factors

c. Some mental disorders demonstrate alterations in adrenal rhythm, temperature patterns, and sleep patterns

V. The Nursing Process

A. Provides the boundaries for psychiatric–mental health nursing and a scientific method for the delivery of nursing care

B. The steps of the nursing process

1. Assessment: establishing a database about a client, family, or community

NCLEX!

a. Observation is extremely important in assessing clients with mental illness; clients are observed in terms of their behavior, affect, cognition, interpersonal relationships, and physiology

b. The psychosocial assessment includes the client's and family's definition of the problem(s), history of the present problem(s), family and social history, spiritual considerations, cultural assessment, physical assessment, and strengths and competencies

c. The neuropsychiatric assessment provides more specific information about the client's appearance, activity, speech, emotional state, cognitive functioning, and perception

NCLEX!

2. Diagnosis: identifying the client's healthcare needs and selecting goals of care; psychiatric–mental health nursing diagnoses are applicable to individuals, families, groups, and communities; they include the etiologies and standard nursing interventions; see Box 1-2 for list of psychosocial nursing diagnoses

3. Outcome identification: establishing criteria for measuring achievement of desired outcomes; client outcomes are specific behavioral measures by which the nurse, clients, and significant others determine progress toward a goal

Box 1-2

NANDA-Approved Nursing Diagnoses in Psychiatric–Mental Health Nursing

Communicating
Impaired verbal communication

Relating
Impaired social interaction
Social isolation
Risk for loneliness
Ineffective role performance
Impaired parenting (also Risk for)
Sexual dysfunction
Interrupted family processes
Caregiver role strain (also Risk for)
Dysfunctional family processes: Alcoholism
Parental role conflict
Ineffective sexuality patterns

Valuing
Spiritual distress (also Risk for)
Readiness for enhanced spiritual well-being

Choosing
Ineffective coping
Impaired adjustment
Defensive coping
Ineffective denial
Disabled family coping
Compromised family coping
Readiness for enhanced family coping
Readiness for enhanced community coping
Ineffective community coping
Ineffective therapeutic regimen management
Noncompliance [or Nonadherence] (specify)
Ineffective family therapeutic regimen management
Ineffective community therapeutic regimen management
Effective therapeutic regimen management
Decisional conflict (specify)
Health-seeking behaviors (specify)

Moving
Fatigue
Disturbed sleep pattern
Deficient diversional activity
Delayed growth and development
Risk for delayed development
Relocation stress syndrome

Perceiving
Disturbed body image
Chronic low self-esteem
Situational low self-esteem (also Risk for)
Disturbed personal identity
Disturbed sensory perception (specify: visual, auditory, kinesthetic, gustatory, tactile, olfactory)
Unilateral neglect
Hopelessness
Powerlessness (also Risk for)

Knowing
Knowledge deficit (specify)
Impaired environmental interpretation syndrome
Acute confusion
Chronic confusion
Disturbed thought processes
Impaired memory

Feeling
Acute pain
Chronic pain
Dysfunctional grieving
Anticipatory grieving
Chronic sorrow
Risk for other-directed violence
Risk for self-mutilation
Risk for self-directed violence
Post-trauma syndrome
Rape-trauma syndrome
Rape-trauma syndrome: Compound reaction
Rape-trauma syndrome: Silent reaction
Risk for post-trauma syndrome
Anxiety
Death anxiety
Fear
Risk for falls
Self-mutilation
Risk for suicide

Used by permission from North American Nursing Diagnosis Association. (1999). *Nursing diagnoses: Definitions and classification, 1999–2000.* Philadelphia: NANDA.

4. Planning: designing a strategy to achieve the goals established for client care
   a. In psychiatric–mental health nursing, safety needs often are more of a priority than physiological needs; clients must be assessed for exhaustion, poor judgment, self-mutilation, and violence and suicide potential

NCLEX!

   b. Ideally, goals are planned with client input, but some clients may be too ill to participate in this process; they must be included as soon as they are psychically and mentally able to participate

5. Implementation: initiating and completing actions necessary to accomplish the defined goals; nurses assume several roles in assisting clients to grow and adapt, such as socializing agent, teacher, role model, advocate, counselor, role player, and milieu manager

6. Evaluation: determining the extent to which the goals of care have been achieved

   a. Formative evaluation is an ongoing process for maintaining, modifying, or expanding the nursing care plan

   b. Summative evaluation is a terminal process; summative evaluations are written in the form of discharge summaries

   c. All steps in the nursing process pertinent to the client must be documented in the client's record; some of the most critical documentation involves falls, seclusion, restraints (both physical and chemical), and suicidal or violent behaviors

VI. Therapeutic Relationship

A. A *therapeutic relationship* is a nurse-client interaction that focuses on client needs and is goal-specific, theory-based, and open to supervision

B. The therapeutic relationship has three phases: introduction, working, and termination

1. The introduction phase of the therapeutic relationship includes establishing a contract, discussing confidentiality, assessing thoroughly, and developing the preliminary nursing care plan

2. During the working phase, the care plan is implemented through the process of therapeutic alliance

   a. Client **transference** is the unconscious process of displacing feelings for significant people in the past onto the nurse in the present relationship

   b. Countertransference is the nurse's emotional reaction to clients based on feelings for significant people in the past

3. The primary goal of the termination phase of the therapeutic relationship is to review the client's progress and plans for the immediate future

4. The physical component of the relationship includes all procedures and technical skills that nurses do for clients

5. The psychosocial component involves qualities such as positive regard, nonjudgmental attitude, acceptance, warmth, empathy, and authenticity

6. The spiritual component is the feeling of connectiveness with clients and the respect for the diversity of spiritual needs among clients

7. The power component includes beliefs and about external and internal locus of control

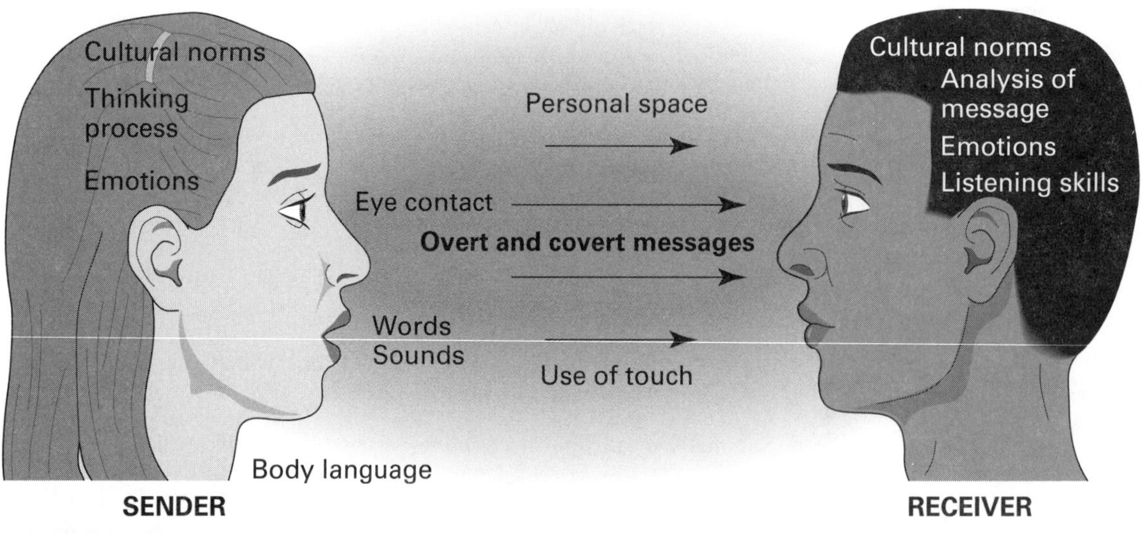

Figure 1-2 **The communication process.**

VII. Therapeutic Communication

A. ***Therapeutic communication*** is the process of influencing the behavior of others by sending, receiving, and interpreting messages; feedback and consideration of the context complete the cycle; see Figure 1-2 for a diagram of the therapeutic communication process

B. **Therapeutic communication** is the foundation of interpersonal relationships and is a key process needed to use the nursing process

NCLEX!

1. Communication includes spoken words, paralanguage, the thinking process, emotions, nonverbal behavior, and the culture of the individuals sending and receiving the message

NCLEX!

2. Nonverbal communication includes body language, eye contact, personal space, and the use of touch

3. Listening means paying attention to what the person is saying, acknowledging feelings, holding back on what the nurse has to say, avoiding interruption, and controlling the urge to give advice

NCLEX!

4. Characteristics of effective helpers include a nonjudgmental approach, acceptance, warmth, empathy, authenticity, congruency, patience, trustworthiness, self-disclosure, and humor

NCLEX!

5. Techniques that facilitate effective communication include broad openings, giving recognition, minimal encouragement, offering self, accepting, making observations, validating perceptions, exploring, clarifying, placing the event in time or sequence, focusing, encouraging the formulation of a plan of action, suggesting collaboration, restating, reflecting and summarizing; see Table 1-4 for examples of therapeutic communication techniques

NCLEX!

6. Techniques that contribute to ineffective communication include stereotypical comments, parroting, changing the topic, disagreeing, challenging, requesting

Table 1-4

Effective Communication Techniques

Technique	Examples
Broad opening	"What would you like to work on today?" "What is one of the best things that happened to you this week?"
Giving recognition	"I notice you're wearing a new dress. You look very nice." "What a marvelous afghan that is going to be when you finish."
Minimal encouragement	"Go on." "Ummm." "Uh-huh."
Offering self	"I'll sit with you until it's time for your family session." "I have at least 30 minutes I can spend with you right now."
Accepting	"I can imagine how that might feel." "I'm with you on that [nodding]."
Making observations	"Mr. Robinson, you seem on edge. You are clenching your fist and grinding your teeth." "I'm puzzled. You're smiling, but you sound so resentful."
Validating perceptions	"This is what I heard you say. . . . Is that correct?" "It sounds like you are talking about sad feelings. Is that correct?"
Exploring	"How does your girlfriend feel about your being to the hospital?" "Tell me about what was happening at home just before you came in the hospital."
Clarifying	"Could you explain more about that to me?" "I'm having some difficulty. Could you help me understand?"
Placing the event in time or sequence	"Which came first. . . ?" "When did you first notice. . . ?"
Focusing	"Could we continue talking about you and your dad right now?" "Rather than talking about what your husband thinks, I would like to hear how you're feeling right now."
Encouraging the formulation of a plan of action	"What do you think you can do the next time you feel that way?" "How might you handle your anger in a nonthreatening way?"
Suggesting collaboration	"Perhaps together we can figure out . . ." "Let's try using the problem-solving process that was presented in group yesterday."
Restatement	*Client:* Do you think going home will be difficult? *Nurse:* How difficult do you think going home will be?
Reflection	*Client:* I keep thinking about what all my friends are doing right now. *Nurse:* You're worried that they aren't missing you? *Client:* He laughed at me. My boss just sat there and laughed at me. I felt like such a fool. *Nurse:* You felt humiliated?
Summarizing	"So far we have talked about . . ." "Our time is up. Let's see, we have discussed your family problems, their effect on your schoolwork, and your need to find a way to decrease family conflict."

Source: Fontaine, K. L. (1999). Communicating and teaching. In K. L. Fontaine & J. S. Fletcher (Eds.), *Mental health nursing* (4th ed.). Menlo Park, CA: Addison-Wesley, p. 102.

an explanation, false reassurance, belittling expressed feelings, probing, advising, imposing values, and double/multiple questions; see Table 1-5 for examples of ineffective communication techniques

Table 1-5

Ineffective Communication Techniques

Technique	Examples
Stereotypical comments	"What's the matter, cat got your tongue?" "Still waters run deep."
Parroting	*Client:* I'm so sad. *Nurse:* You're so sad.
Changing the topic	*Client:* I was so afraid I was going to have another panic attack. *Nurse:* What does your husband think about your panic attacks?
Disagreeing	"I don't see any reason for you to think that way." "No, I think that is a silly response to your mother."
Challenging	"Is that a valid reason to become angry?" "You weren't really serious, were you?"
Requesting an explanation	"Why did you react that way?" "Why can't you just leave home?"
False reassurance	"Don't worry anymore." "I doubt that your mother will be angry about your failing math."
Belittling expressed feelings	"That was four years ago. It shouldn't bother you now." "You shouldn't feel that all men are bad." "It's wrong to even think of your mother like that."
Probing	"I'm here to listen. I can't help you if you won't tell me everything." "Tell me what secrets you keep from your wife."
Advising	"You sound worried. I think you'd better talk to your doctor or your rabbi." "I think you should divorce your husband."
Imposing values	*Client:* [With head down and low tone of voice.] I was going to go on the cruise, but my mother is coming to stay with me. *Nurse:* You must be looking forward to her arrival.
Double/multiple questions	"What makes you feel that you should stay? How would you get along if you left? Would you rent an apartment or move in with a friend?"

Source: Fontaine, K. L. (1999). Communicating and teaching. In K. L. Fontaine & J. S. Fletcher (Eds.), *Mental health nursing* (4th ed.). Menlo Park, CA: Addison-Wesley, p. 104.

VIII. Older Adults

A. Etiology

1. Between 15 to 25 percent of older adults living in the community have symptoms of mental disorders

2. Almost 20 percent of the population over 65 years of age experience significant anxiety that may be related to anxiety disorders or to medical illness

3. Although depression is common, it may not be recognized in older adults and may be confused with dementia

4. Older adults with Parkinson's disease and cerebral vascular accidents are at risk for a concurrent depression

5. Alcohol abuse is a problem for 10 to 15 percent of older adults, and it is often underdiagnosed

6. As the aging population grows, there will be an inevitable increase in age-related mental disorders such as dementias

7. Aging causes a decrease in a number of neurotransmitters, which may be a factor in mood disorders among older adults

8. **Ageism** is a process of systematic stereotyping and discrimination against older people simply on the basis of their age; it contributes to the incidence of depression among older adults

You are working with an 82-year-old client who is experiencing dementia. She is oriented to self only. She wanders the halls and is often found in other clients' rooms both lying in their beds and going through their clothes. Many of the clients have become angry with her and have threatened to hurt her if she does not stop stealing from them. Based on this data, what are the top three nursing diagnoses for this client?

B. Assessment

1. It is imperative to carefully assess older adults to differentiate between dementia, delirium, and depression

2. Older adults may have loss of hearing that may lead to incorrect or bizarre responses when they are unable to hear questions clearly

3. Assess the older adults' ability to accomplish physical and instrumental activities of daily living (e.g., shopping, cooking, financial management, etc.)

C. Nursing diagnoses: related to the behavioral, affective, cognitive, sociocultural, and physiological changes that occur with aging and life events; see Box 1-3 for nursing diagnoses for older adults with mental health problems

D. Interventions

1. Older adults are more prone to the side effects and toxic effects of many medications

   a. Many times medications are given at half the normal adult doses

   b. The key to starting older adults on psychopharmacologic medication therapy is to reduce the dose and progress any increases in dosage slowly

Box 1-3

Psychosocial Nursing Diagnoses for Older Adults

- Chronic confusion related to changes in brain function; being in an unfamiliar environment.
- Chronic low self-esteem related to lack of acceptance of the retirement role; continuous feelings of despair.
- Chronic sorrow related to loss of life partner and possessions; isolation from social support.
- Disturbed body image related to multiple physiological losses; changes in body composition.
- Disturbed sexuality patterns related to poor body image; loss of life partner, ageism.
- Fear related to the inevitability of mortality.
- Hopelessness related to isolation from significant others; overwhelming stress.
- Impaired adjustment related to retirement from active work responsibilities; non-supportive relationships with significant others.
- Impaired memory related to disturbed mood; changes in brain function.
- Ineffective coping related to unsuccessful attempts at forming a philosophy of life; multiple losses.
- Powerlessness related to inadequate finances and economic burdens; inadequate societal provisions for older adults.
- Relocation stress syndrome related to having to sell family home and moving into an assisted living facility.
- Risk for isolation related to loss of social support; multiple losses.
- Spiritual distress related to the inability to find meaning in life; hopelessness and despair in the life review.

2. Physical restraints increase agitation, confusion, incontinence, pressure sores, feelings of anger and fear, and even death from accidental strangulation
3. Electroconvulsive therapy (ECT) is highly successful for treating mood disorders among treatment-resistant older adults
4. Reminiscence therapy can raise self-esteem and increase social intimacy

IX. Cultural Considerations

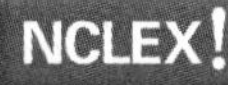

A. ***Culture*** is a pattern of learned behavior based on values, beliefs, and perceptions of the world; culture is taught and shared by members of a group or society

1. A **subculture** is a smaller group within a large cultural group that share values, beliefs, behaviors, and language

NCLEX!

2. **Ethnicity** is ethnic affiliation and a sense of belonging to a particular cultural group

NCLEX!

3. **Ethnocentrism** is the belief that one's own culture is more important than, and preferable to, any other

B. Culture and mental health

1. Ideas about mental health, mental illness, psychiatric problems, and treatments are based on cultural values and understanding
2. What is considered normal or abnormal depends on the specific cultural viewpoint

NCLEX!

C. ***Values:*** a set of personal beliefs about what is meaningful and significant in life

1. They provide general guidelines for behavior and are standards of conduct in which people or groups of people believe
2. Every society has basic values about the relationship between humans and nature, sense of time, a sense of productivity, and interpersonal relationships
3. Predominant American values have historically tended to represent European American, middle-class, Judeo-Christian, male values; nursing as a discipline tends to have the same values as middle-class American or European American background

D. Attitudes and perceptions

1. Natural biases refer to how nurses' points of view cause them to notice some things and not others
2. **Negative bias** is a refusal to recognize that there are other points of view
3. Generalizations are a way of organizing information; arising out of natural biases, they are changeable starting places for comparing typical behavioral patterns with what is actually observed

NCLEX!

4. **Stereotypes** are also a way of organizing information; arising out of negative biases, they are images frozen in time that cause us to see what we expect to see, even when the facts differ from our expectations; stereotypes can be favorable or unfavorable, and either kind is potentially harmful
5. **Prejudice** is negative feelings about people who are different from oneself

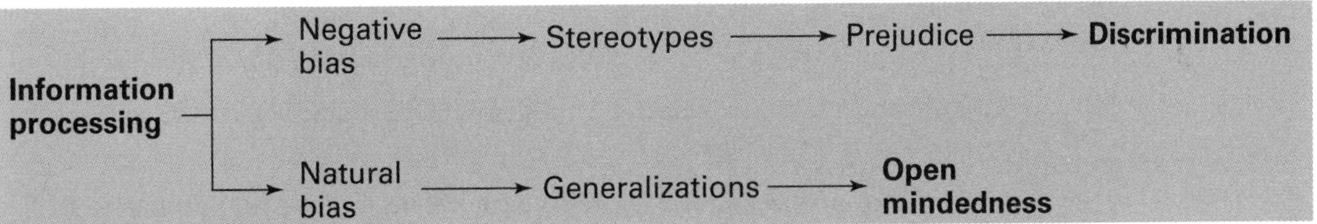

Figure 1-3 **Pathways to open-mindedness and discrimination.**

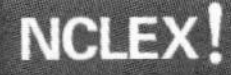

6. **Discrimination** is prejudice that is expressed behaviorally; examples are racism, ageism, heterosexism, and sexism

NCLEX!

7. Open-mindedness is a positive outcome in an attempt by the nurse to be more sensitive to diverse cultural groups and being willing to support clients in their own cultural beliefs and practices; see Figure 1-3 for diagram of pathways to open-mindedness or discrimination

E. Caring for a culturally diverse population

1. Effective advocacy for culturally diverse groups depends on a balance of knowledge, sensitivity, and skills
2. Nurses must understand their own ethnocentrism and acquire knowledge about other cultural groups
3. Sensitivity includes examining how our own attitudes, values, and prejudices affect our own nursing practice
4. Communication is an important skill in caring for clients from diverse backgrounds; it includes learning clients' level of fluency in spoken and written English, and determining the most important style of communication
5. Becoming culturally competent and confident in managing diversity requires practice and patience

X. Legal and Ethical Issues

A. Client autonomy and liberty: must be ensured by treatment in the least restrictive setting by active client participation in treatment

NCLEX!

B. Voluntary admission: occurs when a client consents to confinement in the hospital and signs a document indicating as much

NCLEX!

C. Commitment, or involuntary admission: may be implemented on the basis of dangerousness to self or others; some states also have the criterion of prevention of significant physical or mental deterioration for involuntary admission

NCLEX!

D. Competency: a legal determination that a client can make reasonable judgments and decisions about treatment and other significant areas of personal life

1. An adult is considered competent unless a *court* rules the client incompetent; in such cases, a guardian is appointed to make decisions on the person's behalf
2. Clients who are committed are still capable of participating in healthcare decisions

E. Informed consent: a client's right to be given enough information to make a decision, to be able to understand the information, and to communicate their decision to others; in an emergency situation with no time to obtain consent without endangering health or safety, a client may be treated without legal liability

F. **Adherence to the principle of confidentiality:** extremely important in the practice of psychiatric nursing

1. There are federal rules regarding chemical dependence confidentiality; staff members are not allowed to disclose any admission or discharge information
2. Some states require written consent before human immunodeficiency virus (HIV) tests may be performed; states have laws regarding when HIV test results or the diagnosis of acquired immunodeficiency syndrome (AIDS) may be disclosed
3. The duty to disclose is the healthcare professional's obligation to warn identified individuals if a client has made a credible threat to harm someone

G. **Nursing ethics**

1. Nurses are required to make numerous ethical decisions every day; client differences in values, culture, and lifestyles often present nurses and other healthcare providers with an ethical dilemma
2. Competent care involves knowing what and how to perform skills, being open to criticism, and a willingness to seek appropriate education when there are known knowledge deficits
3. The perspective of principalism in ethics ignores the socioeconomic and cultural contexts and is too abstract to have practical application in clinical practice
4. Nursing is based on ethics of care, including medical indications, client preferences, quality of life, and contextual factors

XI. NCLEX Test-Taking Tips for Psychiatric–Mental Health Nursing Questions

A. **NCLEX questions for psychiatric–mental health nursing:** primarily test on two levels—application and analysis

1. Application: the process of using information to know why a phenomenon occurs; effective application relies on the use of understood memorized facts to verify intended action; application is the progression from facts to nursing action; Box 1-4 gives an example of an application question

Box 1-4

Application Question

A client who is hospitalized for panic disorder is experiencing increased anxiety. The client exhibits selective inattention and tells the nurse, "I'm anxious now." The nurse determines that the degree of the client's anxiety is:

1. mild.
2. *moderate.* *
3. severe.
4. panic.

*The nurse must know the facts related to levels of anxiety. The nurse must be able to differentiate the correct level of anxiety the client is experiencing in order to implement appropriate nursing actions.

Box 1-5

Analysis Question

A hospitalized client with depression asked the nurse, "Do you think I should go home this weekend?" The nurse uses the technique of reflection when the nurse responds:

1. *"Should you go home for the weekend?"**
2. "Home means . . . ?"
3. "It sounds as if you haven't decided whether or not to go home this weekend."
4. "Do you think you are ready to go home this weekend?"

* The nurse must know the relationship of reflection in order to distinguish the cause and effect between it and the other communication techniques used in the situation.

2. Analysis: the ability to use abstract or logical forms of thought to show relationships and to distinguish the cause and effect between the variables in a situation; Box 1-5 gives an example of an analysis question
3. The components of a NCLEX test question include the basic parts of a background statement, a stem and a list of four options; most psychiatric–mental health nursing NCLEX test questions have two or more right answers; therefore, the question usually targets a BEST answer; the key to answering the questions is to understand the *what* or the *how* the question is attempting to elicit
   a. When answering a NCLEX test question, first read the background statement, noting key concepts or conditions, and then read the stem again noting key words
   b. Attempt to answer the question *before* reviewing the list of four options; if an option matches your hypothesized answer, that is the most likely correct response; if none of the options matches your hypothesized answer, then re-review the question noting the key concepts and words
   c. With physiological NCLEX-type questions, when all answer choices are equal in importance, the *priority* or the correct answer will most likely follow the rule of the "ABCs"—Airway, Breathing, Circulation; in psychological NCLEX-type questions, when all answer choices are equal in importance, the *priority* or the correct answer will most likely follow the rule of the "SEAs"—Safety, Expressing feelings, Assisting with problem-solving
   d. Questions that elicit an effective response by the nurse (refer back to Section VII, Therapeutic Communication) follow these general rules:
      1) Do not solve the clients' problems; the nurse's role is to assist clients in solving their own problems
      2) Correct responses often challenge clients to examine their own thoughts or feelings
      3) Often the correct response is to restate the client's comments or to reflect back to the client the content and/or feelings behind the client's comments
      4) Do not change the subject or topic; if the client brings up an unsettling topic, then the client is ready to discuss or address the issue

5) The nurse's role is *not* to make the client feel better, happier, or less worried; rather, it is to have clients develop an understanding of their own feelings and thoughts as well as to assist clients in forming their own solutions to problems

6) Do not discount the client's feelings or thoughts; a client who verbalizes sadness is not going to become less sad or happy because the nurse simply states "Don't worry," or "Don't be sad," or "Cheer up, it could be worse."

7) Feelings are not good or bad, they just *are;* it's the behaviors the client exhibits that make the situation good or bad; for example, anger is not a "bad" feeling; anger can motivate a client to change a stressful situation or to get out of a dangerous circumstance; however, an angry client who threatens to harm others or does harm to others may be placed in jail

Case Study

A nurse approaches a depressed female client on a psychiatric unit. The nurse sits down close to the client, introduces herself, compliments the client on her appearance, and asks, "Are you doing okay today?" The client leans away, maintains a rigid posture, avoids eye contact, and nods her head yes. The nurse leans back to give the client her space and crosses her arms over her chest to create a less threatening posture. After several minutes of silence, the nurse explains to the client that she has an hour that she can spend with her today. Following another long period of silence, the nurse says, "I guess you're not in the mood to talk today, so I'll see you tomorrow." The nurse leaves after spending 25 minutes with the client.

1. What actions by the nurse demonstrate respect for the client?
2. What actions by the nurse, if any, did not represent therapeutic communication skills and could decrease the client's confidence and trust in the nurse?
3. How would you interpret the client's body language and silence during this first session?
4. How could the nurse's interaction with the client have been improved?
5. Why do you think the nurse decided to leave after 25 minutes?

For suggested responses, see page 305.

Posttest

1 A client was quite upset the entire time she was pregnant and made it clear that she did not want her unborn child. However, after the birth, she becomes overly protective and refuses to let anyone else near the infant. The nurse recognizes this as the use of which defense mechanism?

(1) Denial
(2) Projection
(3) Reaction formation
(4) Displacement

2 In assisting a post-abortion client in dealing with the procedure, which approach by the nurse would be *best?*

(1) Reassuring her that she has made the best decision
(2) Encouraging her to use an effective method of birth control
(3) Encouraging expression of feelings of loss and disappointment
(4) Helping her to seek out spiritual help

3 A client expressed feelings of hopelessness and helplessness about her husband's illness and her inability to care for him. Of the following issues, which would be the *best* for the client to focus on first?

(1) Her husband's present illness
(2) Her past losses of significant others
(3) Her loneliness and isolation in her new surroundings
(4) Her future loss of her husband

4 While assessing the defense mechanisms used by the client, the nurse recognizes the client's use of defense mechanisms as adaptive when the:

(1) Mechanism used decreases anxiety.
(2) Client seeks isolation to avoid stress.
(3) Anxiety is expressed in behaviors.
(4) Client can identify the stressor.

5 A female client comes with the nurse for an evaluation with a therapist. As they sit down and prepare for the interview, the client turns to the therapist, looks at him sternly and says, "I didn't think you would even want to see or talk to me." The therapist responds, "How could this be since I do not even know who you are?" The nurse understands that the client's thinking is an example of which of the following defense mechanisms?

(1) Denial
(2) Projection
(3) Reaction formation
(4) Rationalization

6 The nursing intervention for action-level defense mechanisms, such as conversion and regression, is to:

(1) Teach the client to deal with impulses by taking constructive action.
(2) Encourage the client to continue such defense mechanisms, as they are adaptive.
(3) Listen to the client and encourage expression of feelings.
(4) Orient client to reality and encourage participation in social activities.

7 A nurse who practices subtle stereotyping or countertransference can expect the cultural assessment to:

(1) Be sensitive to the unmet needs of the culture.
(2) Be open and honest, reflecting the client's concerns.
(3) Reinforce the nurse's prejudices about the culture.
(4) Facilitate the treatment process.

8 The nurse should do which of the following as a primary nursing strategy for dealing effectively with the spiritual needs of clients?

(1) Refer clients to appropriate clergy.
(2) Clarify own spiritual beliefs and values.
(3) Use a spiritual assessment tool.
(4) Discuss own religiosity with the client.

9 During a team meeting, the nurse develops the outcomes of care for a depressed client. Which of the following is an appropriately stated outcome?

(1) Client will feel less depressed.
(2) Client's score on depression scale will decrease.
(3) Client will have significantly more insight into his problems.
(4) Client will feel supported as he deals with grief issues.

10 **Among the following symptoms reported by a grieving older adult, which should concern the nurse the *most?***

(1) Occasional shortness of breath
(2) Expressed thoughts of being better off dead
(3) Guilt about what was done at the time of a loved one's death
(4) A morbid preoccupation with worthlessness

See pages 27–28 for Answers and Rationales.

Answers and Rationales

Pretest

1 **Answer: 4** ***Rationale:*** Option 4 is seeking clarification after the nurse was unable to understand the client. Option 1 is exploring, option 2 is placing events in time or sequence, and option 3 is focusing.
Cognitive Level: Analysis
Nursing Process: Analysis; ***Test Plan:*** PSYC

2 **Answer: 2** ***Rationale:*** Countertransference is the nurse's emotional reaction to clients based on feelings for significant people in the nurse's past (option 2). Transference is the unconscious process of displaying feelings for significant people in the past onto the nurse in the present relationship (option 1). Denial is a defense mechanism used by individuals in an attempt to screen or ignore unacceptable realities by refusing to acknowledge them (option 3). Reaction formation is a defense mechanism that causes people to act exactly opposite to the way they feel (option 4).
Cognitive Level: Application
Nursing Process: Assessment; ***Test Plan:*** PSYC

3 **Answer: 4** ***Rationale:*** Advising clients prevents them from taking responsibility and using the problem-solving process. "Why" questions (option 1) demand an explanation for clients to defend themselves. Disagreeing with the client's actions denies clients the right to think and feel as they do (option 2). Belittling ignores the importance of the problem to the client (option 3).
Cognitive Level: Application
Nursing Process: Analysis; ***Test Plan:*** PSYC

4 **Answer: 3** ***Rationale:*** Feedback provides the opportunity for the nurse to offer clients information about their verbal and nonverbal responses. Giving advice (option 1) is an ineffective communication technique because the nurse should avoid giving advice by encouraging clients to solve their own problems. Exploring feelings (option 2) and explaining behavior (option 4) may be a part of the therapeutic communication and feedback, but the *primary* purpose of feedback is to offer clients information about themselves.
Cognitive Level: Application
Nursing Process: Assessment; ***Test Plan:*** PSYC

5 **Answer: 1** ***Rationale:*** Mental health is growing toward potential with an inner feeling of satisfaction. Mere absence of disease does not equal mental health (option 2). Dissatisfaction with a part of life is leaning toward the mentally unhealthy end of the continuum (option 3). Being healthy has a general feeling of vitality, not boredom (option 4).
Cognitive Level: Application
Nursing Process: Assessment; ***Test Plan:*** PSYC

6 **Answer: 2** ***Rationale:*** In supportive therapy the nurse takes on a noncondemning manner to promote client independence and productivity as much as possible. The nurse does not take on the role of beneficent authority (option 1). Negative emotions are discouraged initially (option 3) until the relationship has developed, and evaluating feelings of inferiority requires long-term therapy (option 4).
Cognitive Level: Application
Nursing Process: Implementation; ***Test Plan:*** PSYC

7 **Answer: 4** ***Rationale:*** The client's problem is clearly focused on the death of her father; subsequently, she would be a good candidate for short-term, focused psychotherapy. There is no indication of irreversible psychological trauma (option 1); her symptoms do not suggest the need for long-term therapy (option 2); and although the client is tearful and anxious, she is not overtly depressed (option 3).
Cognitive Level: Application
Nursing Process: Assessment; ***Test Plan:*** PSYC

8 **Answer: 1** ***Rationale:*** Clarifying the client's intention communicates to the client that all behaviors have meaning and gives the nurse the opportunity to set boundaries. Leaving the situation (option 2) or continuing to interact with the client without

acknowledging the comment (option 4) may reinforce the behavior as being acceptable. Refusing to interact with the client (option 3) harms the nurse–client relationship and should only be an option after the nurse has clearly set boundaries with the client.
Cognitive Level: Application
Nursing Process: Implementation; ***Test Plan:*** PSYC

9 **Answer: 2** ***Rationale:*** The hypothalamus is located in the diencephalon and is responsible for regulating temperature, appetite, and the integration of the autonomic nervous system. The thalamus (option 1) is also located in the diencephalon, and its functions are concerned primarily with sensation. The cerebrum's (option 3) primary functions include higher-order thinking, abstract reasoning, visual function, judgment, memory, and sensory function. The cerebellum (option 4) is primarily responsible for balance and coordination.
Cognitive Level: Application
Nursing Process: Assessment; ***Test Plan:*** PSYC

10 **Answer: 2** ***Rationale:*** Insufficient serotonin activity in the CNS is responsible for depression, not excessive serotonin (option 1). Excessive dopamine activity in the CNS (option 3) is responsible for schizophrenic disorders, and insufficient dopamine activity in the CNS (option 4) has not been shown to have a role in depression.
Cognitive Level: Application
Nursing Process: Evaluation; ***Test Plan:*** PSYC

Posttest

1 **Answer: 3** ***Rationale:*** Reaction formation is a mechanism that causes people to act exactly opposite to the way they feel. Denial (option 1) is an attempt to screen or ignore unacceptable realities by refusing to acknowledge them. Projection (option 2) is a process in which blame is attached to others or the environment for unacceptable desires, thoughts, shortcomings, and mistakes. Displacement (option 4) is the transferring or discharging of emotional reactions from one object or person to another object or person.
Cognitive Level: Analysis
Nursing Process: Analysis; ***Test Plan:*** PSYC

2 **Answer: 3** ***Rationale:*** Feelings of loss and guilt are normal following an abortion or loss; resolution of these feelings is essential to avoid future mental health issues. Telling the client that this was the best decision (option 1) is providing her with false reassurance. Although counseling the client about the use of effective birth control methods may be appropriate, it is not the time to discuss future prevention teaching (option 2) at this time. Seeking out spiritual help (option 4) is imposing the nurse's own personal choices on the client. First, the nurse should assess the client's spiritual needs.
Cognitive Level: Analysis
Nursing Process: Implementation; ***Test Plan:*** PSYC

3 **Answer: 2** ***Rationale:*** The nurse should help the client identify her coping strategies and her experience with past losses in order to identify the client's strengths and past coping strategies. This helps the client draw on experiences of the past to help her cope and look at events rationally. Focusing on the client's husband's current illness (option 1) will only keep the client stuck in hopelessness and helplessness. Focusing on loneliness and isolation (option 3) and the future loss of her husband (option 4) may be appropriate, but the nurse and client need to *first* examine how the client has coped with past losses.
Cognitive Level: Analysis
Nursing Process: Implementation; ***Test Plan:*** PSYC

4 **Answer: 1** ***Rationale:*** The purpose of defense mechanisms is to reduce anxiety levels and allow the client to function adequately. Seeking isolation to avoid stress (option 2) is an unhealthy adaptive strategy. Anxiety is expressed in behavior (option 3); however, that behavior can be harmful to clients or others. Recognition of a stressor (option 4) is important but may not be useful in the client's adaptive use of defense mechanisms.
Cognitive Level: Analysis
Nursing Process: Assessment; ***Test Plan:*** PSYC

5 **Answer: 2** ***Rationale:*** Projection is a process in which blame is attached to others or the environment for unacceptable desires, thoughts, shortcomings, and mistakes. This client does not feel the therapist will care about her. Denial (option 1) is an attempt to screen or ignore unacceptable realities by refusing to acknowledge them. Reaction formation (option 3) is a mechanism that causes people to act exactly opposite to the way they feel. Rationalization (option 4) is the justification of certain behaviors by faulty logic and ascription of motives that are socially acceptable but did not, in fact, inspire the behavior.
Cognitive Level: Analysis
Nursing Process: Assessment; ***Test Plan:*** PSYC

6 **Answer: 1** ***Rationale:*** Conversion and regressive behavior impair the client's ability to function in society. Teaching the client constructive ways to cope

would be helpful. These defense mechanisms are not adaptive and impair the client's function (option 2). Listening to the client's expression of feelings (option 3) and orienting the client to reality (option 4) are therapeutic but will not assist the client in coping with maladaptive defense mechanisms and may only increase the client's anxiety level.
Cognitive Level: Comprehension
Nursing Process: Implementation; *Test Plan:* PSYC

7 **Answer: 3** *Rationale:* Stereotyping arises out of negative biases; stereotypes are images frozen in time that cause us to see what we expect to see, even when the facts differ from our expectations. Countertransference is the nurse's emotional reaction to a client based on feelings for significant people in the nurse's past. These would only reinforce the nurse's prejudices about the culture and cause the nurse to be insensitive, not sensitive, to the client's needs (option 1). When governed by stereotyping or countertransference, the nurse is unable to be open and honest (option 2) and unable to facilitate effective treatment (option 4).
Cognitive Level: Analysis
Nursing Process: Assessment; *Test Plan:* PSYC

8 **Answer: 2** *Rationale:* The *first* priority of nurses in assisting clients to manage any area of their lives is to understand themselves and clarify their own spiritual beliefs and values. Referring clients to appropriate clergy (option 1) may be an effective intervention, but the nurse has adequate skills in meeting many spiritual needs of clients. Use of a spiritual assessment tool (option 3) is important but should be used after the nurse has done self-exploration. Discussing the nurse's own religious beliefs (option 4) is inappropriate and projects the nurse's own religious beliefs onto the client.
Cognitive Level: Analysis
Nursing Process: Evaluation; *Test Plan:* PSYC

9 **Answer: 2** *Rationale:* The most appropriate outcome is one that is measurable. Using a scale or depression score is a measurable outcome. The client's feeling of being less depressed (option 1) is less accurate in turns of agreed upon criteria of "less." Having insight into one's problems (option 3) does not necessarily cause a decrease in depression, and it may even initially increase depression. Support for the client as he deals with grief issues (option 4) will not necessarily decrease depression.
Cognitive Level: Application
Nursing Process: Planning; *Test Plan:* PSYC

10 **Answer: 2** *Rationale:* An older adult who expresses thoughts of death has priority over other choices—safety is always a priority. Everyone experiences grief differently. Older adults often normally experience grief somatically (option 1). Guilt about actions or lack of action at the time of a loved one's death (option 3) is not uncommon. A morbid preoccupation with worthlessness (option 4) is a concern, but safety takes priority.
Cognitive Level: Analysis
Nursing Process: Assessment; *Test Plan:* PSYC

References

American Psychiatric Association (2000). *Diagnostic and statistical manual of mental disorders* (4th ed.). Washington, DC: American Psychiatric Association.

Beck, A. (1976). *Cognitive therapies and the emotional disorders.* New York: International Universities Press.

Ellis, A. (1973). *Humanistic psychotherapy: The rational-emotive approach.* New York: The Julian Press.

Erikson, E. (1963). *Childhood and society.* New York: W. W. Norton.

Fontaine, K. L. (1999). Communicating and teaching. In K. L. Fontaine & J. S. Fletcher (Eds.), *Mental health nursing* (4th ed.). Menlo Park, CA: Addison-Wesley, pp. 5, 9–12, 21–22, 30–31, 89–113, 506–507.

Fontaine, K. L. (1999). Introduction to mental health nursing. In K. L. Fontaine & J. S. Fletcher (Eds.), *Mental health nursing* (4th ed.). Menlo Park, CA: Addison-Wesley, pp. 3–36.

Fontaine, K. L. (1999). Legal and ethical issues. In K. L. Fontaine & J. S. Fletcher (Eds.), *Mental health nursing* (4th ed.). Menlo Park, CA: Addison-Wesley, pp. 532–440.

Freud, S. (1936). *The problem of anxiety.* New York: W. W. Norton.

Frisch, N. & Frisch, L. (1998). *Psychiatric mental health nursing.* Albany, NY: Delmar.

Isaacs, A. (2001). *Mental health and psychiatric nursing* (3rd ed.). Philadelphia: Lippincott.

Kavanagh, K. H. (1999). The role of cultural diversity in mental health nursing. In K. L. Fontaine & J. S. Fletcher (Eds.),

Mental health nursing (4th ed.). Menlo Park, CA: Addison-Wesley, pp. 55–67.

Keltner, N., Schwecke, L. & Bostrom, C. (1999). *Psychiatric nursing* (3rd ed.). St. Louis: Mosby.

Menninger, K. (1963). *The vital balance.* Newark, NJ: Viking Press.

Moller, M. & Fontaine, K. L. (1999). Neurobiology and behavior. In K. L. Fontaine, & J. S. Fletcher (Eds.), *Mental health nursing* (4th ed.). Menlo Park, CA: Addison-Wesley, pp. 69–85.

Murray, C. & Lopez, A. (1990). *The global burden of disease and injury series, volume 1: A comprehensive assessment of mortality and disability from diseases, injuries, and risk factors in 1990 and projected to 2020.* Retrieved July 7, 2001 from the Internet at *http://www.nimh.nil.gov/ publicat/burden.cfm.*

Peplau, H. (1952). *Interpersonal relations in nursing.* New York: G. P. Putnam's Sons.

Piaget, J. (1974). *The origins of intelligence in children.* New York: International Universities Press.

Shives, L. (1998). *Basic concepts of psychiatric–mental health nursing* (4th ed.). Philadelphia: Lippincott-Raven.

Skinner, B. F. (1953). *Science and human behavior.* New York: Macmillan.

Sullivan, H. S. (1953). *Interpersonal theory of psychiatry.* New York: W. W. Norton.

Townsend, M. (1999). *Essentials of psychiatric–mental health nursing* (4th ed.). Philadelphia: F. A. Davis, pp. 101–114.

Townsend, M. (2001). *Nursing diagnoses in psychiatric nursing: Care plans and psychotropic medications* (5th ed.). Philadelphia: F. A. Davis.

CHAPTER 2

Crisis Intervention and Suicide

Mark D. Soucy, MS, RN, CS

CHAPTER OUTLINE

OBJECTIVES

- List five characteristics of a crisis situation.
- State four goals for crisis intervention and stabilization.
- Outline the steps involved in crisis intervention.
- Formulate six intervention strategies for clients experiencing a crisis.
- Describe six common myths of suicide.
- Identify at least two groups at high risk for suicide.
- Describe the therapeutic milieu for a client on suicide precautions.

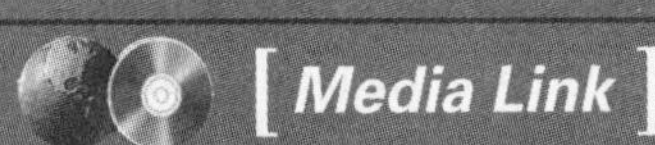

Use the CD-ROM enclosed with this text, or log onto the address given to access the free, interactive Companion Website created for this series. The CD-ROM and Companion Website accompanying this book offer additional practice opportunities and information—NCLEX Review, Case Studies, Glossary, In Depth with NCLEX, and more.

www.prenhall.com/hogan

REVIEW AT A GLANCE

coping *a conscious attempt to manage stress and anxiety; may be physical, cognitive or affective*

crisis *an experience of being confronted by a stress in which the individual is unable to cope or solve problems*

equilibrium *a state of balance; a condition in which contending forces are equal*

helplessness *a state that may arise when a client has a condition in which he or she is dependent on an outside source for life support*

hopelessness *a subjective state in which an individual sees limited or no alternatives or personal choices available and is unable to mobilize energy on own behalf*

suicide *the intentional and voluntarily taking of one's life*

Pretest

1 A client who is unable to cope with the sudden loss of a job and who is feeling confused and unable to make decisions is said to be experiencing which of the following?

(1) Adventitious crisis
(2) Maturational crisis
(3) Situational crisis
(4) Social crisis

2 In assessing a client in crisis, it is important for the nurse to first assist the client to identify:

(1) The client's feelings.
(2) The realistic nature of the event.
(3) Others who might be affected by the event.
(4) An immediate action plan.

3 A client was admitted to the hospital with suicidal ideations and a plan to harm himself. His wife recently died after a very brief illness, and he sees no reason to go on living. He says that his wife was his best friend, and they did everything together. He feels alone in the world and yet allows no one into his life. Which of the following nursing diagnoses *best* categorizes this problem?

(1) Helplessness related to the death of his wife
(2) Ineffective individual coping related to loneliness
(3) Post-trauma response related to suicidal plan
(4) Social isolation related to the loss of his wife and failure to establish meaningful relationships

4 A client came into the crisis center for assistance after he was involved in clean-up efforts following a shooting at a local high school. The client says he has been feeling very anxious since his involvement in these efforts. The nurse working with the client chooses which of the following to help him cope with the experience?

(1) Arrange for his priest to visit with him.
(2) Advise him to avoid going near the school for at least 90 days.
(3) Send him to the Emergency Department for further evaluation because he is experiencing a crisis situation, which is an emergency.
(4) Create an opportunity for to him to talk about his experience, ask him about how he has coped thus far, and explore enhanced coping skills.

5 When working with the client in crisis, which of the following is *most* important?

(1) Obtaining a complete assessment of the client's past history
(2) Remaining focused on the immediate problem
(3) Determining whether the client may have had a part in the emergence of the crisis
(4) Assisting the client to identify what is similar about this crisis to other crises in the client's life

6 A 35-year-old client with a diagnosis of bipolar disorder, mixed and borderline personality disorder was brought to the Emergency Department after taking a handful of pills and calling 911. The nurse overheard a staff member saying of the client, "Oh, here she comes again. If she was serious about committing suicide, she'd have done it by now." The nurse considers which of the following when preparing to see the client?

(1) Clients with personality disorders rarely kill themselves.
(2) People who talk about suicide or have a history of suicidal behavior are at serious risk of self-harm and each event must be taken seriously.
(3) The nurse should not reinforce manipulative behaviors, therefore the nursing assessment must be brief and exploration of suicidal ideations must be kept to a minimum.
(4) The nurse should anticipate that the client will be admitted directly to the inpatient unit.

7 The client is transferred to the psychiatric inpatient unit of a general hospital from the surgical ICU after being treated for a self-inflicted gunshot wound. The nurse schedules time to meet with the client on a one-to-one basis with which of the following goals in mind?

(1) The client will explore current life events that led to the suicide attempt.
(2) The client will initiate contact with the nurse spontaneously.
(3) The client will identify past suicidal ideations and behavior.
(4) The client will begin group therapy as soon as he is able to ambulate and remain seated for 50 minutes.

8 A client admitted to the psychiatric inpatient unit following expressed suicidal ideations tells the nurse the next day that she feels fine, is at peace, and wants to go home now. The nurse understands that the client:

(1) Has resolved her feelings and is no longer at risk for self-harm.
(2) Is probably ready to be discharged to home since the suicidal intent has been resolved.
(3) Remains at risk, may have sufficient psychic energy to act out on the suicidal ideation, and requires further assessment.
(4) Has reached a realistic self-appraisal of the serious nature of her suicidal intentions.

9 The *priority* nursing diagnosis for a client with suicidal ideations and intent is:

(1) Risk for violence, self-directed.
(2) Ineffective individual coping.
(3) Hopelessness.
(4) Defensive coping.

10 A female client is placed on one-to-one observation, and as the nurse follows her into the bathroom, she objects strongly, yelling, "I'm sick of being followed around and watched like a small child who can't be trusted." The *best* response for the nurse would be:

(1) "I understand you are angry, but I must be able to see you at all times to make sure you are safe."
(2) "Stop yelling at me! I can't change the rules for clients who talk about suicide as you have done."
(3) "Well, you are better; I'll wait outside the bathroom and you can close the door until you are finished."
(4) "You should stop being angry and uncooperative and focus on happy things."

See pages 45–46 for Answers and Rationales.

I. Overview of Crisis

A. Definition of *crisis:* an experience of being confronted by a stress in which the individual is unable to cope/problem-solve

1. Change or loss threatens the individual's **equilibrium:** a state of balance; a condition in which contending forces are equal

2. Anxiety and tension accompany the experience, making it more difficult to cope
3. Hopelessness and/or helplessness results in a state of disorganization where previous experience and coping fail to enable the individual to problem-solve; **coping** is a conscious attempt to manage stress and anxiety; may be physical, cognitive, or affective
4. **Hopelessness:** a subjective state in which an individual sees limited or no alternatives or personal choices available and is unable to mobilize energy on own behalf
5. **Helplessness:** a state that may arise when a client has a condition in which he or she depends on an outside source for life support
6. Loss of equilibrium ensues

NCLEX!

7. Crises are generally time limited, lasting from 4 to 6 weeks during which time there is a potential for either increased psychological vulnerability or personal growth

B. Developmental phases of crisis

1. Initial increase in tension as the stimulus continues and further discomfort is experienced
2. Failure to succeed in coping with the stimulus while continuing to experience distress
3. Additional tension forces mobilization of internal and external resources whereby emergency problem-solving efforts are attempted; the problem may be redefined or the individual may resign himself or herself and give up certain aspects of his or her goal that the client perceives as unattainable
4. If the problem remains unresolved and cannot be ignored, tension builds and major disorganization results

C. Characteristics of crisis

1. The stimulus is beyond the person's usual experience
2. Previously developed coping mechanisms are ineffective
3. Anxiety, tension, and disorganization ensue
4. The individual perceives a threat to own integrity and/or established goals

NCLEX!

5. Maturational crises involve normal life transitions that evoke changes in individual self-perception in role, status, and integrity

NCLEX!

6. Situational crises involve an external event that disturbs the individual's equilibrium (loss, change) and threatens consistency between self-behaviors and values or beliefs

NCLEX!

7. Adventitious crises involve external events such as natural disasters or other events of catastrophic proportion that are unpredictable and often engender fear, confusion, and loss of consistency with internalized beliefs/values and behavior; these may also be called a community crisis
8. Cultural crises accompany culture shock while adapting or adjusting to a new culture or returning to one's own culture after being assimilated into another

List at least two kinds of crises.

D. Balancing factors determining the client's response to crisis

1. The individual's perception of the event
2. Past experience in coping with stress
3. Established coping strategies
4. Availability of support persons

E. Goals for treatment

1. The client will remain free of self-harm
2. The client will identify the specific problem
3. The client will verbalize feelings related to the event
4. The client will analyze the event/problem and express perceptions of the event
5. The client will identify and seek help from support systems
6. The client will explore alternatives for coping with the crisis
7. The client will participate in choosing an action plan
8. The client will implement an action plan
9. The client will experience less anxiety and tension
10. The client will verbalize enhanced self-esteem

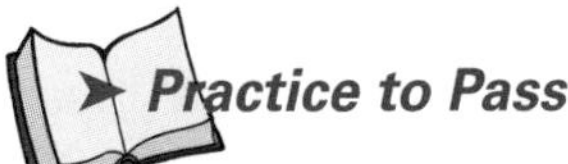

What are the balancing factors determining the client's response to a crisis situation?

II. Nursing Process during Crisis

A. Assessment

1. Identify the history of the presenting problem
   a. Focus on the immediate problem—not on past history
   b. Determine client's perception of problem—how threatened are they?
   c. Assess client's cognitive appraisal—identify any faulty thinking
2. Identify current feelings
   a. Assist client to express current feelings
   b. Validate current feelings and assist client to accept them
   c. Acknowledge that the client ultimately makes own decisions
3. Assess client's support systems
   a. Identify available resources in whom client trusts
   b. Identify spiritual and religious beliefs
4. Assess for potential for self-harm
   a. Ask directly if the client has had any thoughts of hurting or killing him- or herself
   b. Determine if the client has thought of plans or made plans to harm self
   c. Determine if the client has the means to harm/kill self (guns in house, access to medications with potential for overdose)

List at least five biological responses to stress or a crisis.

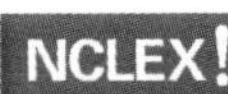

NCLEX!

d. Determine if the client can contract with the nurse to maintain safety and to identify an action plan if suicidal ideation increases or the client feels he or she will act on ideas to harm self

B. Nursing diagnoses/analysis useful in crisis

1. Nursing diagnoses related to safety/self harm
   - **a.** Risk for self-directed violence
   - **b.** Risk for self-mutilation
2. Nursing diagnoses related to coping
   - **a.** Ineffective individual coping
   - **b.** Ineffective family coping
   - **c.** Hopelessness
   - **d.** Impaired adjustment
   - **e.** Powerlessness
   - **f.** Post-trauma response
   - **g.** Altered role performance
   - **h.** Situational low self-esteem
   - **i.** Spiritual distress
3. Nursing diagnoses related to cognitive, perceptual, and communication problems
   - **a.** Acute confusion
   - **b.** Impaired verbal communication
   - **c.** Decisional conflict
   - **d.** Sensory/perceptual alterations (specify, illusions, cognitive distortions, etc.)
   - **e.** Altered thought process: visual hallucination, auditory hallucination, ideas of reference, delusions, inability to make decisions
4. Nursing diagnoses related to behavioral responses
   - **a.** Impaired social isolation
   - **b.** Social isolation
   - **c.** Powerlessness
   - **d.** Potential self care deficits

C. Planning and implementation for clients in crisis

1. Specific treatment modalities
   - **a.** Mutual goal planning; often the nurse must use a directive approach
   - **b.** Goals are set based on the assessment and nursing diagnoses
   - **c.** Overarching goals include establishing a relationship with the client, identifying the problem, identifying and reducing the client's perceptual distortions, enhancing self-esteem, alleviating anxiety, promoting engagement of

support systems (family and friends), reinforcing healthy coping, and validating the client's ability to problem-solve

d. Examine client's feelings that may block ability to cope adaptively

e. Teach the client how to ask for help from others

f. Identify previously acquired adaptive coping strategies and assist the client to modify and expand these coping strategies to the new stress

g. Teach and encourage the use of expression of feelings, comfort strategies, and self-care activities

h. Focus on problem resolution in a step by step, concrete way, first focusing on alternatives and then selecting and acting on appropriate ones

i. Consider involving the client in a crisis group, which helps clients feel less isolated and engage in group problem-solving to identify alternatives

j. Involve family in crisis intervention, as other members of the family often experience the crisis

D. Evaluation/outcomes for clients in crisis

1. Evaluation of outcomes is measured by comparing actual outcomes to the goals of treatment and client response to nursing interventions

a. The client will remain free of self-harm

b. The client has clearly identified the problem

c. Perceptual distortions have been identified and resolved

d. The client verbalizes a stable sense of self-esteem and perceives the ability to work on the problem

e. Anxiety has been reduced by identification and implementation of effective coping strategies

f. Unhealthy coping mechanism is identified and explored if client is willing

g. The client acknowledges his or her need for help and asks for help

h. The client identifies and verbalizes his or her feelings

i. The client demonstrates self-care behaviors

j. The client verbalizes an action plan

k. The client has begun to implement the action plan

E. Potential for growth

1. The client identifies and practices new coping skills that may be useful in the future in dealing with stressful and potentially traumatic events

2. The client verbalizes a renewed or enhanced sense of self-worth

III. Psychopharmacology as Treatment during Crisis

A. Treatment with pharmacologic interventions should not interfere with crisis intervention strategies such as crisis intervention

B. A crisis is not a psychiatric illness, nor a prolonged condition, therefore pharmacologic interventions are not the intervention of choice

C. **Pharmacologic agents** may be used to treat target symptoms that interfere with the client's ability to function but should *not* be used as a substitute for crisis intervention

D. **Anxiolytics of the benzodiazepine group** such as alprazolam (Xanax), clonazepam (Klonopin), diazepam (Valium), lorazepam (Ativan), etc. may be used to treat anxiety, panic, and sleep disturbances that accompany a crisis

E. **Other agents** such as the antidepressant trazadone (Desyrel) may be used for the management of insomnia

F. **Neuroleptic medications:** the atypicals, such as olanzapine (Zyprexa), risperidone (Risperdal), quetiapine (Seroquel) and typical agents such as haloperidol (Haldol), etc.), may be used to treat psychotic symptoms that emerge; however, psychosis does not commonly follow the experience of a crisis unless the client has a preexisting psychotic disorder

IV. Overview of Suicide

A. ***Suicide:*** the intentional and voluntary taking one's life

B. **Suicide is the 8th-leading cause of death** among all age groups and the 3rd-leading cause of death in young people

1. Whites are more likely to die from suicide than non-whites
2. Men are 3 to 4 times more likely to commit suicide than women and the elderly are 4 times more likely to kill themselves than younger people
3. Gay teens are at increased risk of suicide

C. **Adolescent and young adult suicide:** suicide is the 3rd-leading cause of death in adolescents and the second most common cause of death in college students; in the past 25 years there has been a 25 percent increase in suicides among adolescents

D. **Clients contemplating suicide** often perceive themselves as isolated; this isolation may be in physical distance or by way of interpersonal discord; there are often experiences of helplessness, loss of self-esteem with feelings of worthlessness, and hopelessness, the latter being most predictive of suicide

E. **Often the desire to be free from pain or to be dead is accompanied by depression and anger**

F. **Warning signs** that may indicate risk for suicidal ideations and self-injurious behavior include changes in personal habits such as appetite, sleep patterns, personal appearance, personality, use of alcohol and other drugs, as well as bodily complaints, self-depreciating comments, making wills and/or giving away personal/meaningful belongings

G. **Academic/occupational warning signs** include truancy/absenteeism, decline in academic/occupational performance, boredom, apathy, disruptive classroom or work behavior and anger/hostility toward authority figures

H. **Family and social relationship warning signs** include decreased interactions with peers and friends; a change in the people the client is spending time with, and either a greater lack or absence of romantic relationships

I. **The single most predictive psychiatric disorder for suicide is the presence of a mood disorder**

J. Common myths of suicide

1. People who talk about suicide won't actually commit suicide
2. People who are serious about suicide will show warning signs or give clues
3. Young children do not commit suicide
4. An improvement in mood means the risk for suicide is over
5. Only people who are depressed commit suicide
6. A written or verbal safety contract is a guarantee that the client will not kill himself or herself

K. Conscious and unconscious suicidal intention

1. Conscious suicidal ideations include an awareness on the part of the client of the potential outcomes or results of suicidal behavior, awareness of other's response to suicidal threats or attempts, awareness of the lethality index of a chosen method, and an awareness of rescue possibilities
2. Unconscious suicidal ideation may be more difficult to assess
   - **a.** The desire to cause self-harm or self-destruction may be beyond the client's conscious awareness
   - **b.** The client may engage in high-risk behaviors that are a way of acting out the unconscious desire to harm themselves (e.g., drinking and driving and engaging in potentially lethal activity)
   - **c.** Careful attention must be paid to direct and indirect ways in which the client may be communicating unconscious suicidal ideations

V. Nursing Process for Suicide

A. Suicide assessment

1. During the initial assessment, question the client about any thoughts or feelings related to harming or killing himself or herself; determining suicidal ideations, how the client has sought help, what kind of plan the client has made, the mental status of the client, the client's available support systems, and the client's lifestyle are all part of the nursing assessment
   - **a.** Ask questions like "Have you had any thoughts about life not being worth living?" (passive suicidal ideations)
   - **b.** Move from general to specific questions like: "Have you had any ideas about killing yourself?"
     - 1) It is a misnomer that the client will volunteer this information without being asked
     - 2) The nurse must be comfortable asking these questions directly and in a matter-of fact way
   - **c.** If the client answers yes, ask the client, "Have you thought of/or made any plans on how you might harm or kill yourself?"
   - **d.** Levels of lethality may be assessed, in part, based on answers to these questions; further assessment includes asking about access to means to self-harm, (i.e., do you have a gun in your home?) and evaluation of the lethality of the means (e.g., guns vs. pills)

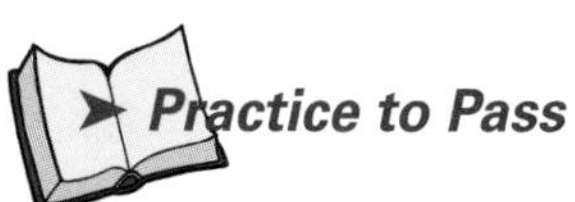

List at least 10 clues to a client's potential for suicide.

e. Take a careful history of previous self-harming behaviors by asking the client such questions as, "Have you ever tried to harm yourself or kill yourself in the past?"

f. Complete a mental status assessment to determine such things as evidence of alterations in thought process, impulsiveness, perceptual distortions, insight and judgment

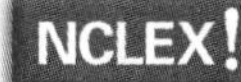

2. Clients may lack the emotional or psychic energy to act on suicidal ideations as a result of some of the negative or neurovegetative symptoms they experience; thus the nurse must be aware that a sudden sense of peace or wellness reported by the client may indicate that the client has sufficient psychic energy to carry out a suicidal act

B. Nursing diagnosis pertaining to suicide

1. Risk for self-directed violence
2. Ineffective individual coping
3. Hopelessness
4. Powerlessness
5. Chronic low self-esteem
6. Altered thought process
7. Social isolation
8. Defensive coping

C. Goal setting for clients at risk for suicide

1. The client will remain safe and free of self-harm
2. The client will verbalize suicidal ideations and discuss these with nursing staff

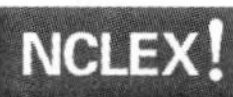

3. The client will develop a safety plan with the nursing staff and other members of the treatment team that identifies steps to keep himself or herself safe and ask for help before acting out a suicidal/self harm thought(s)
4. The client will verbalize a decrease or absence in suicidal ideations
5. The client will verbalize a desire to live and reasons for living

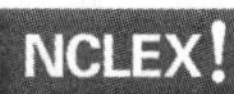

6. The client will identify an aftercare plan following discharge from the hospital that includes a commitment to follow up with psychotherapy and adherence to psychopharmacologic interventions
7. The client will identify a support system outside the hospital

D. Nursing interventions to reduce risk of suicide

1. Inpatient treatment is indicated if the client is felt to be at high risk for self-directed violence
2. Inpatient interventions include providing a safe milieu in which the client's ability to act out on suicidal ideations is minimized

a. While the client may be admitted to the milieu voluntarily, the unit is self-contained and doors are commonly locked; nursing staff regulate the flow of traffic on and off the unit

NCLEX!

b. Depending on the degree of suicidal ideation and lethality assessed, place the client on constant observation for the first 24 hours or until the degree of suicidal risk is lessened

NCLEX!

c. Place the client on q 15-minute checks thereafter

d. Maintain an awareness of the client's whereabouts constantly

e. Develop rapport with the client and foster a therapeutic relationship with the client

f. On admission to the unit, assess the client's personal belongings and remove any items that could be used by the client to harm him- or herself (drugs, potentially sharp objects, cords, and neck ties) and keep them in a safe place

NCLEX!

g. Keep the unit free of materials that can be readily used by clients to harm themselves (i.e., metal or glass objects that may be altered to create a sharp edge, light fixture or call bell cords); keep windows locked, count silverware, and check the client's belongings when returning from a pass; check gifts and other items brought in by family members/friends for safety before being given to the client

h. Work with the client to develop a safety plan and assess the client frequently

i. Meet with the client one-to-one to explore the client's feelings and help the client work toward re-engagement with significant others and fulfilling life activities

j. Give the client a roommate to reduce opportunity for solitude

k. Make sure that the client swallows oral medications and is not holding the medication in the oral cavity to hoard medications for a later overdose

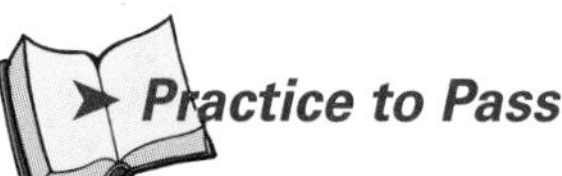

What are some precautions used in ensuring suicidal prevention of a hospitalized client?

l. Work with the client's participation to identify an aftercare plan that includes a commitment on the client's part to attend aftercare appointments, maintain contact with social support systems, and identify a safety plan with emergency contact numbers and an action plan should suicidal ideations return

m. Realize that despite use of all proper precautions, a client may still take own life after hospitalization (if unable to do so during); the ultimate decision to live belongs with the client

E. Evaluation/outcomes for clients comtemplating suicide; the client will:

1. Remain safe and free from self-directed violence
2. Verbalize the absence or decreased intensity and severity of suicidal ideations, with absence of plan and intent
3. Verbalize a desire to live and state several reasons for living
4. Agree to maintain a "no-self harm contract" with the nursing staff and other treatment staff for specified periods of time
5. Identify a safety plan should suicidal ideations worsen, intent reemerge, or the when the client feels unsafe, that provides for asking for help before acting out
6. Meet other goals incorporated in the treatment plan relative to other problems identified

VI. Psychopharmacology as Treatment to Prevent Suicide

A. **Pharmacologic interventions** used in the presence of suicidal ideations are aimed at treating the underlying mood disorder, other psychiatric disorder, or coexisting psychiatric disorders

B. **Since there is a high correlation between mood disorders and suicide,** adequate treatment of these mood disorders is essential in the overall treatment of clients at risk for suicide

C. **Depressive disorders** are treated with antidepressants; because of the relatively low risk of lethal overdose with the selective serotonin reuptake inhibitors (SSRIs), in addition to their relatively low side effect profile, these agents are often first-line drugs in the treatment of depression

D. **The SSRIs are:**

1. Citalopram (Celexa)
2. Paroxetine (Paxil)
3. Fluoxetine (Prozac)
4. Sertraline (Zoloft)

NCLEX!

E. **While effective in the treatment of depression,** tricyclic antidepressants can be highly lethal in overdose and are not a first-line agent; when used, the quantity of tablets/capsules dispensed at any given time should be kept at a minimum and may need to be managed by a family member; the tricyclics are:

1. Amitriptyline (Elavil)
2. Clomipramine (Anafranil)
3. Desipramine (Norpramin)
4. Doxepin (Sinequan)
5. Imipramine (Tofranil)
6. Nortriptyline (Pamelor)
7. Trimipramine (Surmontil)

F. **Other agents** such as the tetracyclics and atypical antidepressants are also helpful in treating depressive disorders and include:

1. Bupropion (Wellbutrin)
2. Nefazadone (Serzone)
3. Trazadone (Desyrel)
4. Venlafaxine (Effexor)
5. Mirtazipine (Remeron)

NCLEX!

G. **Monoamine oxidase inhibitors (MAOIs)** are useful in treating depressive disorders; however, there are serious drug and food interactions that make these agents presenting particularly challenging; they can be used if clients will comply with a tyramine-free diet (noncompliance can lead to hypertensive crisis); they are:

1. Tranylcypromine (Parnate)

2. Phenelzine (Nardil)
3. Isocarboxazid (Marplan)

H. Bipolar disorders: characterized by cycling of moods with episodes of mania and depression are also associated with suicide; they are treated with a class of drugs known as mood stabilizers:

1. Lithium
2. Valproic acid (Depakote)
3. Zyprexa (Olanzapine), a neuroleptic
4. Tegretol (Carbamazepine)

I. Clients with other psychiatric disorders are also at risk for suicide and may be treated with anxiolytics, neuroleptics, and other psychotropic agents; any psychotropic medication can be dangerous in overdose, thus a careful assessment must be made with proper client and family teaching about each drug (see psychopharmacology section)

Case Study

An 82-year-old male client with a history of major depression was brought to the Emergency Department by his son. The client recently lost his wife of 53 years, moved into an assisted living facility, and had to give up the family pet in order to move. The client had ingested an unknown quantity of sleeping medication and was found unresponsive by his son and daughter-in-law. After stabilization in the Emergency Department, the client is referred to the mental health unit for hospitalization.

❶ What are some risk factors of this client to suicide?

❷ List the top three nursing diagnoses.

❸ List at least five nursing interventions for suicidal clients.

❹ Identify at least two outcome expectations for this client.

❺ What are precautions the nurse should take to ensure the client is safe?

For suggested responses, see page 305.

Posttest

1 In working with a client in crisis, the nurse recognizes that there are four balancing factors that determine if an individual will enter a crisis state. Which of the following is a balancing factor?

(1) How the person perceives the event
(2) How the person feels about the event
(3) How close the person is to the event
(4) How many times the person has been exposed to the event

2 The nurse working with a client using crisis intervention understands that crisis intervention is different from traditional Freudian therapy in that crisis intervention focuses on:

(1) Unconscious processes that are the goal of personality change.
(2) An immediate problem as perceived by the client with a short-term goal of problem resolution.
(3) Past experiences with a goal of self-actualization.
(4) Pathology as the underlying reason for inadequate coping.

3 When caring for a client in crisis the nurse assists the client in asking for help from others by role modeling because clients in crisis:

(1) Often are overwhelmed, feel isolated, and may be unable to ask for help on their own.
(2) Lose their ability to act autonomously.
(3) Have an external locus of control.
(4) Feel guilty.

4 A 50-year-old client comes to the outpatient crisis unit after several people in his family have been involved in an auto accident. He is somewhat disorganized, anxious, and jumps from one subject to the next. The nurse uses which of the following as the most effective approach?

(1) Allows the client to continue in his disjointed efforts to discuss the events that preceded accident
(2) Sends the client to the chapel to gather his thoughts
(3) Assists the client to focus on the problem, providing direction for him to identify the problem and immediate alternatives
(4) Requests a one-time anxiolytic for the client to alleviate his anxiety

5 A 23-year-old client who's life partner died recently from complications of AIDS has just found out that he is HIV-positive. He has been referred to the outpatient crisis unit from his doctor's office because he "shut down" after finding out his HIV status. The nurse meets with the client, provides comfort measures, and begins the assessment. An *immediate* priority is to evaluate if the client:

(1) Is at risk for self-directed violence.
(2) Has an altered thought process.
(3) Has a psychiatric provider.
(4) Has a fear of dying.

6 A young client in his 20s frequently engages in high-risk behaviors including driving his car at excessive speeds, drinking excessively, and engaging in high-risk sexual behaviors. The nurse assessing this client suspects that:

(1) His substance abuse leads to these behaviors.
(2) He may be experiencing unconscious suicidal ideations.
(3) He is in an arrested stage of growth and development.
(4) He has an antisocial personality disorder.

7 The nursing staff of the psychiatric inpatient unit maintains a safe milieu by monitoring the whereabouts of clients at all times. A client with suicidal ideations and feeling unable to contract for his or her own safety is considered at high risk for self-directed violence. The nursing staff must be prepared to implement:

(1) Checks every 15 minutes.
(2) Constant observation.
(3) Having a roommate assigned to the client.
(4) Having the client wear a special ID bracelet.

8 A 52-year-old client who was admitted to the hospital 5 days ago with major depression and suicidal ideations is now preparing for discharge. Which of the following statements by the client demonstrates she has met one of her outcome/evaluation measures? "When I go home:

(1) I'll finally get some sleep."
(2) I'll be able to take care of my plants again."
(3) I have a list of people that I can call if I start to feel poorly."
(4) I'll cook for myself."

9 When working with a depressed client with suicidal ideation, the nurse understands that the client may be overwhelmed by personal problems. Keeping this in mind, the nurse assists the client in coping by:

(1) Encouraging the client to make a list of problems from most urgent to least urgent.
(2) Supporting the client to put off problem-solving until outpatient therapy has begun.
(3) Encouraging the client to work on problems only in group therapy.
(4) Taking a directive approach and advising the client on how to set priorities.

10 In teaching the family of a client with suicidal ideations how to help care for the person at home, the nurse includes which of the following priority interventions with the family?

(1) Explain to the family that after discharge they are responsible for keeping the client safe.
(2) Inform the family about warning signs the client may exhibit that indicate the client may be struggling and to eliminate guns and other weapons from the home.
(3) Teach the family about basic psychological processes and how to intervene when appropriate.
(4) Teach the family crisis intervention strategies.

See pages 46–47 for Answers and Rationales.

Answers and Rationales

Pretest

1 **Answer: 3** ***Rationale:*** A situational crisis is one that is often sudden and unavoidable. The stressful event threatens a person's physical, emotional, or social integrity. An adventitious crisis (option 1) occurs from an accidental or sporadic event. A maturational crisis (option 2) occurs because of a situation occurring from the maturing process, such as in adolescents or older adults. A social crisis (option 4) is a crisis that occurs within a social context.
Cognitive Level: Application
Nursing Process: Assessment; ***Test Plan:*** PSYC

2 **Answer: 1** ***Rationale:*** It is helpful for the client to identify the feelings he or she has about the crisis in order to feel validated and begin work on the problem. The realistic nature of the event (option 2), others impacted by the event (option 3), and a plan of action (option 4) all are important next steps once the client has identified his or her own feelings.
Cognitive Level: Analysis
Nursing Process: Assessment; ***Test Plan:*** PSYC

3 **Answer: 4** ***Rationale:*** In order to deal with crisis, clients must identify and be able to rely on others in their world whom they find supportive and who will be there after the immediate crisis is over. There is not enough data to support the other nursing diagnoses (options 1, 2, and 3).
Cognitive Level: Analysis
Nursing Process: Analysis; ***Test Plan:*** PSYC

4 **Answer: 4** ***Rationale:*** Assessing current coping and assisting in the enhancement of coping skills will enable the client to gain problem solving in his present circumstance and afford new coping for the future. Arranging for a priest (option 1) may be an effective intervention, but the nurse must first assess whether the client would find this intervention beneficial. Avoiding the school for 90 days (option 2) may or may not be either effective or possible and referring the client to Emergency Department (option 3) is too early at this time.
Cognitive Level: Analysis
Nursing Process: Planning; ***Test Plan:*** PSYC

5 **Answer: 2** ***Rationale:*** The nurse must remain focused on the immediate problem as there is not enough time and no need to delve into the complete past history (option 1). The client's role in the current crisis (option 3) is not relevant at this time, although it may be more important in learning to prevent future crisis situations. Assisting the client to identify what is similar about this crisis to other crises (option 4) may be a usual next step.

Cognitive Level: Application
Nursing Process: Implementation; *Test Plan:* PSYC

6 **Answer: 2** *Rationale:* The majority of people who commit suicide communicate intent either verbally or nonverbally. All expressions of suicidal intent must be taken seriously and each episode must be evaluated individually. Clients with personality disorders (option 1) are at greater risk of committing suicide than the general public. This client is at serious risk of suicide and a complete assessment must be performed (option 3). The client may or may not be admitted to the inpatient unit (option 4).
Cognitive Level: Application
Nursing Process: Assessment; *Test Plan:* PSYC

7 **Answer: 1** *Rationale:* A priority goal for the client, once safety has been assured, is to explore life events leading to the decision to die. This can then be followed by reviewing current feelings in the hopes that the client will now want to live. The other goals (options 2, 3, and 4) are not relevant to the client's current needs.
Cognitive Level: Application
Nursing Process: Planning; *Test Plan:* PSYC

8 **Answer: 3** *Rationale:* People who have completed suicide frequently showed an improvement in mood and energy prior to their deaths. Improved mood and energy may mean the client has resolved ambivalent feelings about suicide and has decided to kill him- or herself.
Cognitive Level: Application
Nursing Process: Assessment; *Test Plan:* PSYC

9 **Answer: 1** *Rationale:* The first priority in caring for the client with suicidal ideation is maintaining safety. Ineffective individual coping (option 2), hopelessness (option 3), and defensive coping (option 4) are appropriate only after safety has been assured.
Cognitive Level: Analysis
Nursing Process: Assessment; *Test Plan:* PSYC

10 **Answer: 1** *Rationale:* Acknowledging the client's feelings of frustration and reaffirming the need for safety is the priority. Telling the client to stop yelling (option 2) and telling the client to stop being angry (option 4) ignore and discount the client's feelings. The client must be observed at all times to ensure her safety (option 3).
Cognitive Level: Analysis
Nursing Process: Implementation; *Test Plan:* PSYC

Posttest

1 **Answer: 1** *Rationale:* The four balancing factors that determine entry into a crisis state are how the person perceives the event, past experience in coping, available coping mechanisms, people who can be supportive to the person. Options 2, 3, and 4 are not balancing factors.
Cognitive Level: Comprehension
Nursing Process: Planning; *Test Plan:* PSYC

2 **Answer: 2** *Rationale:* Crisis intervention assists a client in resolving an immediate problem that the client perceives as overwhelming. Issues from the client's personality (option 1), past experiences (option 3), and pathology (option 4) are not dealt with until the crisis is resolved.
Cognitive Level: Comprehension
Nursing Process: Implementation; *Test Plan:* PSYC

3 **Answer: 1** *Rationale:* It is natural for clients in crisis to feel isolated and withdrawn. Clients frequently need help communicating with others directly, especially if they place a high value on independence. Role modeling by the nurse helps the client to learn this skill. Options 2, 3, and 4 are incorrect.
Cognitive Level: Application
Nursing Process: Implementation; *Test Plan:* PSYC

4 **Answer: 3** *Rationale:* The nurse keeps the client focused and provides direction to avoid fragmentation of the client's efforts (option 1). Sending the client to a chapel (option 2) is not appropriate at this time. Nonpharmacological strategies should be attempted prior to pharmacological strategies (option 4).
Cognitive Level: Application
Nursing Process: Implementation; *Test Plan:* PSYC

5 **Answer: 1** *Rationale:* While some clients will not talk about thoughts of self-harm, they will usually talk about suicidal thoughts when asked. Safety is priority and suicidal clients should not be left alone. Altered thought process (option 2), psychiatric providers (option 3), and feelings toward dying (option 4) are important assessments areas after the client's safety has been ensured.
Cognitive Level: Analysis
Nursing Process: Assessment; *Test Plan:* PSYC

6 **Answer: 2** *Rationale:* Unconscious suicidal behavior is often expressed by extreme risk-taking behaviors. Options 1, 3, and 4 are incorrect.
Cognitive Level: Analysis
Nursing Process: Assessment; *Test Plan:* PSYC

7 Answer: 2 ***Rationale:*** Providing safety and preventing violence on an inpatient unit involves one-to-one supervision for the client as warranted, based on an assessment of current lethality level. Checks every 15 minutes (option 1) may not be safe enough for this client. Assigning a roommate (option 3) and wearing a special ID bracelet (option 4) do not ensure client safety.
Cognitive Level: Application
Nursing Process: Implementation; *Test Plan:* PSYC

8 Answer: 3 ***Rationale:*** One desired outcome is for the client to have enhanced social support. The client should be sleeping better by discharge (option 1). Taking care of her plants (option 2) and cooking for herself (option 4) do not necessarily indicate the client's level of recovery.
Cognitive Level: Analysis
Nursing Process: Evaluation; *Test Plan:* PSYC

9 Answer: 1 ***Rationale:*** Nurses help reduce the client's feelings of being overwhelmed by helping clients prioritize concerns and problems. Supporting the client to put off problem-solving (option 2) is not advisable. Working on problem-solving within a group setting (option 3) is one of many ways to solve problems. Being directive and setting the priorities for the client (option 4) should be avoided.
Cognitive Level: Application
Nursing Process: Implementation; *Test Plan:* PSYC

10 Answer: 2 ***Rationale:*** After determining the degree of family availability, teach the family about critical warning signs to watch for and how to keep the environment safe, thus minimizing the risk for self-directed violence at home. The family members have shared responsibility for the client's safety (option 1). Teaching families about basic psychological processes (option 3) and crisis intervention (option 4) may be appropriate after making the home environment safe.
Cognitive Level: Analysis
Nursing Process: Implementation; *Test Plan:* PSYC

References

Aguilera, D .C. (2000). Crisis intervention. In K. M. Fortinash & P. A. Holoday-Worret (Eds.), *Psychiatric-mental health nursing* (2nd ed.). St. Louis: Mosby, pp. 590–603.

American Psychiatric Association (2000). *Diagnostic and statistical manual of mental disorders* (4th ed.). Washington, DC: American Psychiatric Association.

Barbee, M. A. & Bricker, P. (2000). Suicide. In K. M. Fortinash & P. A. Holoday-Worret (Eds.), *Psychiatric-mental health nursing* (2nd ed.). St. Louis: Mosby, pp. 652–677.

Fontaine, K. L. (1999). Suicide. In K. Fontaine & J. Fletcher (Eds.), *Mental health nursing* (4th ed.). Menlo Park, CA: Addison-Wessley, pp. 413–427.

CHAPTER 3

Infancy, Childhood, Adolescence, and Developmental Disabilities

Pamela Gaurkee, RN, BSN

CHAPTER OUTLINE

OBJECTIVES

- Discuss at least three causative factors pertaining to disorders of infancy, childhood, and adolescence.
- Differentiate assessment techniques used in evaluating infants, children, and adolescents.
- List four nursing diagnoses associated with psychiatric disorders in infancy, childhood, and adolescence.
- Formulate four intervention strategies unique to disorders of infancy, childhood, and adolescence.
- Identify five characteristics commonly seen in developmental disorders.
- Explain the dynamics of autistic behavior.
- Formulate four intervention strategies frequently used for children with developmental disorders.
- Describe at least five factors that may contribute to development of an eating disorder.
- Differentiate between anorexia nervosa and bulimia nervosa.

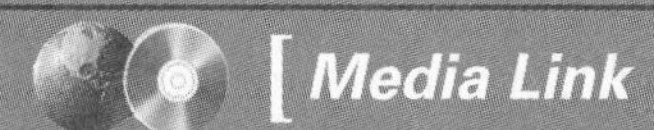

Use the CD-ROM enclosed with this text, or log onto the address given to access the free, interactive Companion Website created for this series. The CD-ROM and Companion Website accompanying this book offer additional practice opportunities and information—NCLEX Review, Case Studies, Glossary, In Depth with NCLEX, and more.

www.prenhall.com/hogan

Review at a Glance

eating binges *episodes of continuous eating even when not hungry*

encopresis *fecal incontinence*

enuresis *incontinence of urine, especially nocturnal bedwetting*

purging *the act of self-vomiting to empty the stomach after eating*

Pretest

1 The nurse is evaluating the progress of a client with an admission diagnosis of bulimia. Which of the following behaviors would indicate the client is making positive progress?

(1) The client's conversations focus on food.
(2) The client identifies healthy ways of coping with anxiety.
(3) The client spends time alone in own room following each meal.
(4) Family contact around meals is minimal.

2 A 13-year-old child is brought to the clinic with a history of conduct disorder. In obtaining a nursing history, which of the following behaviors would suggest support for the diagnosis?

(1) The parents have very high expectations of the child.
(2) There is inconsistent limit-setting with very harsh discipline.
(3) The parents are very involved with the child.
(4) The child has no siblings.

3 A client comes into the clinic for genetic counseling. She fears having another child with autism. The *most* appropriate response by the nurse is:

(1) "There is no way to predict if you will have an autistic child before conception."
(2) "Autism does not run in families."
(3) "There is a genetic tendency for autism to run in families."
(4) "You have a 50/50 chance of having a child without autism."

4 Primary nursing interventions effective for the impulsive, egocentric, and aggressive behaviors of children with conduct disorders are:

(1) Limit setting and consistency.
(2) Open communication and flexible approach.
(3) Open expression of feelings.
(4) Assertiveness training.

5 The nurse assesses for which of the following common anxiety disorders among children?

(1) Obsessive-compulsive disorder
(2) Simple phobia
(3) Separation anxiety disorder
(4) Post-traumatic stress disorder (PTSD)

6 In planning the care for a young child with oppositional defiant disorder, the psychiatric nurse would include:

(1) Reminiscence therapy.
(2) Emotive therapy.
(3) Behavior modification.
(4) Cognitive retraining.

7 A 3-year-old client has been diagnosed with attention deficit/hyperactivity disorder (ADHD). Which medication is most likely to be prescribed?

(1) Amitriptyline (Elavil)
(2) Paroxetene (Paxil)
(3) Methylphenidate (Ritalin)
(4) Pemoline (Cyclert)

8 One of the outcomes of play therapy is to enable children to:

(1) Act out feelings in a constructive manner.
(2) Learn to talk openly about themselves.
(3) Learn how to give and receive feedback.
(4) Learn problem-solving skills.

9 Community-based peer helping programs provide adolescents *primarily* with:

(1) Recreational activities.
(2) Career-oriented activities.
(3) Problem-solving practice skills.
(4) The opportunity to help others.

10 The school nurse who is planning a community education program would include information that one childhood psychiatric disorder that appears to be genetically transmitted is:

(1) Anxiety.
(2) Sleepwalking.
(3) Enuresis.
(4) Mania.

See page 60 for Answers and Rationales.

I. Overview

A. Although children and adolescents may experience some of the same mental disorders as adults, their symptoms are often determined by their developmental level; other disorders may arise in childhood and continue on through adulthood

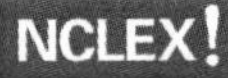

B. In evaluating disorders in children and adolescents, it is important to keep these points in mind:

1. The diagnosis does not define the person
2. All behavior has meaning
3. Behavior does not define the person
4. Identify the source of the primary problem
    a. The person being assessed (infant, child, or adolescent)
    b. The caregiver (parent or family)
5. What need the behavior is fulfilling
    a. Attention from significant other(s) (parent, family, caregiver)
    b. Avoidance of task or situation
    c. Expression of some "inexpressible" thing (something the client has no words for)
        1) Pain
        2) Fear
        3) Hunger
        4) Cold/hot
        5) Upper-respiratory tract infection, urinary tract infection, constipation
        6) Response to internal stimuli
        7) Withdrawal from "reality"
6. Whether the behavior is dangerous to self or other
7. Maladaptive behavior(s) are learned and take time to "unlearn" or replace with socially acceptable behavior(s)

II. Potential Causative Factors

A. Newborns/infants

1. Genetic: inborn anomalies passed from parent to newborn/infant
2. Medical
   a. Perinatal exposure to viruses
   b. Injury during the birth process
3. Environmental
   a. Income status, living situation
   b. Access to health care
   c. Level of education of parent/family
   d. Prenatal and/or perinatal exposure to drugs and/or alcohol or other toxins

B. Children: in addition to all of the above:

1. Postnatal injury
2. Postnatal exposure to chemicals/toxins

C. Adolescents: in addition to all of the above:

1. Self-medication
2. Substance abuse

D. Developmental theory is basic to the understanding of infant, childhood, and adolescent disorders; deviation from developmental norms is an important assessment screen and a sign of potential problems

III. Assessment

A. Bio-psycho-social-spiritual assessment of client/patient is imperative

B. Bio: biological assessment

1. Complete medical workup
2. Medication used in the past, successful or not
3. Onset of or worsening of symptoms
4. Description of symptoms
5. Allergies
6. Cyclical quality to symptoms
7. Family history of medical illnesses
8. Goal of intervention for client
9. Goal of intervention for parent/family

C. Psycho: psychological or psychiatric assessment

1. Understanding of the disorder
2. Medications used in the past, successful or not

3. Family history of psychiatric disorder(s)
4. Coping mechanisms present, past, successful or not
5. Support system
6. Onset of or worsening of symptoms
7. Psychiatric evaluation
8. Cyclical quality to symptoms
9. Goal of intervention for client
10. Goal of intervention for parent/family

D. **Social:** social setting, social network, and social interactions assessment

1. Support system
2. Family constellation
3. Social contacts for client
4. Social contacts for parent/family

E. **Spiritual:** spiritual assessment (not necessarily religious)

1. What is important to client
2. What gives meaning to life of client
3. What is important to parent/family
4. What gives meaning to life of parent/family

IV. Nursing Diagnoses/Analysis

NCLEX!

A. **Anxiety** related to separation from parents; school phobia; unrealistic concerns over past behaviors and future events

B. **Fear** related to unfamiliar people and situations

C. **Impaired social interactions** related to problems with peers; antisocial behaviors

NCLEX!

D. **Low self-esteem** related to low achievement in school; beliefs that others do not understand them; frequent criticism from self and others

NCLEX!

E. **High risk for violence** directed at others related to aggression; antisocial behaviors

NCLEX!

F. **High risk for self-directed violence** related to poor impulse control leading to accidents; repetitive behavior such as head banging; risk-taking behaviors; poor judgement and poor concentration; suicide or self-inflicted harm

G. **Impaired physical mobility** related to unusual motor behavior

H. **Impaired thought process** related to loose association; poor concentration

I. **Impaired verbal communication** related to an inability to formulate words; labile mood

J. **Impaired family processes** related to intensified parent-child conflict; dysfunctional family communication

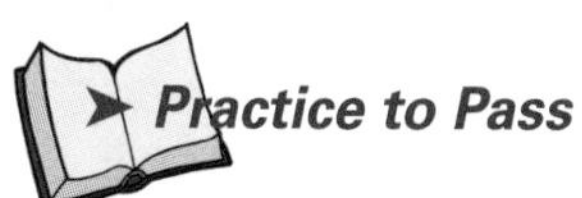

Which medication is most often prescribed for ADHD and why?

V. Planning and Implementation

A. Psychopharmacological interventions

1. Children suffering from major depression may be prescribed amitriptyline (Elavil), imipramine (Tofranil), nortriptyline (Aventyl), venlafaxine (Effexor), and bupropion (Wellbutrin); lithium and carbamazepine (Tegretol) are combined in managing symptoms of bipolar disorder

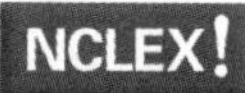

2. Children experiencing ADHD usually are prescribed methylphenidate (Ritalin) or dextroamphetamine (Dexedrin); less so pemoline (Cyclert) because it takes 6 to 8 weeks to become effective

B. Multidisciplinary interventions

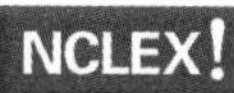

1. Play therapy is used to establish rapport with children, reveal feelings they are unable to verbalize, enable them to act out their feelings in a constructive manner, understand their relationships and interactions with others, and teach adaptive socialization skills

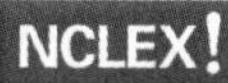

2. Group therapy gives children and adolescents the opportunity to learn to talk openly about themselves, practice active listening, give and receive feedback, learn to help others, and learn new ways of relating to others
3. Parents may be involved in a parallel group to learn growth and development stages, give and receive support, increase parenting skills, and explore their own needs and problems

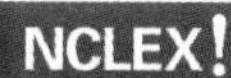

4. Art therapy is a way for children to express what is contained in the unconscious
5. Guided imagery or visualization can facilitate coping and increase sense of self-esteem

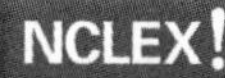

6. Behavior modification identifies behaviors that are unacceptable, those that are acceptable, and consequences for undesirable behavior
7. Community-based programs to improve mental health of children and adolescents include adult mentor plans, youth organizations, and peer-assistance programs

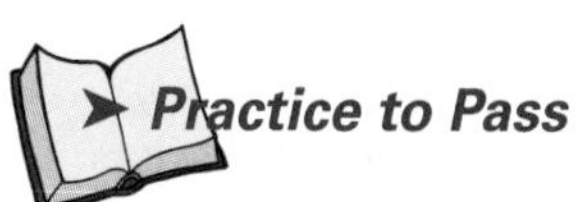

What are some common side effects and toxic effects of CNS stimulants?

8. Family therapy can facilitate healthy functioning in the family

C. Nursing interventions

1. Avoid asking multiple questions of children and adolescents; they respond better to active listening and undivided attention

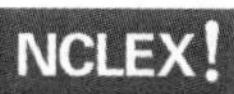

2. Focusing on positive characteristics and behaviors will assist clients to improve their self-esteem

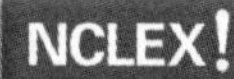

3. Social skills training includes self-expression skills, using support systems, seeing the perspective of others, helping others, assertiveness techniques, social problem-solving techniques
4. Through the use of problem-solving, older children and adolescents can locate information, design solutions, predict consequences, implement strategies, and confirm the outcomes

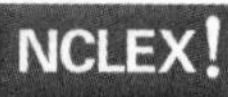

5. Homework assignments increase clients' active participation in the therapeutic process

VI. Evaluation

A. Successfully meeting the outcome criteria depends on individualizing strategies according to cognitive level, emotional and social development, and physical abilities

NCLEX!

B. Plan and discuss termination of the nurse–client relationship in advance

VII. Specific Disorders

A. Obsessive-compulsive disorder (OCD): like adults with OCD, children with OCD try to hide symptoms from others

B. Younger children with post-traumatic stress disorder (PTSD) may repeatedly act out specific themes of the trauma

C. General anxiety disorder (GAD): characterized by unrealistic concerns over past behavior, future events, and personal competency

NCLEX!

1. Social phobia is a persistent fear of such things as formal speaking, eating in front of others, using public restrooms, and speaking to authorities

NCLEX!

2. Separation anxiety is more common in children than in adolescents; the child may need to remain close to the parent(s), and their worries focus on separation themes
3. Selective mutism is the steady failure to speak in specific social situations where speaking is expected

NCLEX!

D. Depression

1. Depression in infants may be exhibited with frozen facial expression, weepy and withdrawn behaviors, weight loss or failure to thrive, and an increased incidence of infections

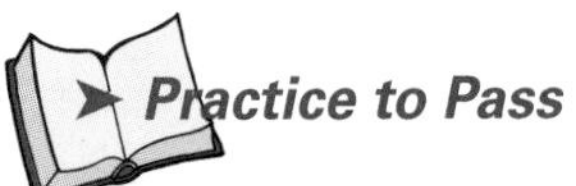

What are some problem behaviors associated with mood disorders in school-aged children?

2. Depression in toddlers may be noted by sad or expressionless face; they may experience delays or regression in developmental skills; they may become apathetic or more clingy; and may have an increase in nightmares
3. Depression in preschoolers may be exhibited by a loss of interest in newly acquired skills, frequent negative self-statements, thoughts of self-harm, or **enuresis** (incontinence of urine, especially nocturnal bed wetting), **encopresis** (fecal incontinence), anorexia, or binge eating
4. School-age children who are depressed may have problems with depressed, irritable, or aggressive moods; academic difficulties; eating and sleeping disturbances; self-criticism; and suicidal ideation and plans

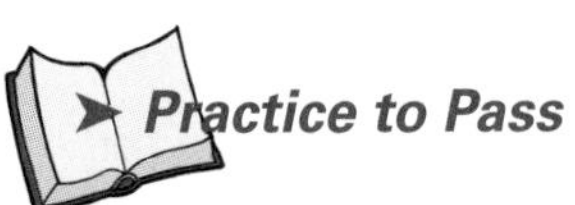

What are some problem behaviors associated with mood disorders in adolescents?

5. Adolescents who are depressed exhibit antisocial behavior, aggression, intense labile moods, difficulties at school, withdrawal, hypersomnia, and very low self-esteem
6. Seasonal affective disorder (SAD) is more frequent after puberty, especially in girls
7. Bipolar disorder is frequently misdiagnosed as ADHD, conduct disorder, or schizophrenia when it occurs in adolescents

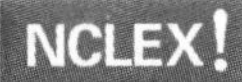

E. Attention deficit/hyperactivity disorder (ADHD)

1. Children with ADHD have impulsive behavior and seek immediate gratification

2. Children with ADHD have labile emotions, and they have difficulty maintaining interpersonal relationships

NCLEX!

3. They have extremely short attention span, which may be accompanied by learning disabilities

4. The exact cause of ADHD is unknown, but it likely involves genetic factors, anatomical abnormalities, neurotransmission problems, and environmental factors

F. Oppositional defiant disorder (ODD) and conduct disorder (CD)

1. Children with ODD are disruptive, argumentative, hostile, and irritable; they have social problems with peers and adults and impaired academic functioning

2. Children with CD engage in antisocial behavior that violates the rights of others: physical aggression, cruelty, stealing, robbing, arson; relationships with peers and adults are manipulative and used for personal advantage

G. Autistic disorder

NCLEX!

1. Children with autistic disorder spend hours in repetitive behavior, have bizarre motor and stereotypical behaviors, have severely impaired communication, and are often mentally retarded

2. Age at onset is usually prior to age 3 (most frequently noted between 18 and 36 months); it is a lifelong disorder

3. Parents often report the infant does not want to cuddle, makes no eye contact, is indifferent to affection or touch, and has little change in facial expression

4. Other associated behavioral problems may include hyperactivity, aggressiveness, temper tantrums, hypersensitivity to touch or hyposensitivity to pain, and self-injuring behaviors such as head-banging or hand-biting

NCLEX!

5. Children with autism will exhibit ritualistic behavior and prefer rigid, unchanging routines, and they are likely to act out if these routines are changed

6. Communication with others is greatly impaired because client may be mute, may utter sounds only, or may repeat words or phrases over and over

7. Thus, these children fail to develop interpersonal relationships, which leads to social isolation that is heightened by difficulties with communication and possible mood disorder

H. Tic disorders

1. Tic disorders involve sudden, rapid, recurrent, stereotyped movements, and/or sounds

NCLEX!

2. They are more noticeable or severe during times of stress but are less pronounced or reduced in intensity when focused intently on an activity, such as watching television, reading, or playing a video game

3. They can be classified into one of three disorders

   a. Tourette's disorder: is characterized by multiple motor tics and one or more vocal tics that occur either simultaneously or at different times; there is not a tic-free period for more than 3 months; the diagnosis implies that symptoms have occurred for at least 1 year or more

   b. Chronic motor or vocal tics: involves either vocal or motor tics, but not both; the diagnosis implies that symptoms have occurred for at least 1 year or more

   c. Transient tic disorder: a tic disorder that does not last longer than 12 months

4. Generally the severity and frequency of symptoms decline as the child progresses through adolescence into adulthood

I. Eating disorders

1. People with anorexia lose weight by dramatically decreasing their food intake and sharply increasing their amount of physical exercise

NCLEX!

2. People with bulimia remain at near-normal weight and develop a cycle of minimal food intake, followed by binge-eating, and then purging

3. The two disorders have many features in common, and a person can revert from one disorder to the other

4. Obesity

   a. Psychosocial factors contributing to the development of obesity include learned patterns of eating, overeating to manage negative feelings, and viewing food as a reward

   b. Leptin, produced by a gene for obesity, travels to the brain, where it affects appetite and metabolic rate

   c. Obese people are no more prone to emotional problems than are people of normal weight; it is the internalization of the culture's hatred and rejection that contributes to the psychological problems of obese people

5. Anorexia and bulimia

NCLEX!

   a. Behaviors associated with anorexia and bulimia are compulsions and rituals about food and exercise, phobic responses to food, **eating binges** (episodes of continuous eating even when not hungry), **purging** (the act of self vomiting to empty the stomach after eating), and the abuse of laxatives and diuretics

   b. Affective characteristics include multiple fears, dependency, and a high need for acceptance and approval from others

   c. Cognitive characteristics include selective abstraction, overgeneralization, magnification, personalization, superstitious thinking, dichotomous thinking, distorted body image, self-depreciation, and perfectionist standard of behavior

   d. In American society, thinness is equated with attractiveness, success, and happiness; this is a contributing factor to eating disorders

   e. Eating disorders are considered to be culture-reactive syndromes in the Western world

NCLEX!

   f. Physiological characteristics include fluid and electrolyte imbalances, decreased blood volume, cardiac arrhythmias, elevated BUN, constipation, esophagitis, potential rupture of the esophagus or stomach, tooth loss, swollen salivary glands, Russell's sign, menstrual problems, and weight loss

g. Concomitant disorders include depression, social phobias, panic attacks, obsessive-compulsive symptoms, and substance abuse

h. Neurobiological factors in the development of eating disorders include 5-HT dysregulation, low levels of endorphins, and a genetic predisposition

i. Intrapersonal theorists consider low self-esteem, problems with identity formation, anxiety intolerance, and maturational problems to be factors in the development of eating disorders

What are two appropriate nursing diagnoses for clients with eating disorders?

j. Cognitive theorists believe that cognitive distortions and dysfunctional thoughts contribute to disordered eating patterns

k. The family system of a person with an eating disorder may be enmeshed; family members may have difficulty with conflict resolution and have high ambitions for achievement and performance

l. Feminist theorists consider that women's preoccupation with their bodies results from the cultural ideal of thinness, and that their identity and self-esteem depend on physical appearance

m. Antidepressant medication is more helpful in treating bulimia than anorexia

Case Study

You are working in a community mental health center. A mother complains that her 10-year-old boy has become unmanageable, and she no longer knows how to cope with his behavior at home. At home, the boy is a bully, insisting on having his way. He takes toys from his siblings, causing arguments and crying, but seldom plays with the toy for more than a few minutes. He has difficulty staying in his chair at school, misses important information, and disrupts other children while they are working.

❶ What data would be helpful to you in making an accurate assessment of the boy's problem?

❷ If the boy is experiencing conduct disorder, what specific behaviors would you inquire about that differentiate it from ADHD?

❸ What indications do you have that the boy is not suffering from a pervasive development disorder, such as autistic disorder?

❹ You can anticipate that the boy's practitioner will place him on a CNS stimulant for ADHD. Why is this the best choice of psychopharmacological intervention for ADHD?

❺ Select two interventions that you feel could be helpful in managing the boy's problems.

For suggested responses, see pages 305–306.

Posttest

1 According to Piaget's theory, one characteristic of the preoperational period is:

(1) Object permanence.
(2) Animism.
(3) Conservation.
(4) Moral idealism.

2 In providing community education to a group of parents, the nurse evaluates teaching as being effective when the group states that common behavioral signs of autism are:

(1) Highly creative, imaginative play.
(2) Early development of language.
(3) Overly affectionate behavior toward parents.
(4) Indifference to being held or hugged.

3 The main emphasis of nursing interventions for the child with phobias is to:

(1) Have the child face his or her fear.
(2) Decrease fear and anxiety.
(3) Protect the child from fears.
(4) Allow the child to express fears.

4 The nurse considering community education about mental health would focus on which of the following, which is responsible for a majority of adolescent deaths?

(1) Suicide
(2) Homicide
(3) AIDS
(4) Accidents

5 In teaching a group of young girls about eating disorders, the nurse would evaluate the sessions as effective if the participants state that anorexia nervosa is best defined as an eating disorder that occurs:

(1) Only in young girls who are depressed.
(2) Primarily in young girls who perceive themselves to be grossly overweight.
(3) In young girls and does not have serious consequences.
(4) In young boys and girls alike.

6 In bulimia nervosa, the client typically responds to increased levels of anxiety by:

(1) Rigidly controlling what he or she eats.
(2) Binging and purging.
(3) Overeating.
(4) Consuming alcohol.

7 In assessing an adolescent client for depression, the nurse recognizes depression in adolescents is often:

(1) Similar in symptomatology to depression in adult clients.
(2) Often masked by aggressive behaviors.
(3) Situational and not as serious as depression in adults.
(4) A sign that the child should be hospitalized.

8 A teenager is being evaluated for anorexia nervosa. Which of the following symptoms would suggest anorexia nervosa?

(1) The client has episodes of overeating and progressive weight gain.
(2) The client expresses a positive self-image.
(3) The client has had severe weight loss caused by self-imposed dietary restrictions.
(4) The client refuses to discuss the topic of food.

9 When talking with adolescent clients, the nurse should:

(1) Assert adult authority at all times.
(2) Interact with client as a friend.
(3) Be firm and not react to provocation.
(4) Be flexible and allow for occasional exceptions to rules.

10 Aside from treating depression, antidepressants are often effective in treating:

(1) Autistic disorders.
(2) Insomnia.
(3) Eating disorders.
(4) Thought disorders.

See page 61 for Answers and Rationales.

Answers and Rationales

Pretest

1 **Answer: 2** ***Rationale:*** Helping the client deal with anxiety would be a positive way of dealing with the eating disorder. Focusing on food (option 1) and spending time alone in his or her own room following a meal (option 3) are not therapeutic interventions when working with eating disorders. The client's contact with family (option 4) should be fostered.
Cognitive Level: Application
Nursing Process: Evaluation; ***Test Plan:*** PSYC

2 **Answer: 2** ***Rationale:*** Inconsistent limit setting with very harsh discipline is often characteristic of families with children suffering from conduct disorders. Having high expectations imposed on the child (option 1) and being overly involved in the child's activities (option 3) may cause anxiety for the child but does not generally result in negative acting-out. Being an only child (option 4) does not suggest conduct disorder.
Cognitive Level: Analysis
Nursing Process: Assessment; ***Test Plan:*** PSYC

3 **Answer: 3** ***Rationale:*** Autism is a lifelong disorder and is most likely the result of multiple etiologies. There is a strong genetic tendency. Factors to be considered include genetics, infectious disease, metabolic disease, and structural abnormalities of the brain. There is no data to support a 50/50 chance of having a child with or without autism.
Cognitive Level: Application
Nursing Process: Implementation; ***Test Plan:*** PSYC

4 **Answer: 1** ***Rationale:*** Behavior modification is quite effective with children and adolescents. The child is told what is expected, what is not acceptable, and the consequences for undesirable behaviors. Open communication is effective, but a flexible approach may be confusing to the child (option 2). Open expression of feelings (option 3) and assertiveness training (option 4) are useful techniques; however, they are more effective within a controlled environment.
Cognitive Level: Comprehension
Nursing Process: Implementation; ***Test Plan:*** PSYC

5 **Answer: 3** ***Rationale:*** Separation anxiety may develop at any age, although it is most common in children, with the peak onset between 7 and 9 years old. Obsessive-compulsive disorder (option 1), simple anxiety (option 2), and PTSD (option 4) are less common in children.
Cognitive Level: Application
Nursing Process: Assessment; ***Test Plan:*** PSYC

6 **Answer: 3** ***Rationale:*** Behavior modification is quite effective with children and adolescents. The child is told what is expected, what is not acceptable, and the consequences for undesirable behaviors. Reminiscence therapy (option 1) is more effective with memory disorders. Emotive therapy (option 2) and cognitive retraining (option 4) are more effective with psychotherapy and older children.
Cognitive Level: Analysis
Nursing Process: Planning; ***Test Plan:*** PSYC

7 **Answer: 3** ***Rationale:*** Central nervous system stimulants such as Ritalin are the most frequently used medications for ADHD. These medications increase the ability to focus attention by blocking out irrelevant thoughts and impulses. Antidepressants (options 1 and 2) may be used, but venlafaxine (Effexor) and fluvoxamine (Luvox) seem to be the most effective. Cyclert (option 4) is used for ADHD, and may have fewer side effects, but is used less often because it takes up to 8 weeks to take effect.
Cognitive Level: Application
Nursing Process: Analysis; ***Test Plan:*** PSYC

8 **Answer: 1** ***Rationale:*** Play therapy is especially useful for children under 12 because their developmental level makes them less able to verbalize thoughts and feelings. Learning to talk openly about themselves (option 2), learning how to give and receive feedback (option 3), and learning problem-solving skills (option 4) are not the intended goals of play therapy. Those skills require more structured group and individual activities.
Cognitive Level: Comprehension
Nursing Process: Evaluation; ***Test Plan:*** PSYC

9 **Answer: 1** ***Rationale:*** Community-based programs can help improve the mental health of children and adolescents. Although activities include career-orientation (option 2), practicing problem-solving (option 3), and opportunities to help others (option 4), the primary purpose is largely recreational.
Cognitive Level: Comprehension
Nursing Process: Analysis; ***Test Plan:*** PSYC

10 **Answer: 3** ***Rationale:*** Childhood disorders that appear to be genetically transmitted include enuresis,

autism, mental retardation, some language disorders, Tourette's syndrome, and attention deficit/hyperactivity disorder (ADHD). Anxiety (option 1), sleepwalking (option 2), and mania (option 4) do not appear to be genetically transmitted for children.
Cognitive Level: Application
Nursing Process: Planning; *Test Plan:* PSYC

Posttest

1 **Answer: 2** *Rationale:* Animism is one characteristic that occurs in the preoperational period. Options 1, 3, and 4 occur in other periods of development.
Cognitive Level: Knowledge
Nursing Process: Analysis; *Test Plan:* PSYC

2 **Answer: 4** *Rationale:* Children with autistic disorders exhibit ritualistic behavior and are highly indifferent to the show of affection by anyone. Autistic children's play is often ritualistic and repetitive. Many autistic children have mental retardation.
Cognitive Level: Application
Nursing Process: Evaluation; *Test Plan:* PSYC

3 **Answer: 2** *Rationale:* The primary focus of anxiety disorders for children is to decrease fear and anxiety. Having the child face his or her fear (option 1) is often unrealistic related to the developmental level. Decreasing the fear, not protecting from fear (option 3), is the aim of treatment. Allowing the child to express his or her fears (option 4) may be useful but does not necessarily lead to decreased anxiety or fears.
Cognitive Level: Analysis
Nursing Process: Implementation; *Test Plan:* PSYC

4 **Answer: 1** *Rationale:* Because of their lack of development, many adolescents have a fatalistic perspective of the future. Suicide is many times the only option they see to manage their pain or problems. Homicides (option 2), AIDS (option 3), and accidents (option 4) occur less often in adolescents.
Cognitive Level: Application
Nursing Process: Planning; *Test Plan:* PSYC

5 **Answer: 2** *Rationale:* Anorexia nervosa occurs more often in young girls who perceive themselves to be grossly overweight. Although anorexia most often occurs in young girls, boys may be affected as well. Untreated anorexia can lead to death.
Cognitive Level: Application
Nursing Process: Evaluation; *Test Plan:* PSYC

6 **Answer: 2** *Rationale:* Binging and purging are characteristics of bulimia nervosa, and the client will increase use of this form of coping during increased levels of anxiety. Clients with anorexia, not bulimia, tend to rigidly control their food intake (option 1). Although bulimic clients do overeat (option 3) and consume alcohol (option 4) during high anxiety times, the binging and purging are more frequent characteristics.
Cognitive Level: Comprehension
Nursing Process: Analysis; *Test Plan:* PSYC

7 **Answer: 2** *Rationale:* Depression in adolescents is often masked by aggressive and/or assaultive behaviors. Symptoms are usually different from adults in that adolescents often exhibit intense mood swings, academic difficulties, antisocial behavior, and hypersomnia (option 1). However, depression in adolescents can have the same consequences as adults and should be treated seriously (option 3). Not all depressed children require hospitalization (option 4).
Cognitive Level: Analysis
Nursing Process: Assessment; *Test Plan:* PSYC

8 **Answer: 3** *Rationale:* Diagnostically a client suffering from anorexia nervosa has a weight loss of 15 percent or greater of their normal body weight because of self-imposed dietary restrictions and/or excessive exercise regimes. Clients with anorexia nervosa usually experience progressive weight loss (option 1), negative self-image (option 2), and are usually obsessed with the topic of food (option 4).
Cognitive Level: Analysis
Nursing Process: Assessment; *Test Plan:* PSYC

9 **Answer: 3** *Rationale:* Many times, an adolescent will challenge authority in order to confirm boundaries. To remain firm and not be reactive is the best intervention. Asserting adult authority at all times (option 1) may be counterproductive. It is important to be respectful and friendly with the adolescent (option 2), but you are the nurse. Avoid occasional exceptions to rules (option 4) because it will only confuse the adolescent.
Cognitive Level: Application
Nursing Process: Implementation; *Test Plan:* PSYC

10 **Answer: 3** *Rationale:* Antidepressants have been effective in the treatment of some clients with eating disorders. Antidepressants have not been found effective with autistic disorders (option 1) or thought disorders (option 4). Insomnia (option 2) is only one possible sign of depression; antidepressants are not effective in treating insomnia in isolation.
Cognitive Level: Comprehension
Nursing Process: Analysis; *Test Plan:* PSYC

References

American Psychiatric Association. (2000). *Diagnostic and statistical manual of mental disorders* (4th ed.). Washington, DC: American Psychiatric Association.

Boyd, M. A. & Nihart, M. A. (1998). *Psychiatric nursing contemporary practice.* Philadelphia: Lippincott.

Carson, V. B. (2000). *Mental health nursing: The nurse-patient journey* (2nd ed.). Philadelphia: W. B. Saunders.

Fontaine, K. L. (1999). Eating disorders. In K. L. Fontaine & J. S. Fletcher (Eds.), *Mental health nursing* (4th ed.). Menlo Park, CA: Addison-Wesley, pp. 205–232.

Fortinash, K. M. & Holoday-Worret, P. A. (2000). *Psychiatric mental health nursing.* St. Louis: Mosby.

Keltner, N. L., Schwecke, L. H., & Bostrom, C. E. (1999). *Psychiatric nursing* (3rd ed.). St. Louis: Mosby.

NANDA. (2001). *Nursing diagnoses: Definitions and classification 2001–2002.* Philadelphia: North American Nursing Diagnosis Association.

O'Brien, P. G., Kennedy, W., & Ballard, K. (1999). *Psychiatric nursing: An integration of theory and practice.* St. Louis: Mosby.

Roebrig, M. J. (1999). Disorders of children and adolescents. In K. L. Fontaine & J. S. Fletcher (Eds.), *Mental health nursing* (4th ed.). Menlo Park, CA: Addison-Wesley, pp. 484–500.

Stuart, G. W. & Laraia, M. T. (2001). *Principles and practice of psychiatric nursing* (7th ed.). St. Louis: Mosby.

Townsend, M. (1999). *Essentials in psychiatric mental health nursing* (4th ed.). Philadelphia: F. A. Davis, pp. 591–608.

Townsend, M. C. (2000). *Psychiatric mental health nursing* (3rd ed.). Philadelphia: F. A. Davis.

CHAPTER 4

Mood Disorders

Lee Murray, MSN, RN, CS, CADAC

CHAPTER OUTLINE

Overview/Classification
Etiology
Assessment
Nursing Diagnoses/Analysis
Planning and Implementation
Evaluation/Outcomes
Specific Disorders

OBJECTIVES

- Discuss at least three etiological theories of mood disorders.
- Differentiate between the primary behavioral characteristics of depressive disorders and manic disorders.
- Identify four specific treatment modalities used in the treatment of mood disorders.
- State examples of at least five nursing diagnoses frequently used in the management of clients experiencing mood disorders.

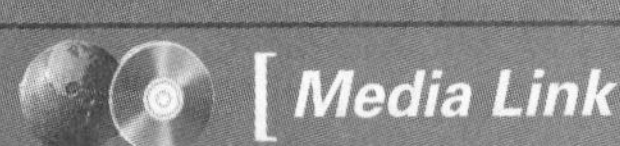

Use the CD-ROM enclosed with this text, or log onto the address given to access the free, interactive Companion Website created for this series. The CD-ROM and Companion Website accompanying this book offer additional practice opportunities and information—NCLEX Review, Case Studies, Glossary, In Depth with NCLEX, and more.

www.prenhall.com/hogan

Review at a Glance

affect *the outward expression of emotions ranging from joy, sorrow, anger, and so on*

ambivalence *experiencing two opposing feelings, thoughts, drives, or intentions at the same time*

anergia *lack of activity*

anhedonia *loss of pleasure; loss of interest in pleasurable activities previously enjoyed*

bipolar disorder *a mood disorder characterized by variations in mood between depression and elation, also called manic-depressive disorder*

bipolar I disorder *a mood disorder characterized by a single manic episode with no past major depressive episodes*

bipolar II disorder *a mood disorder characterized by at least one major depressive episode and past hypomanic episodes but not a full manic episode*

catastrophize *to exaggerate all failure in one's life*

circadian rhythms *correlation of a person's activities, behaviors and external environmental stimuli for a 24-hour period*

cyclothymic disorder *a mood disorder characterized by a mood range from moderate depression to hypomania, which may or may not include periods of normal mood*

dysthymic disorder *a mood disorder similar to major depression but remaining mild or moderate in severity*

electroconvulsive therapy *the introduction of an electric current through one or two electrodes attached to the temple; used for the treatment of major depression*

group therapy *persons coming together to receive psychotherapy*

major depression *a mood disorder characterized by a loss of interest in life events or situations; usually lasts at least 2 weeks; also known as unipolar disorder*

manic-depressive disorder *a mood disorder characterized by variations in mood between depression and elation, also called bipolar disorder*

mood *a prolonged emotional state that effects a person's life and personality*

schizoaffective disorder *a combination of the signs and symptoms of schizophrenia and those of the mood disorders*

seasonal affective disorder (SAD) *depression that occurs in the fall and winter months, while during the spring and summer the client experiences normal mood or hypomania*

unipolar disorder *a loss of interest in life and a depressed mood which moves from mild to severe and lasts at least 2 weeks; also known as major depression*

Pretest

1 The client is scheduled for electroconvulsive therapy (ECT). You will inform the client that after the procedure there may be:

(1) An immediate increase in the client's ability to recall recent events.
(2) Some memory deficit of the period before ECT was begun.
(3) Slowing of the client's physical abilities for the remainder of the day of treatment.
(4) No recall of long-term events.

2 The client has been diagnosed with bipolar I disorder. Lithium carbonate (Lithium) 300 mg q.i.d. has been prescribed. After 3 days of lithium therapy, the client says, "My hands are shaking." Your best response to the client is:

(1) "These fine motor tremors can be an early effect of the lithium. The tremors should subside after the first few weeks of taking the lithium."
(2) "You do not have to worry about that yet. If it is still happening next week, then we will worry about your hands shaking."
(3) "The tremors are an early warning sign of lithium toxicity, but you need to continue to take the medication. We will continue to monitor your blood to be sure you are taking enough lithium to treat your bipolar I disorder."
(4) "You can expect hand tremors when you begin to take lithium. They will go away soon. Why are you so concerned about such a small tremor?"

3 The client is being admitted to the inpatient psychiatric unit. You determine that which of the following *must* be present in order to be diagnosed with major depression?

(1) Suicidal thoughts or plans of suicide reported over at least the last 2 weeks
(2) History of one depressive episode within the last 2 years
(3) Loss of appetite for more than 3 days
(4) Loss of interest in previously enjoyed activities

4 A client has bipolar disorder and is in a state of mania. He is in an inpatient setting and tells the nurse that he is here because he said he would stay but now has decided to leave the unit later today. The nurse will *first:*

(1) Notify the police about the client's intention.
(2) Develop a plan with the client's wife.
(3) Develop a contract for safety with the client.
(4) Notify the supervisor on the nursing unit.

5 While teaching about sertraline (Zoloft), you explain to the client that in order for the medication to be effective it should be taken:

(1) Twice daily.
(2) Only with food.
(3) Before meals.
(4) As prescribed.

6 A client had coronary bypass surgery 3 days ago. He says he is feeling very sad and does not have much of an appetite. He is also complaining of difficulty falling asleep but, once asleep, he usually can sleep at least 6 hours. You conclude the client may have:

(1) A mild depression.
(2) Too much time to think.
(3) Severe depression.
(4) A normal reaction to recent surgery.

7 In order to help the client understand dysthymia, you explain that the signs and symptoms of depression must be present for:

(1) At least 2 weeks.
(2) At least 1 month.
(3) At least 2 years.
(4) More than 1 year.

8 The nurse would assist the client to set which of the following as an appropriate goal while being hospitalized in the acute stage of mania?

(1) Participate in unlimited television privileges daily to keep busy.
(2) Participate in the drama group daily.
(3) Be able to express all feelings as they arise.
(4) Be able to maintain adequate distance when interacting with others.

9 The nurse should consider the irregularities in which of the following body systems before an accurate diagnosis of mood disorder can be assigned?

(1) Integumentary
(2) Cardiovascular
(3) Respiratory
(4) Endocrine

10 During a manic episode, a client talks about self-harm. The nurse must plan care so that the client:

(1) Has a room that is observable from the nurses' station.
(2) Has constant supervision until the risk for suicide is ruled out.
(3) Receives all medications intramuscularly rather than orally until the threat of suicide has passed.
(4) Will notify the family immediately of self-harm intent.

See page 93 for Answers and Rationales.

I. Overview/Classification

A. *Mood*

NCLEX!

1. A prolonged emotional state that affects a person's life and personality
2. Change of mood is a normal and expected life occurrence; each individual feels a range of emotions regularly during daily life, such as joy, happiness, sadness, depression, anger, and fear
3. When individuals go to a movie they may become more aware of mood changes because of the influence of the unfolding story and how it affects their mood during a short period of time

B. ***Affect***

1. How individuals present feelings and mood is affect

2. Individuals give verbal and nonverbal cues of how they feel and what their mood is at the present time

3. They demonstrate mood, thoughts, and feelings as behavior

C. When there are no changes in mood or the change is too pronounced or interferes with daily living, working, attention in school, or regular involvement in social activities, the individual may be experiencing a mood disorder

D. The *mood disorders* are characterized by changes in mood that range from depression to elation (see Figure 4-1)

1. The *Diagnostic and Statistical Manual of Mental Disorders, fourth edition, Text Revision (DSM-IV-TR)* (2000) describes the diagnosis of **major depression** (also called **unipolar disorder**) as a person experiencing a loss of interest in life and a depressed mood that moves from mild to severe and lasts at least 2 weeks

   a. Other major features of major depression can include disturbances in eating, sleeping and functioning at work, home, and/or school; most individuals also withdraw and become less sociable

   b. Individuals with a major depression may also experience delusions and/or hallucinations and are diagnosed with severe depression with psychotic features

2. **Dysthymic disorder**

   a. A mood disorder classified as chronic

   b. There is a depressed mood that fluctuates with a normal mood

   c. The symptoms in dysthymic disorder are less severe than in major depression

Figure 4-1

Mood disorders and ranges.

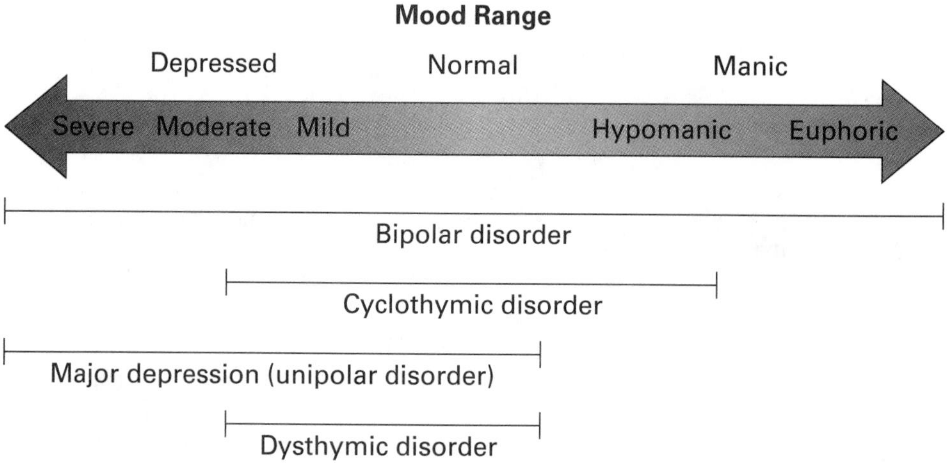

3. **Bipolar disorder** (also called **manic-depressive disorder**)

   a. Is assigned when an individual has moods alternating between depression and elation

   b. Clients currently are assessed by more specific criteria than in the past

   c. The categories of bipolar disorder are defined as follows:

      1) **Bipolar I disorder** is characterized by the occurrence of one or more manic episodes and one or more depressive episodes

      2) **Bipolar II disorder** is characterized as less severe and has one or more *hypomanic* (mild mania) episodes and one or more depressive episodes

      3) Bipolar disorder is further classified as mixed (i.e., the individual has rapidly alternating moods), manic (i.e., the individual is currently in a manic state), or depressed (i.e., the individual is in the depressed phase, but there is also a history of manic episodes)

4. **Cyclothymic disorder**

   a. Is also a mood disorder

   b. The client demonstrates a range of mood changes between moderate depression and hypomania

   c. This disorder lasts for at least 2 years

   d. There is usually no sign of a normal range in clients with cyclothymic disorder

5. **Seasonal affective disorder (SAD)**

   a. Client exhibits a depressed mood that occurs in the fall and winter months

   b. During the spring and summer the client experiences normal mood or hypomania

   c. There is a direct correlation with light and the production of melatonin in clients with SAD

6. **Schizoaffective disorder**

   a. Is a combination of the signs and symptoms of schizophrenia and those of the mood disorders

   b. Symptoms

      1) Delusions

      2) Hallucinations

      3) Disorganized speech

      4) Disorganized behavior

      5) Negative symptoms (**anergia**—lack of activity; **anhedonia**—loss of pleasure, asocial behavior, attention deficits, avolition, blunted affect)

      6) Other symptoms include communication difficulties, difficulty with abstractions, passive social withdrawal, poor grooming and hygiene, poor rapport, poverty of speech

      7) Major depressive symptoms or manic symptoms or mixed symptoms

7. Co-occurring disorders
    a. Persons who suffer from mood disorders may also suffer from a physical and/or psychological co-morbid disorder
    b. Physical disorders can include pain, physical illness, stroke, dementia, diabetes, coronary artery disease, cancer, chronic fatigue syndrome, and fibromyalgia
    c. Psychiatric disorders can include alcohol and other drug disorders, anxiety disorders, eating disorders, obsessive-compulsive disorders (OCD), somatization disorders, and personality disorders
8. Suicide and mood disorders
    a. 15 percent of the population who experience major depressive disorders die by suicide
    b. Epidemiological evidence suggests that there is a fourfold increase in death rates in individuals who suffer from a major depressive disorder and are over age 55
    c. Individuals with major depressive disorder admitted to nursing homes are said to be more likely to commit suicide during the first year after admission
9. In the United States, many individuals with mood disorders go undiagnosed or are misdiagnosed because their symptoms are seen as part of a medical disorder and not explored as a mood disorder or psychological entity

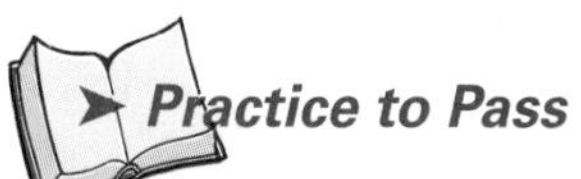

A client is on suicide precautions. She states she does not want anyone with her when she is in the bathroom. What would be your best response?

II. Etiology

A. Biological causative theories of depressive disorders

1. Alterations in neurochemical functioning
    a. Have been very prominent in the literature in the past few years
    b. During the "Decade of the Brain" (1990s) researchers have studied correlations between the central nervous system's neurotransmitter levels and depressive disorders
    c. The biogenetic amines most often identified as relevant in depression are dopamine, serotonin, and norepinephrine
    d. Also indicated are the dysregulation of acetylcholine and gamma-aminobutyric acid (GABA)
    e. More specifically studies investigating these neurotransmitters have found that there can be an alteration in the amount of specific neurotransmitters or a change in neurosynaptic receptor sites in the brain
    f. The result of these changes can be a significant change in mood
2. Genetic predisposition
    a. Is currently believed to be a significant contributor to depression in offspring of individuals who have suffered from major depression
    b. Studies conducted with twins show significantly high incidences of depression when one or both parents have been diagnosed with major depression

3. Endocrine or hormonal change

 a. Strongly affect an individual's mood and emotions

 b. Irregularities in the thyroid (such as insufficient secretion of thyroxin) are seen as especially important in relation to major depression

 c. There is also evidence of a strong correlation with depression and the hypothalamic-pituitary-adrenal (HPA) axis that mediates the stress response; studies indicate that malfunction of this system leads to hypersecretion of cortisol and subsequent increase in depressive symptoms

4. **Circadian rhythms**

 a. Individuals exhibiting changes in circadian rhythms are at increased risk for developing depressive symptoms and major mood disorders as well

 b. Circadian rhythms are responsible for an individual's daily regulation of sleep–wake cycles, arousal and activity patterns, and hormonal secretions

 c. In depressed individuals, these regulatory mechanisms are altered, which can generate alterations in sleep–wake patterns, changes in rapid eye movement (REM) sleep and dreaming patterns, insomnia, frequent waking and/or more intensified dreaming; these changes may be caused by changes in biological functioning, nutritional status, and/or hormones

B. Psychological theories

1. Are derived from the psychoanalytic, cognitive, interpersonal, and behavioral perspectives

2. Psychoanalytic perspective

 a. Freud believed depression occurs because of an ego or object loss in early life

 b. He also believed the loss had a profound effect on the development of mental difficulties in later life

 c. Freud explained depression as an anger turned inward

 d. The loss of a person or object was usually the *trigger* of the depression

 e. In order to help clients regain or attain an improved mental health status, Freud developed psychoanalysis to help the client gain insight into the meaning of thoughts, feelings and actions

 f. Freud believed insight could help the person gain/regain his/her mentally healthy state

3. Cognitive perspective

 a. Cognitive theorists believe that depression is the outcome when an individual perceives all stressful situations as negative

 b. The person sees most situations in a negative light because of early life experiences of loss of significant people in his or her life and spends most of life believing that life is negative

 c. Cognitive therapy aims to help individuals learn how to perceive the world in a positive light and teach them how to relearn thinking and decision making based on positive rather than negative processing

d. The process of relearning is slow but has an outcome that helps the individual change his or her moment-to-moment thinking from a negative frame of reference to a positive outlook

e. In essence, the client expels negative perceptions and distortions and replaces them with positive experiences and tools

4. Behavioral perspective

a. Behavioral therapists believe that individuals develop depression when feelings of helplessness, unworthiness, and powerlessness are the norm during the developmental years

b. Once learned these attitudes are used to evaluate life situations and the individual finds most of life outcomes negative

5. Sociological perspective

a. Sociological theorists use the medical, social learning, stress, and antipsychiatric models to explain the development of depression

b. The medical model theorists believe that depression is treatable using medications, changes in nutrition, and ECT treatments

c. Social learning theorists believe that the individual becomes depressed because of repetitive reinforced learned negative attitudes and outlook

d. Variations of the learned theory include stress theory and antipsychiatric theory

1) Stress theorists believe that the individual becomes depressed because of an inability to incorporate life experiences, perceptions, social support, biopsychosocial powerlessness, and occurrences of stress into life

2) In contrast, antipsychiatric theorists believe that depression is not an abnormal state but rather a reaction to oppression and socioeconomic inequality

A client states, "I can't believe my mother gave me her depression!" Is this statement accurate, and what is your best response to the client?

III. Assessment

A. **Intake assessment** of individuals with a mood disorder should be conducted in 15- to 20-minute segments at one time

1. Individuals who have mood disorders either do not have enough energy to talk for long periods of time or are not able to focus their attention for extended periods of time; clients with mania may not be able to sit still for long periods of time nor can they focus on the present because of elevated mood and flight of ideas

2. An intake assessment helps the clinician formulate a differential diagnosis based on DSM-IV-TR criteria; the assessment can establish whether a client suffers from a mood disorder or a normal process such as grieving (see Chapter 14)

B. **The assessment documentation** should always include both biological and nonbiological methodology; before beginning an in-depth psychological assessment, the clinician should establish:

1. A history of onset of symptoms

2. Any history of alcohol or other drug use and recent or current use of prescription or over-the-counter medications

3. Physical examination to rule out the possibility of a current pathophysiology
4. Levels of suicidality
5. Available support systems in the client's life
6. Level of stressors currently perceived by the client

C. **Focused psychological assessment tools** for a client with a mood disorder should be based on the following characteristics:

1. Behavioral assessment is an examination of a person's ability to act, react, and interact
    a. The behavioral characteristics usually exhibited by depressed individuals are withdrawal from others and decreasing interest in life activities that can become so severe that the person may not take care of basic needs, such as activities of daily living
    b. With a manic disorder, the individual may display an interest in all activities around him/her; the individual becomes more talkative, more gregarious, and displays independence with all aspects of life
2. An affective assessment is the examination of mood, levels of guilt, sadness, gratification, and emotional attachment
3. Cognitive assessment focuses on self-evaluation, expectations, self-criticism, decision-making ability, flow of thoughts, body image, and delusions or hallucinations that the client is experiencing
4. Social assessment is usually based on the individual's ability to interact and participate in life activities such as work, social interactions and ongoing interpersonal relationships, and also includes a client's ability to have an intimate relationship with another

NCLEX!

5. Cultural assessment is the examination of the client's cultural norms and how the present characteristics are viewed in his/her culture
    a. Some cultures recognize depression as a moral weakness or an invasion of the body by evil spirits
    b. Therefore an individual who demonstrates these characteristics can be more devastated and feel even more powerless if there is a cultural stigma attached to their depression or euphoric display of behavior
    c. This can contribute an added burden to the dimension of their already compromised sense of well-being
6. Physiological assessment includes changes in appetite (increase or decrease), sleep (amount, quality duration), activity levels, bowel activity and physical appearance

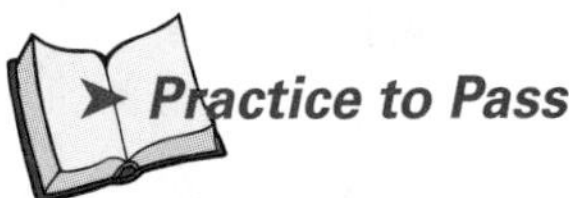

Assessment of a client with a mood disorder is often done in 15- to 20-minute segments. Discuss the rationale behind these timed segments.

D. **Other assessment tools** that can be used to help determine a diagnosis of mood disorders

1. Beck Depression Inventory (BDI)
2. Geriatric Depression Scale (GDS)
3. Zung Self-Rating Depression Scale (SDS)

IV. Nursing Diagnoses/Analysis

A. High risk for violence, self-directed related to depressed mood, feelings of worthlessness, hopelessness, and suicide ideation or plan

NCLEX!

1. The client's safety is the nurse's number-one priority

NCLEX!

2. The danger for self-harm is more prominent as the client begins to regain strength and hope; therefore, frequently assess client for levels of hopeful-/hopelessness, self-esteem, and be alert for signs and symptoms of thoughts or plan for suicide

NCLEX!

3. History of violence is *always* important in determining seriousness of the client's present risk for self-harm
4. The client often displays **ambivalence** (experiencing two opposing feelings, thoughts, drives, or intentions at the same time) or expresses sadness, dejection, hopelessness or loss of pleasure or purpose in life
5. There are overt attempts to harm self (cheeks and hoards medications, self-mutilation, attempts to hang self)

NCLEX!

6. The nurse must be alert for overt signs of hopelessness: refusal to eat; withdrawal from the milieu; resisting or refusing medications; inability to see future for self; suddenly gives away possessions; refusal to sign a "no self-harm" contract

B. High risk for violence, directed at others related to poor impulse control and labile effect

1. Clients with bipolar disorder may exhibit emotional difficulties, irritability, impulsive behavior, delusional thinking, and angry response when ideas are refuted/wishes denied

NCLEX!

   a. The client's safety is the nurse's most important priority
   b. Assist client to identify alternative behaviors that are acceptable to client and staff
   c. Encourage client, during calm moments, to recognize antecedents/precipitants to agitation and loss of control

NCLEX!

   d. Always give realistic positive feedback and encouragement to client
2. The danger of risk to harm others is *always* present with a client who is in a manic state
   a. Some of the more prominent risk factors include: history of harm to self/others during the manic phase; history of another's death as a result of the client's abuse; history of substance use/abuse; overt attempts to harm self or others; demonstrated aggressive behaviors/mannerisms such as hitting, kicking objects, clenched fists, rigid posture, angry facial features; demonstrated inability to exercise self-control; stated feeling confined or crowded
   b. Key nursing actions include the following:

NCLEX!

      1) Decrease the environmental stimuli when client becomes agitated

NCLEX!

      2) Continually monitor client's ability to tolerate frustration and/or individual situations

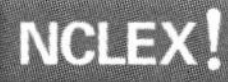

3) Provide a safe environment, removing objects and barriers to prevent accidental/purposeful injury to self or others

4) Increase environmental stimulation gradually

5) Offer alternatives when available (e.g., "There is no coffee available, how about a glass of juice?")

6) Communicate with respect with client; speak clearly in a nonjudgmental tone

7) Always try to convey realistic positive feedback, especially as client attempts to handle frustration in a positive manner

C. **Ineffective individual coping** related to lack of energy, inability to concentrate or make decisions

1. If the depressed or manic client is unable to meet activities of daily living, unable to concentrate or remain in the present, cannot accomplish problem-solving functions or has little or no energy to do so, assist the client to:

   a. Maintain activities of daily living

   b. Carry out problem solving

   c. Maintain a safe environment until the client is able to resume self-care

2. Clients with depression or mania

   a. May express their needs by: expressing their inability to cope (e.g., "I can't do this"); demonstrating frequent bouts of crying for no obvious reason

   b. May become easily overwhelmed or demonstrate problem-grouping (stating several problems together)

   c. May fail to meet basic grooming and hygiene needs

   d. May demonstrate impaired judgment and insight (e.g., "I was doing okay before I came in here") or totally isolate self from others

   e. May verbalize self-depreciating thoughts (e.g., "I'm no good") or delusions (e.g., "I will die soon"; "I don't deserve to live")

3. Key nursing actions

   NCLEX!

   a. Provide a safe environment for the client

   NCLEX!

   b. Observe the client closely, especially after the antidepressant medication(s) begins to raise the client's mood, after any sudden dramatic behavioral change, or during unstructured time on the unit

   NCLEX!

   c. Encourage the client to focus on strengths rather than weaknesses

   NCLEX!

   d. Encourage identification of individuals who are supportive and encouraging to the client

   NCLEX!

   e. Assist the client to learn strategies that will effect more positive thinking (cognitive, behavioral, imagery)

   f. Encourage the client to express feelings and needs

   g. Inform family and friends that the client may direct anger toward them, but that he or she is learning more effective coping skills to deal with feelings

h. Assist the client to gradually become involved with activities on the unit

i. Encourage client to socialize as tolerated with staff, other clients on the unit, and with family members in a structured environment

D. **Nutrition, altered, less/more than body requirements** related to inappropriate nutritional intake to meet metabolic needs; lack of interest in eating/food or choosing nutritional foods; aversion to eating; dysfunctional eating pattern (e.g., eating in response to internal cues other than hunger)

NCLEX!

1. For clients with mania this nursing diagnosis can be vital

   a. A client in the manic phase can be preoccupied with racing thoughts, anxious feelings, ineffective coping with internal or external stimuli

   b. There can be an aversion to eating because of paranoid thoughts, such as food is contaminated or someone is trying to poison them

   c. All of these can lead to a serious weight loss

2. Some of the frequently demonstrated signs and symptoms associated with the manic state include:

   a. At least 20 percent loss of ideal body weight

   b. Is easily distracted from eating

   c. Unable to sit through routine meals

   d. Appears wary or frightened when offered food

   e. Pale mucous membranes and conjunctivae

   f. Capillary fragility

   g. Loose, dry skin turgor/decreased subcutaneous fat

   h. Poor muscle tone

   i. Fluid and electrolytes below normal levels

   j. Hyperactive bowel sounds

   k. Nausea/GI upset from increasing lithium levels

3. Nursing interventions during manic episodes

   a. Offer frequent carbohydrate and protein-rich snacks

   NCLEX!

   b. Offer nutritious finger foods and sandwiches

   NCLEX!

   c. Offer easy-to-carry drinks that are high in vitamins, minerals, and electrolytes

   d. Assess fluid and electrolyte status, especially sodium and lithium levels

   e. Continually assess urinary output

   f. Assess daily bowel movements for frequency and consistency

   g. Assess for abdominal pain or discomfort

   h. Administer high-fiber foods unless contraindicated

   i. Offer frequent liquids and snacks to maintain hydration

4. Clients with depression may demonstrate a nutritional pattern that relates more to their depressed mood
   a. Lack of interest in eating; poor or no appetite
   b. Aversion to food
   c. Dysfunctional eating patterns
   d. Poor choices of food
   e. Recent weight loss/gain
   f. Poor muscle tone
   g. Decreased subcutaneous fat/muscle mass
   h. Pale conjunctivae and mucous membranes
   i. Weight gain
5. Nursing interventions during depression
   a. Monitor and record daily intake and output
   b. Explain to client the importance of maintaining an adequate intake of food and fluids to prevent malnutrition

NCLEX!

   c. Determine client's daily caloric intake needs
   d. Monitor body weight, depending on the seriousness of the depression and weight problem and response to being weighed
   e. As possible, obtain and offer client desirable small amounts of food frequently throughout the day
   f. Monitor laboratory studies as indicated (such as serum albumin, prealbumin, glucose, electrolytes, nitrogen balance)

E. **Sleep pattern disturbance** related to biochemical alterations (decreased serotonin) or psychological stress, lack of recognition of fatigue/need to sleep, hyperactivity

1. Mania
   a. In clients with mania, sleep disturbances can be evidenced by a denial by the client of a need to sleep
   b. The client can also demonstrate changes in behavior and performance, increasing irritability, restlessness, and dark circles under the eyes
   c. The client may experience interrupted nighttime sleep or one or more nights without sleep
   d. Nursing interventions
      1) Identify with client the environmental stimuli that might prevent or interrupt sleep
      2) Restrict intake of caffeine
      3) Offer small snack/warm milk at bedtime or when awake during the night

4) Encourage activities in morning and early afternoon, and restrict activities during the evening and prior to bedtime

5) Encourage routine bedtime relaxation techniques

6) Collaboratively administer medications as indicated

2. Depression

a. In clients with depression, the signs and symptoms may include difficulty in falling asleep, difficulty remaining asleep, experiencing early-morning awakening, or awakening later than desired

b. The client may indicate not feeling rested, or demonstrate hypersomnia or using sleep as an escape

c. Nursing interventions

1) Identify nature of sleep disturbance and variations from usual pattern (difficulty falling asleep, remaining asleep, or waking early and unable to return to sleep)

2) Assess what client does when awakened or when client is unable to fall asleep, and make a plan with the client to change pattern as necessary

NCLEX!

3) Identify previous nighttime rituals that may have been effective and reestablish when possible

4) Decrease intake of caffeine especially later in afternoon or nighttime

5) Restrict evening fluids, and have client void before retiring

6) Provide a light bedtime snack such as warm milk, if client is agreeable and it is not otherwise contraindicated

7) Encourage use of bedtime relaxation techniques

NCLEX!

8) Reduce environmental stimuli (lights, noises, television, radios, etc.)

9) Encourage use of alternative therapies as client recovers to make available more effective illness-prevention techniques

10) Collaboratively administer hypnotic or sedative medications only if other methods fail

F. Spiritual distress related to a sense of no purpose or joy in life; lack of connectedness to others; misperceived shame and guilt

1. With spiritual distress, the client finds a disruption in the life principle that pervades a person's entire being and that integrates and transcends his or her biological and psychosocial nature

2. The client demonstrates a sense of despair and reports feelings of abandonment by God and may even choose not to practice usual religious rituals

3. The client may also report ambivalent feelings (doubts) about beliefs and express a sense of spiritual emptiness and show signs of emotional detachment from self and others

4. Nursing interventions

a. Allow the client to express feelings and thoughts about religious doubt or fears of abandonment

You are formulating a nursing care plan for a client with a diagnosis of ineffective individual coping. Identify five short-term goals (while inpatient) and five long-term goals (to be accomplished by discharge).

b. Explore with the client alternative or past effective religious or spiritual practice or ritual as an illness-prevention measure

c. Eliminate or reduce causative and contributing factors of illness if possible

d. Encourage client to discuss thoughts and feelings with clergy or chaplain when possible

V. Planning and Implementation

A. Specific treatment modalities

1. Electroconvulsive therapy (ECT)

a. ECT is used for the treatment of depression because multiple studies have shown it to be highly effective in helping clients with severe depression who are resistant with other types of treatment modalities, including the use of medications such as tricyclic antidepressants and monoamine oxidase (MAO) inhibitors

b. The procedure involves the application of pulses of electrical energy to the forehead and temporal area of the scalp, sufficient to cause a brief convulsion or seizure; usually carried out under anesthesia

c. A series of ECT are usually carried out over a short period of time

d. The effects of ECT are usually very positive for the treatment of depression

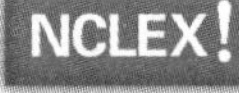

e. The side effects are low and seem to be limited to short-term, temporary memory deficits; deaths have been reported in clients who undergo ECT, but they are infrequent; risks related to anesthesia are present

2. Antidepressant medications

a. Table 4-1 presents an overview of antidepressants, their usual dosage ranges, common adverse effects, and associated nursing responsibilities

Table 4-1 Medications Commonly Used to Treat Depression

Drug Class and Name: Generic (Trade)	Usual Adult Dosage Range (mg/day)	Most Common Adverse Effects*	Nursing Responsibilities
Tricyclic antidepressants (TCAs)			
Amitriptyline (Elavil)	75–300	1 (++), 2 (++++), 3 (++++), 4 (++++), 5 (+++)	• Educate the client early about potential side effects • Inform client that side effects will diminish with time and, if necessary, there are management alternatives that can be implemented • Advise client that response will take some time and continued efficacy is essential • Inform client that first-time treatment for major depression should continue for 6 to 12 months • Warn client of a possible significant weight gain • Monitor for improvement. If no change or minimum change after 2 to 4 weeks it may be necessary to change the medication
Clomipramine (Anafranil)	75–300	1 (++), 2 (++++), 3 (++++), 4 (++++) , 5 (++++)	
Desipramine (Norpramin)	75–300	1 (++), 2 (++), 3 (++), 4 (+++), 5 (++)	
Doxepin (Senequin)	75–300	1 (++), 2 (+++), 3 (++++), 4 (++), 5 (++)	
Imipramine (Tofranil)	50–150	1 (+++), 2 (+++), 3 (+++), 4 (++++), 5 (++)	
Maprotiline (Ludiomil)	50–100	1 (++), 2 (+++), 3 (+++), 4 (+++), 5 (+++)	
Nortriptyline (Pamelor)	25–100	1 (+), 2 (++), 3 (+++), 4 (+++), 5 (++)	
Protriptyline (Vivactil)	10–60	1 (++), 2 (+++), 3 (+), 4 (++++), 5 (++)	
Trimipramine (Surmontil)	50–150	1 (+++), 2 (+++), 3 (++++), 4 (++++), 5 (++)	

(continued)

Table 4-1 Medications Commonly Used to Treat Depression (*continued*)

Drug Class and Name: Generic (Trade)	Usual Adult Dosage Range (mg/day)	Most Common Adverse Effects*	Nursing Responsibilities
Selective serotonin reuptake inhibitors (SSRIs)			
Fluoxetine (Prozac)	20–80	Stimulation, skin rash, weight loss	• Inform client to take medication as prescribed; abrupt discontinuation of the drug is contraindicated • Continuously monitor client for side effects or adverse effects, particularly in the area of sexual dysfunction; client may be reluctant to discuss
Fluvoxamine (Luvox)	50–100	3 (++) and can cause nausea, and vomiting, insomnia, dry mouth, headache, and constipation; monitor liver function early in treatment	
Paroxetine (Paxil)	20–50	Can cause headache and weight gain, or mild stimulation	
Sertraline (Zoloft)	50–200	7 (occurs in approx. 9 to 21 percent of males), and can cause headache, tremor, stimulation, insomnia, agitation, nervousness, nausea, and diarrhea	
Monoamine oxidate inhibitors (MAOIs)			
Phenelzine (Nardil)	45–75	1 (++), 3 (+), 6 (even mania), 8	• Educate client concerning a tyramine restricted diet • Caution client about side effects and adverse effects of the MAOIs • Educate client about careful use of over-the-counter or other prescription medications and be sure client understands the seriousness of the effects • Monitor efficacy of drugs and continuously reeducate client concerning abrupt discontinuation of medication or not taking medications as prescribed
Tranylcypromine (Parnate)	20–30	1 (++), 8 and can cause stimulation	
Atypical antidepressants			
Bupropion (Wellbutrin)	200	1 (+), 2 (++), 3 (produces stimulation not sedation), 4 (+), 5 (++++)	• Instruct client about the side effects and adverse effect of the medication, especially seizure risks at higher drug doses • Instruct client concerning the importance of taking this and all medication as prescribed
Trazodone (Desyrel)	150	1 (+++), 3 (+++), 4(+), 5 (+), priapism (painful and continuous penile erection)	• Instruct client to take medication as prescribed and monitor for any adverse or side effects • Instruct client to report any signs of sexual dysfunction, especially priapism, immediately

*See Table 4-2 for details.
Note: (+) indicates mild reaction and (++++) indicates severe reaction.

b. Tricyclic antidepressants (TCAs)

1) Imipramine (Tofranil), the first antidepressant medication used to treat depression, was introduced in the late 1950s and is still used effectively in the treatment of depressive disorders

2) TCAs block monoamine (norepinephrine and serotonin) reuptake, thus intensifying the effects of the norepinephrine and serotonin

3) TCAs can elevate mood, increase activity and alertness, decrease a client's preoccupation with morbidity, improve appetite, and regulate sleep patterns

NCLEX!

4) The *initial* mechanism of the TCAs is said to take about 1 to 3 weeks to develop while the *maximum* response is achieved in approximately 6 to 8 weeks

5) Dosing with TCAs is individualized and based on *clinical response* or *plasma drug levels* (must be above 225 ng/mL for antidepressant effects to occur)

6) The normal route for administration of TCAs is by mouth; amitriptyline and imipramine may be given by IM injection; intravenous administration is not used

7) Nine TCAs, all equally effective, are available in the United States

8) Major differences among these preparations can be found in their side effects; for example, doxepin has sedative effects and could be more effectively used with clients who experience insomnia

9) Other uses for the TCAs are to treat clients with chronic insomnia, attention deficit/hyperactivity disorder, and panic disorder

NCLEX!

10) Clients who are elderly, have glaucoma or constipation, or have prostatic hypertrophy (males) can be especially sensitive to anticholinergic effects, making desipramine (a TCA with weak anticholinergic effects) more appropriate for use with these clients

11) Although dosing is individualized, TCAs generally have long half-lives; thus, they can be taken daily at bedtime in a single dose

NCLEX!

12) Once-daily dosing at bedtime has several advantages, including ease of taking as part of daily routine, promotion of sleep-through sedative effect, and reduced intensity of the daytime side effects

13) Table 4-2 lists the most common adverse effects from TCAs and other antidepressant medications

NCLEX!

14) TCAs are still the preferred class of drugs for the treatment of major depression based on cost

NCLEX!

15) A major consideration for clients at risk for suicide who are taking TCA medications is availability of large amounts of TCA medication; clients taking TCAs should always be hospitalized until the danger of suicide has been ruled out, and they should not have access to a large quantity of the medication

c. Selective serotonin reuptake inhibitors (SSRIs)

1) This class of antidepressant medications has the same efficacy as the TCAs, causes fewer side effects than the TCAs or MAO inhibitors, and has a decreased time between the time of *initial* dose and the reporting of initial reduction of the signs and symptoms of the depression

2) SSRIs do not cause hypotension, sedation, or anticholinergic effects, as do the TCAs; the only side effects usually reported are nausea, insomnia, and sexual dysfunction (refer again to Table 4-2 for specific sexual dysfunctions and other mild side effects for each drug)

Table 4-2

Most Common Adverse Effects from Antidepressant Medications

Effect	Identifiers	Notes
1. Orthostatic hypotension*	Major decrease in blood pressure with body position changes	The most serious of the common adverse responses to TCAs Advise client to rise slowly, in stages
2. Anticholinergic*	Block muscarinic cholinergic receptors which produces: • Dry mouth • Blurred vision • Photophobia • Constipation • Urinary hesitancy • Tachycardia	Advise client to use sugarless mints, ice chips for dry mouth Advise client to drink adequate fluid, eat bulk-forming foods, and get exercise to prevent constipation Monitor clients with benign prostatic hyperplasia for increased difficulty with urination
3. Sedation*	A common response to TCAs; the cause is blockade of histamine receptors in the CNS	Clients should be advised to avoid hazardous activities if sedation is present
4. Cardiac toxicity*	TCAs can adversely effect the heart's function: • Decreasing vagal influence (secondary to muscarinic blockade) • Acting directly on the bundle of His to slow conduction	Rare occurrences Clients over 40 or who have a family history of heart disease should have baseline ECG and periodically during treatment
5. Seizures*	Lower seizure threshold	Caution must be taken with clients who have seizure disorders
6. Hypomania*	Mild mania can occur	If hypomania develops, client should be evaluated for drug adverse effect or symptoms of bipolar disorder
7. Sexual dysfunction	• Anorgasm • Delayed ejaculation • Decreased libido	Occurs in about 70% of men and women
8. Hypertensive crisis from dietary tyramine	Although MAOIs normally produce hypotension these drugs can be the cause of severe hypertension if client eats tyramine-rich foods	Always caution clients using MAOIs of the many and serious adverse effects indicated with this class of drugs
9. Drug interactions	Always teach clients the importance of preventing adverse drug effects/drug interactions; see individual classification in Table 4-1 for specific nursing responsibilities	Instruct client to *always* take medications as directed Take over-the-counter medications *only after consulting an appropriate health-care professional* Always teach clients of *any* specific instructions for medications they are taking

*Reported in Table 4-1 as a +, where (+) indicates mild and (++++) indicates more severe reactions reported.

3) All of the SSRIs have been found to be effective in the treatment of obsessive-compulsive disorder (OCD)

4) The mechanism of action for SSRIs is to block the reuptake of serotonin and intensify the transmission at serotonergic synapses; the effects can usually be seen after 1 to 3 weeks and are equivalent to those produced from TCAs

5) The SSRIs are administered orally in liquid or pulvules; for elderly clients or clients with impaired renal function, low doses are given and increases are done cautiously

6) Evaluate clients frequently for safety and desired effect of medication

d. Monoamine oxidase inhibitors (MAOIs)

1) MAOIs are still used to treat major depression but only as a second or third choice

2) There is also the danger of taking MAOIs and other antidepressant medications (refer back to Tables 4-1 and 4-2 for details)

3) MAOIs decrease the amount of monoamine oxidase in the liver, which breaks down the amino acids tyramine and tryptophan

NCLEX!

4) This class of medications has some very dangerous adverse effects such as hypertensive crisis when clients ingest tyramine-rich foods

NCLEX!

5) See Box 4-1 for a listing of foods to avoid or use cautiously while taking MAOIs

e. Atypical antidepressants

1) Bupropion (Wellbutrin) is similar in structure to amphetamines; can suppress appetite; is without the usual cardiotoxic, anticholinergic and antiadrenergic side effects (therefore can be used more readily with elderly clients); the most common adverse effects are as listed in Tables 4-1 and 4-2; daily dose should be limited to 450 mg/day to reduce risk of seizures at higher doses

2) Trazodone (Desyrel) is a second-line agent for the treatment of depression; is usually used in combination with another antidepressant agent; usually is prescribed for treatment of insomnia because of its very pronounced sedative effect; refer to Tables 4-1 and Table 4-2 for common side effects

Box 4-1

Foods to Avoid with Monoamine Oxidase Inhibitors

Foods to Avoid

- All cheeses except cream or cottage
- Meats and fish: aged/cured
- Fruits and vegetables: broad bean pods, tofu, soybean extracts
- Alcohol: draft beer
- Other: sauerkraut, soy sauce, yeast extracts, soups (especially miso)
- Drugs: other antidepressant drugs; nasal and sinus decongestants; allergy, hayfever, and asthma remedies; narcotics (especially meperidine); epinephrine; stimulants; cocaine; amphetamines

Consume with Caution

- Cheeses: mozzarella, cottage, ricotta, cream, processed
- Meats and fish: fresh: chicken liver, meats, liver, herring
- Fruits and vegetables: raspberries, bananas, small amounts only of avocado, spinach
- Alcohol: wine
- Other: monosodium glutamate, pizza, small amounts only of chocolate, caffeine, nuts, dairy products
- Drugs: insulin, oral hypoglycemics, oral anticoagulants, thiazide diuretics, anticholinergic agents, muscle relaxants

3. Mood stabilizer medications

   a. Lithium is the drug of choice for controlling manic episodes in clients with bipolar disorder; is also used for long-term prophylaxis against recurrent mania and depression

      1) Is an inorganic ion that carries a single positive charge; occurs naturally in animal tissues but has no known physiologic function

      2) Is well absorbed following oral administration and distributes evenly to all tissues and body fluids; mechanism of action is not known

      3) Has a short half-life and high toxicity; is excreted by the kidneys

NCLEX!

      4) Instruct clients to maintain a constant sodium intake; sodium depletion will *decrease* renal excretion of lithium, which will cause the drug to accumulate and lead to lithium toxicity

NCLEX!

      5) It is essential that serum lithium be monitored frequently to detect lithium toxicity, since the *therapeutic level* and the *toxic levels* are very close; the therapeutic range is 0.8 to 1.4 mEq/L, while the toxic level is 1.5 mEq/L or greater

      6) In clients with mania, lithium reduces euphoria, hyperactivity, and other symptoms but does not cause sedation; antimanic effects are usually seen in 5 to 7 days after initial doses, although the full effect does not usually occur for 2 to 3 weeks

      7) For many clients, adjunctive therapy with a benzodiazepine can be used to provide the sedation clients need

      8) Antipsychotic medications can also be used short term to rapidly decrease the symptoms of psychoses

NCLEX!

      9) Some adverse effects that have been reported at therapeutic drugs levels are fine hand tremors, gastrointestinal upset, thirst, and muscle weakness

NCLEX!

      10) At toxic levels, more adverse effects are seen, such as: persistent GI upset, coarse hand tremor, confusion, hyperirritability of muscles, ECG changes, sedation, incoordination; at levels in the blood above 2.5 mEq/L, death has resulted

   b. Carbamazepine (Tegretol) and valproic acid (Depakote)

      1) Were originally developed and marketed for treatment of seizure disorders

      2) Recently these drugs have been used with success to treat bipolar disorders; they are usually reserved for clients who cannot tolerate lithium or who have not responded to lithium

4. Group and individual therapies

   a. Have proven to be very effective treatment methodologies for mood disorders; can be done with or without adjunct use of psychopharmacologic agents

   b. Some methodologies that have been used to treat mood disorders and associated psychosocial issues include cognitive, behavioral, interpersonal relationship, psychodynamic, family, and group therapy

c. Cognitive therapy

1) Was introduced in the late 1960s
2) The therapist helps the client address negative cognitive processing
3) Once the underlying cognitive schemata and specific distortions in thinking are identified, the client is asked to identify automatic thoughts, silent assumptions, and arbitrary inferences so that negative thoughts and assumptions can be examined logically, challenged against realistic attributes, and subsequently validated or refuted
4) Cognitive therapy has been effective in treating clients with unipolar mild to moderate depression

d. Behavioral therapy

1) Is often successfully used in conjunction with cognitive therapy for the treatment of mild to moderately depressed outpatients
2) Is an effective treatment for depression, comparing favorably with medication and cognitive therapy
3) There is less information about its effectiveness with clients experiencing mania
4) Behavioral therapy is based on learning theory
5) Abnormal or negative behaviors, such as the symptoms of depression and mania, represent behaviors acquired as a result of negative environmental events that are reinforced
6) The behavioral therapist works with clients to determine specific behaviors to be modified and identify factors that evoke and reinforce these behaviors
7) Using role-modeling, role-playing, and situational analysis, clients are assisted in learning and practicing different adaptive behaviors that elicit positive environmental reinforcement

e. Interpersonal therapy

1) Is based on beliefs that depression develops from pathologic early interpersonal relationship patterns that continue to be repeated in adulthood
2) The emphasis for this therapy is on relationships and social functioning
3) The goal of the therapy is to understand the social context of current problems based on earlier relationships and to provide symptomatic relief by solving or managing current interpersonal problems
4) It has been demonstrated to be effective for clients with mild to moderate depression, although not more so than other types of psychotherapy

f. Psychodynamic therapy

1) Is derived from Freud's psychoanalytic model
2) Depression is derived from early childhood loss of a significant object
3) There is ambivalence about the object, which then affects the libido and produces an intrapsychic conflict during the oral or anal stage of psychosexual development

4) The client's self-esteem is damaged, and there is a repetition of the primary loss pattern occurring throughout life

5) The psychodynamic therapist establishes a relationship with the client and helps uncover repressed experiences, which then leads the client to experience a catharsis of feelings, confront defenses, interpret current behavior, and work through early loss and cravings for love

g. Family therapy

1) Is an assessment, intervention, and evaluation of family functional and dysfunctional patterns of behavior and relating

2) There is a need to examine interactions between parents/adults and children

3) The goal is to help family members identify and change behaviors that maintain depression and dependence among the family members

4) This form of therapy is a specialized area of care and the psychiatric nurse needs additional education in order to practice this type of therapy

h. Group therapy

1) Consists of persons coming together to receive psychotherapy

NCLEX!

2) The phases of group work are orientation, working, and termination

3) Whatever the kind of group, virtually all groups go through phases identical to those described in relation to the nurse–patient relationship

i. Various types of groups identified in the literature include support, self-help, psychoeducational, psychotherapeutic, socialization, and others

j. The psychiatric mental health nurse has the skills and the license to assess and provide care for clients utilizing group process in many settings; frequently combines expertise in group process, therapeutic nurse–patient relationship skills, experience in client education, and personal creativity to establish and manage supportive groups

5. Phototherapy

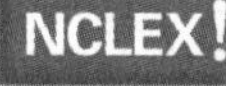

a. A treatment that has effectively been used to lessen symptoms of recurrent seasonal affective disorder (SAD)

b. The exact mechanism of action remains unclear, although it is believed that exposure to *morning light* causes a circadian rhythm shift that regulates the normal relationships between sleep and circadian rhythms

c. Phototherapy treatment consists of a minimum of 2,500 lux of light usually administered on waking in the morning; the clients can be exposed for 30 minutes to several hours, depending on the strength of the light source

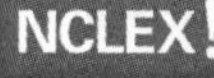

d. An antidepressant effect is usually seen within 2 to 4 days and is complete after 2 weeks

e. Maintenance treatment usually consists of 30 minutes of exposure each day; side effects are usually minimal

B. Nursing modalities

1. Planning and implementation of nursing care for clients with mood disorders is always based on an established nursing theoretical foundation
2. The nursing process combines scientific principles with the most desirable elements of the art of nursing and with the appropriate systems theory
3. This theoretical foundation should be based on criteria such as found in *A Statement on Psychiatric-Mental Health Clinical Nursing Practice and Standards of Psychiatric-Mental Health Clinical Nursing Practice* (ANA, 1994)
4. These standards have provided the impetus and support for individualized and appropriate nursing care to psychiatric mental health clients in all types of settings
5. The nurse establishes a cost-effective, timely plan of care based on client's abilities, needs, resources, and outcome criteria, and identifies the appropriate nursing diagnoses, prioritizes interventions, and selects desired outcomes
6. The care plan documents prioritized nursing interventions based on the multidisciplinary resource data including diagnostic studies, support systems available to the client, response to treatment, financial abilities/restraints, and client's abilities/needs
7. See previously discussed nursing diagnoses for more specific information

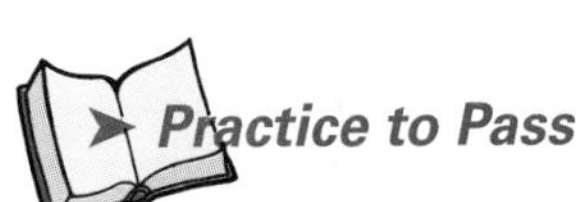

The client is scheduled for his first phototherapy session. Develop a teaching plan to instruct the client about what he needs to know to make an informed decision about participating in the therapy.

VI. Evaluation/Outcomes

A. Outcome criteria for clients suffering from mood disorders include long- and short-term behaviors and responses that indicate improved functioning

B. These are based on nursing diagnoses and are achieved through the implementation of specific nursing interventions

C. Outcome criteria provide the nurse with direction for evaluating the client's response to treatment and nursing care

D. Short- and long-term goals for clients with mood disorders

1. Remain safe and free from harm (NCLEX!)
2. Verbalize suicidal ideations and contract not to harm self or others
3. Verbalize absence of suicidal or homicidal intent or plan
4. Express a desire to live and not to harm self or others
5. Establish a pattern of rest/activity/sleep that enables fulfillment of role and self-care demands
6. Initiate social interactions with others
7. Describe information about his/her disorder, including triggers for relapse and preventive measures in place for relapse prevention (NCLEX!)
8. Identify medications, including action, dosage, side effects, therapeutic effects, and self-care issues (NCLEX!)
9. Report increased communication and problem-solving strategies between client and family/significant others
10. Demonstrate participation/reinstatement of spiritual practices (or a positive change in these)

E. **The nurse evaluates the client's progress** by measuring achievement of identified outcomes

F. **The data for evaluation** is derived from the nurses' interactions with client, observations of client's behavior changes over time, verbalization of feelings and changes in thinking, processing information, and behavior

G. **Once the client is discharged** from an inpatient setting a community care or home care, nurse may evaluate the client's behavior and progress at a community level

H. **With decreasing lengths of stay** in hospital settings, nurses in all settings must continue to evaluate and reevaluate prioritized short- and long-term goals for the client; the nurse must:

NCLEX!

1. Continue to see clear progress related to absence of imminent suicidal intent and a plan for addressing the potential return of suicidal ideation after discharge
2. Observe the client to be more able to perform self-care activities and have some alleviation of the neurovegetative symptoms of depression (irregular patterns of sleep, loss of/increased appetite, fatigue, psychomotor retardation, etc.)
3. Monitor clients with mania for evidence of alleviations of the severe hyperactive behavior of mania, improvement in cognitive functioning/communication, and ongoing understanding of the disorder and the treatment including necessary self-care management
4. Monitor compliance by clients concerning regular ongoing visits to psychiatrists, therapists, group therapy meetings, home care, and community mental health agencies
5. Look for improvement in long-term outcomes such as improved socialization, return to activities of daily living, an increase in activities such as work, school, family roles; the client may be receiving care at a community-care day program as well
6. Monitor for ongoing noticeable reduction in negative thinking, increases in self-esteem, use of new coping strategies, resuming previous levels of functioning (these can take weeks for some clients; there may also be episodes of relapse with exacerbation of symptoms)
7. Assess frequently for depressive episodes, especially in clients who have recently been in a state of mania

NCLEX!

8. Provide careful follow-up after discharge into the community

VII. Specific Disorders

A. Bipolar disorders

1. Are characterized by moods alternating between episodes of depression and episodes of mania or hypomania
2. Are defined by the pattern of manic, hypomanic, and depressed episodes over time
3. The depressed and manic episodes cannot be caused by the effects of a substance, including over-the-counter or prescribed medication, alcohol, illegal drugs, electroconvulsive therapy, or light therapy

4. Various theories have been proposed concerning the cause of mood disorders, but the etiology remains unknown
5. Bipolar disorders can be further described as follows (DSM-IV):
   a. Bipolar I disorder occurs when there is only a single manic episode and no past major depressive episodes; or
   b. Bipolar I episodes can be defined with the most recent episode being a hypomanic episode where the client has experienced at least one previous manic episode; or
   c. The most recent episode is manic and at least one previous depressive, hypomanic, or manic episode has occurred; or
   d. The most recent episode is mixed and at least one past major depressive or hypomanic episode has occurred; or
   e. The most recent episode is depressed mood and the client has experienced at least one past manic episode
   f. Bipolar II disorder is assigned when the client has never exhibited a full manic episode but has experienced at least one prior major depressive and one prior hypomanic episode
6. Manic episodes are episodes of elation where there is an abnormally and persistently elevated, expansive, or irritable mood for at least 1 week and also includes at least three of the following: inflated self-esteem; decreased need for sleep; more than usual talkativeness; racing thoughts; distractibility; increase in goal-directed activity; and excessive involvement in pleasurable activities
7. Hypomania is described as an elevation in mood with increases in activity but not as severe elation as in mania
8. Recent data suggest that the lifetime prevalence of bipolar disorder is about equal for men and women

B. Major depression

1. Is characterized by loss of interest in life and a depressed mood, which moves from mild to severe and lasts at least 2 weeks
2. Other major features of major depression can include disturbances in eating; sleeping; and functioning at work, home, and/or school
3. Most individuals also withdraw and become less socially active over time
4. Further distinctions (DSM-IV)
   a. Depressed mood present for most of the day, nearly every day, as indicated by subjective (client reports) or objective (facial expression, appears tearful) signs and symptoms
   b. Markedly diminished interest or pleasure in all or almost all activities most of the day, nearly every day (as indicated by subjective or observations)
   c. Significant weight loss/gain
   d. Insomnia or hypersomnia
   e. Psychomotor agitation or retardation nearly every day

f. Fatigue or loss of energy nearly every day

g. Diminished ability to think or concentrate, or indecisiveness, nearly every day

h. Recurrent thoughts of death; suicidal ideation with/without a specific plan or a suicide attempt

5. The symptoms cause clinically significant distress/impairment in social, occupational, or other important areas of functioning
6. The symptoms do not meet criteria for a mixed episode
7. The symptoms are not caused by the direct physiologic effects of a substance (drug of abuse, or medication) or a general medical condition (such as hypothyroidism)
8. The symptoms are not better accounted for by bereavement
9. A number of theories have been proposed to account for gender differences in the rates of depression (men 12.7 percent and women 21.3 percent in the general population), but they have not been adequately explained empirically; additional research is needed to determine why women are at higher risk

C. **Dysthymic disorder** differs from major depression in that it is a chronic, low-level depression (refer to Figure 4-1); DSM-IV criteria that must be present for this diagnosis include:

1. Must have had depressed mood and at least three of the following symptoms for most of the day, nearly every day, for at least 2 years: poor appetite/overeating; insomnia/hypersomnia; low energy; low self-esteem; poor concentration/difficulty making decisions; and feelings of hopelessness
2. There cannot have been a manic or hypomanic episode
3. There may have been an episode of major depression before the onset of dysthymia, provided there were at least 6 months with no signs or symptoms of depression
4. After 2 years, the client may be diagnosed with dysthymia, the client may be diagnosed with major depression superimposed on dysthymia if symptoms increase in severity
5. Also the dysthymic disorder cannot be caused by the effects of a substance or medical condition
6. There are usually no psychotic features present in this disorder

D. **In order to have a better understanding of the mood disorders,** it is helpful to identify some of the basic characteristic differences noted between depressive disorder and bipolar disorders

1. Behavioral characteristic differences

a. In major depression there is a progression from a decreased desire to engage in social, work and school activities to an absence of participation in even the most common activities of daily living

1) There is a progressive loss of self-esteem, the individual feels more and more incompetent and less and less motivated

2) Statements such as, "Why bother, I can't anyway" are common

b. In contrast, an individual with bipolar disorder exhibits high energy and productivity

1) There is positive feedback from others

2) As the disease progresses there is decreased ability to concentrate, make judgments, or participate in everyday activities, which leads to frustration and an increasing effort to regain control

3) The individual becomes more and more frustrated and irritable and, in conjunction with a shortened attention span, unrealistic self-confidence and poor judgment, becomes unable to function

4) This is exhibited by engagement in spending sprees, making foolish financial investments, and/or high-risk lifestyle changes

NCLEX!

c. Relationships and interactions change with mood disorders

1) Individuals with depression withdraw from personal and social activities and events

2) Individuals say they feel lonely but often cannot halt the process of withdrawal and isolation

3) In contrast, persons with bipolar disorder are unable to set boundaries, exhibit incessant talkativeness and gregarious behavior that are often an embarrassment when they return to their normal range of mood

2. Affective characteristics

a. Alterations in affect for individuals with depression are broad and deep

1) There is a sense of sadness that becomes more and more pronounced

2) This can be accompanied by guilt that may be expressed as a vague concern or a specific issue

3) Cues to these emotions are statements such as, "I have so much to be thankful for, I shouldn't feel this way"

4) There is also a loss of emotional attachment in depressed individuals that is evidenced by expressions of or indifference toward family and friends

b. On the other hand, individuals with bipolar disorder exhibit mood ranges between cheerful and euphoric

1) For example, they make statements such as, "I feel great!"

2) In the presence of an external negative stimulus, the individual can become irritable, argumentative, hostile, and even combative

3) Once the stimulus is removed, there is usually a return to euphoria

4) In these individuals there is not usually a sense of guilt

5) They respond to another's feelings of hurt or anger with their own anger, laughter, or indifference

NCLEX!

c. Clients with mild or moderate depression exhibit bouts of crying; those in the severe stages of depression may not even have the energy to cry; those with bipolar disorder express feelings of euphoria and "all being wonderful"

d. While depressed individuals exhibit depressed or sad affect, individuals with bipolar disorder usually exhibit a cheerful to euphoric presentation

e. Clients with major depression exhibit anhedonia or a lack of pleasure, while clients with bipolar disorder try to participate in every activity/event available

3. Cognitive characteristics

a. A person's opinion about personal worth and value contributes to his or her sense of self-esteem

NCLEX!

b. The client in a manic state does not suffer from low self-esteem; there is a very grandiose belief about self

c. The client in a depressed state can only seem to focus on the negative, with a presentation of self as a failure and totally incompetent

NCLEX!

d. A client with depression will **catastrophize** or exaggerate all of life as failure, personalizes comments made by others, and believes his or her present and future life is hopeless

NCLEX!

e. The depressed person overgeneralizes, is self-critical and perfectionistic, and anticipates disapproval from others, while the person in a manic state exhibits unwarranted positive expectations, is unable to see potential negative outcomes, and is irate if criticized by others

f. The person in the manic state of bipolar disorder:

1) Will present as easily distractible and impulsive

2) Has flight of ideas

3) Has a belief in self as being very attractive

4) Exhibits delusions of grandeur

5) Exhibits hallucinations in approximately 15 to 25 percent of cases

g. When in the depressed state, an individual will:

1) Exhibit a decreased ability or even an inability for decision making

2) Have a decrease in rate and number of thoughts

3) Have a belief about self as being ugly or unattractive

4) Have somatic delusions

5) Have hallucinations (approximately 15 to 25 percent of cases)

4. Sociocultural characteristics associated with the depressed state include a loss of desire in sexual activities, while for the individual in manic phase there is an increase in activity even to promiscuity

5. Physiological characteristics

NCLEX!

a. A client in the manic state may have difficulty eating because of the inability to physically slow down or sit still; the person in the depressed state will have either an increased or decreased appetite; when in a severe state of depression, a decrease in appetite usually occurs

NCLEX!

b. A client in the manic state will sleep only 1 or 2 hours per night and is usually hyperactive when engaged in activities; sleep can either be increased or decreased in mild to moderate depression, while sleep is usually decreased in severe depression

NCLEX!

c. Reported gastrointestinal activity for those in manic and depressed states is usually constipation

NCLEX!

d. The physical appearance of the person in a manic state usually includes bright clothing, frequent changes in clothing and an exaggerated presentation of the physical self, while those with depressed mood exhibit unkempt presentation and the appearance of little attention to or poor hygiene

Case Study

You are admitting a client to the inpatient unit. The client is in a manic state exhibiting flight of ideas, loose association, poor appetite, irritability, and rapid mood swings between elation and crying spells. The client has been unable to sleep for the past three nights and stays awake pacing the floor.

❶ Identify at least five questions you will ask during your initial interview.

❷ List three main priorities of care for this client.

❸ What are the medication(s) that will probably be prescribed for this client?

❹ If Sleep pattern disturbance related to sensory alterations as evidenced by verbal complaint of difficulty sleeping is one of your nursing diagnoses, identify one short-term outcome and three nursing interventions for the nursing care plan.

For suggested responses, see page 306.

Posttest

1 The nurse should plan to do which of the following in order for a client to have the greatest benefit from treatment on an acute inpatient psychiatric unit?

(1) Establish a nursing care plan for the client.
(2) Utilize a basic standardized nursing care plan and tell the client what the short- and long-term goals are.
(3) With the multidisciplinary team, plan and implement short- and long-term client goals.
(4) With the client, establish and implement a plan of care and evaluate outcomes.

2 The nurse knows that the client attended group therapy from 10:30 A.M. to 11:30 A.M. At 11:45 A.M., the client says, "I am not going to eat lunch; I am going to take a nap." The nurse's best response would be to:

(1) Ask the client to sit for a few minutes to discuss this.
(2) Ask the client if he is angry.
(3) Tell the client that there is a unit schedule that must be followed by everyone.
(4) Ask the client if there is a problem with the food.

3 The nurse is conducting discharge teaching for a client taking tranylcypromine (Parnate). The nurse determines that the client understands the instructions given if the client refrains from eating which of the following favorite foods?

(1) Potato chips
(2) Salami
(3) Chicken
(4) Cheerios oat cereal

4 A client is admitted to a secure psychiatric inpatient unit for the treatment of bipolar I disorder. The nurse begins the intake assessment but the client stands up and begins to walk around the room and shouts, "You can't do this to me! Do you know whom I am?" The *best* action of the nurse at this time focuses on:

(1) Obtaining the assessment information from the client.
(2) Providing the client with adequate food and fluids to maintain homeostasis.
(3) Providing self and client with a safe environment.
(4) Administering the prescribed medications to keep the client from escalating.

5 The nurse observes that a depressed client visited the coffee shop this afternoon and sat at a table with two other clients on the unit. The *best* feedback the nurse can give to the client would be:

(1) "You are doing such a wonderful job interacting with the other clients."
(2) "It is good to see you sitting in the coffee shop with others this afternoon."
(3) "How are you feeling after your visit to the coffee shop with other clients today?"
(4) "Will you go to the coffee shop again tomorrow?"

6 The client is admitted today to the inpatient unit in a manic phase of bipolar I disorder. The nurse would indicate which of the following as the *priority* nursing diagnosis for this client?

(1) Ineffective individual coping
(2) Altered nutrition: less than body requirements
(3) Risk for violence: self-directed
(4) Sleep pattern disturbance

7 The nurse observes that a client is pacing in the hallway, talking rapidly, and gesturing dramatically. The nurse concludes that the client is beginning to demonstrate what kind of behavior?

(1) Psychomotor retardation
(2) Anxiety
(3) Psychomotor agitation
(4) Anger

8 A female client states, "I just want to sleep. I am overweight again. I don't want to eat anymore. All I ever seem to do is sleep right now. Then, I'll be okay for a while. I will go to work and do my grocery shopping, but right now, I don't want to do any of that." The nurse determines that which of the following is the *primary* nursing diagnosis for the client at this time?

(1) Ineffective individual coping
(2) Risk for violence: self-directed
(3) Sleep pattern disturbance
(4) Altered nutrition: less than body requirements

9 The client has a diagnosis of bipolar I disorder. The psychiatrist has prescribed lithium carbonate (Lithium), lorazepam (Ativan), and therapy. Which of the following therapies would be *most* appropriate for this client?

(1) Phototherapy
(2) Electroconvulsive therapy (ECT)
(3) Psychoanalysis
(4) Group therapy

10 A client in an inpatient unit is awake at 1 A.M. and tells the nurse, "I can't sleep because of the light in the hall and the noise from the kitchen. I need to have another sleeping pill." The *most* appropriate nursing intervention is to:

(1) Administer a prn sedative.
(2) Move the client to a quieter room.
(3) Close the door to the client's room.
(4) Allow the client to watch television for 1 hour.

See pages 93–94 for Answers and Rationales.

Answers and Rationales

Pretest

1 **Answer: 2** *Rationale:* There may be some memory deficits for the period before the treatment began. These may disappear or may not. There is no immediate increase in the client's ability for recall nor are there any physical changes noted. ECT is a fast-acting form of therapy.
Cognitive Level: Application
Nursing Process: Implementation; *Test Plan:* PHYS

2 **Answer: 1** *Rationale:* Fine hand tremors can interfere with writing and other motor skills. It is important that the client continue to take the medication as prescribed to maintain a therapeutic level. Helping the client understand that the tremors can subside or disappear after 1 or 2 weeks is helpful, but helping the client reduce stress or caffeine use can also reduce the tremors as well without having to decrease a therapeutic dose. Options 2 and 4 provide no information to client and will not reduce his or her need to know or anxiety. Option 3 is incorrect because tremors are not an early warning of lithium toxicity.
Cognitive Level: Analysis
Nursing Process: Implementation; *Test Plan:* PHYS

3 **Answer: 4** *Rationale:* DSM-IV-TR states that depressed mood or loss of interest in previously enjoyed activities must be present in order to qualify for a diagnosis of major depression. Although each of the other options may be present with depression, this criteria must be met first.
Cognitive Level: Analysis
Nursing Process: Analysis; *Test Plan:* PSYC

4 **Answer: 3** *Rationale:* The client in a state of mania may deny the seriousness of his or her status, have poor judgment, and be in danger of harm. The nurse should try to contract for safety with the client in the manic state. Options 1, 2, and 4 will not provide a direct intervention to ensure client safety.
Cognitive Level: Analysis
Nursing Process: Implementation; *Test Plan:* SECE

5 **Answer: 4** *Rationale:* All medications should be taken as prescribed. There is no rationale for taking sertraline (Zoloft) with or without food or liquids. Sertraline is usually taken in once a day dosages.
Cognitive Level: Application
Nursing Process: Implementation; *Test Plan:* HPM

6 **Answer: 1** *Rationale:* There is a high incidence of depression among hospitalized clients. Usually the more severe the illness the more pronounced the symptoms. There is not enough data to support options 2, 3, and 4.
Cognitive Level: Analysis
Nursing Process: Assessment; *Test Plan:* PSYC

7 **Answer: 3** *Rationale:* DSM-IV indicates that the client must have a depressed mood for at least 2 years. Options 1, 2, and 4 are incorrect time frames.
Cognitive Level: Application
Nursing Process: Implementation; *Test Plan:* PHYS

8 **Answer: 4** *Rationale:* The client in the manic state needs to have clear set boundaries, a decrease in stimulation, and expression of dramatic reactions. The nurse must encourage the client to set and maintain boundaries while interacting with others. Options 1, 2, and 3 will not assist the client in setting these boundaries.
Cognitive Level: Application
Nursing Process: Planning; *Test Plan:* SECE

9 **Answer: 4** *Rationale:* Any client who is being evaluated for a mood disorder should have a workup to rule out the possibility of a pathophysiologic disorder being overlooked. The body systems listed in options 1, 2, and 3 would not have actual irregularities that would indicate the same signs and symptoms as mood disorders.
Cognitive Level: Application
Nursing Process: Assessment; *Test Plan:* PHYS

10 **Answer: 2** *Rationale:* Individuals at high risk for suicide should have constant supervision even though there is a loss of privacy. Just providing a room that can be seen from the nurses' station will not ensure safety for the client. There needs to be a responsible healthcare person assigned to the client. There is no reason to give IM rather than PO medications, but the nurse must be sure that the client has swallowed the medication. The patient's bill of rights indicates that the nurse has no right to notify the family.
Cognitive Level: Analysis
Nursing Process: Implementation; *Test Plan:* SECE

Posttest

1 **Answer: 4** *Rationale:* The nurse needs to establish a plan of care *with* the client. Utilizing a standardized plan of care without individualized short- and long-

term goals is not effective. Before a nurse can establish short- and long-term goals with other healthcare professionals, there needs to be an assessment. The only correct answer is to establish and implement a plan *with the client,* to promote the client's involvement in self-care as possible, being sure to also evaluate outcomes to continuously update the plan and maintain an optimum level of care.
Cognitive Level: Application
Nursing Process: Planning; *Test Plan:* PSYC

2 **Answer: 1** *Rationale:* The client is demonstrating a pattern of behavior that should be investigated. The nurse should take the time to assess the client's feelings, thoughts, and actions. The client may just be tired or may have a need to rest but the nurse needs to be sure that the client is safe and not upset. Asking the client a closed question (option 2) at this time will not be therapeutic nor will telling the client that there is a schedule that no one can deter from (option 3). Asking the client if there is a problem with the food (option 4) is clearly nontherapeutic and will not help the nurse evaluate the present situation.
Cognitive Level: Analysis
Nursing Process: Evaluation; *Test Plan:* PSYC

3 **Answer: 2** *Rationale:* Salami is a cured meat and should be avoided by clients taking tranylcypromine, a monoamine oxidase inhibitor (MAOI). Foods rich in tyramine or tryptophan may induce a hypertensive episode in clients taking MAOI medication. Potato chips (option 1), chicken (option 3), and Cheerios (option 4) are all acceptable foods.
Cognitive Level: Analysis
Nursing Process: Evaluation; *Test Plan:* HPM

4 **Answer: 3** *Rationale:* Providing safety for the nurse and the client is the primary concern immediately after admission while the client is in the manic phase. Obtaining the intake assessment (option 1) data is not a priority. Adequate food and fluids (option 2) and medications (option 4) are important but are not the primary concern.
Cognitive Level: Application
Nursing Process: Implementation; *Test Plan:* SECE

5 **Answer: 2** *Rationale:* Option 2 acknowledges independent positive actions by the client. The feedback is therapeutic and encouraging. Option 1 does not provide a therapeutic response or feedback. The nurse should not ask the questions in options 3 and 4 because they are not feedback.
Cognitive Level: Application
Nursing Process: Evaluation; *Test Plan:* PSYC

6 **Answer: 3** *Rationale:* Whenever there is a danger to the client or another, this is a priority nursing diagnosis. All of the others listed are important as well to the client with mania but the primary concern is safety.
Cognitive Level: Analysis
Nursing Process: Planning; *Test Plan:* PHYS

7 **Answer: 3** *Rationale:* Clients may exhibit psychomotor agitation as described here. Option 1 is opposite of option 3, while anxiety (option 2) and anger (option 4) are words to describe feelings, not behavior.
Cognitive Level: Analysis
Nursing Process: Assessment; *Test Plan:* PSYC

8 **Answer: 1** *Rationale:* This client is exhibiting signs and symptoms of dysthymia. She should be evaluated to determine what is causing her depression. The client must have a physical examination to rule out other causes for the depression and be able to begin to receive treatment to treat the loss of appetite, fatigue, sleep pattern disturbance. She makes no indication of being at risk for self-directed violence.
Cognitive Level: Analysis
Nursing Process: Assessment; *Test Plan:* HPM

9 **Answer: 4** *Rationale:* In addition to one-on-one therapy, clients with maladaptive emotional responses can benefit from family and group therapy. Phototherapy (option 1) is used for individuals with seasonal affective disorder (SAD) and ECT (option 2) is used for treatment of major depression. Psychoanalysis (option 3) is contraindicated for clients with mania.
Cognitive Level: Analysis
Nursing Process: Planning; *Test Plan:* HPM

10 **Answer: 3** *Rationale:* It is not necessary to move the client when closing the door can produce a noninvasive strategy. Before administering a prn sedative the nurse should attempt other nonpharmacological options. Allowing the client to watch television may not be a therapeutic first strategy.
Cognitive Level: Analysis
Nursing Process: Implementation; *Test Plan:* PHYS

References

American Psychiatric Association (2000). *Diagnostic and statistical manual of mental disorders, fourth edition, Text Revision* (DSM-IV-TR). Washington, DC: American Psychiatric Association, pp. 345–410.

Burkhardt, M. A. & Nathaniel, A. K. (1998). *Ethics and issues in contemporary nursing.* Albany, NY: Delmar, pp. 63–77.

Burns, C. (2001). Somatic therapies. In G. Stuart & M. Laraia (Eds.), *Principles and practice of psychiatric nursing* (7th ed.). St. Louis: Mosby, pp. 608–624.

Carpenito, L. J. (2000). *Nursing diagnosis: Application to clinical practice* (8th ed.). Philadelphia: Lippincott, pp. 822–829, 862–864.

Doenges, M. E., Townsend, M. C., & Moorhouse, M. F. (1998). *Psychiatric care plans: Guidelines for individualizing care* (3rd ed.). Philadelphia: F. A. Davis, pp. 4–21, 269–305.

Epocrates qRx version 4.0. Retrieved January 4, 2001 from the World Wide Web: *http://www.epocrates.com/.*

Fontaine, K. L. & Fletcher, S. J. (1999). *Mental health nursing* (4th ed.). Menlo Park, CA: Addison-Wesley, pp. 145–166, 205–280.

Fortinash, K. & Holoday-Worret, P. (2000). *Psychiatric mental health nursing* (2nd ed.). St. Louis: Mosby, pp. 800–814.

Fortinash, K. M. & Holoday-Worret, P. A. (1999). *Psychiatric nursing care plans* (3rd ed.). St. Louis: Mosby, pp. 50–74.

Frisch, N. (1998). Group therapy. In N. Frisch & L. Frisch (Eds.), *Psychiatric mental health nursing.* Albany, NY: Delmar, pp. 685–699.

Frisch, N. C. & Frisch, L. E. (1998). The client experiencing depression. In N. Frisch & L. Frisch (Eds.), *Psychiatric mental health nursing.* Albany, NY: Delmar, pp. 236–267.

Frisch, N. C. & Frisch, L. E. (1998). The client experiencing mania. In N. Frisch & L. Frisch (Eds.), *Psychiatric mental health nursing.* Albany, NY: Delmar, pp. 268–291.

Grendell, R. (2000). Alternative therapies. In K. Fortinash & P. Holoday-Worret (Eds.), *Psychiatric mental health nursing* (2nd ed.). St. Louis: Mosby, pp. 572–588.

Green, C. (2000). *Critical thinking in nursing: Case studies across the curriculum.* Upper Saddle River, NJ: Prentice-Hall, Inc., pp. 251–308.

Hagerty, B. (2000). Mood disorders: Depression and mania. In K. Fortinash & P. Holoday-Worret (Eds.), *Psychiatric mental health nursing* (2nd ed.). St. Louis: Mosby, pp. 258–292.

Keltner, N. (1999). Mood disorders. In N. Keltner, L. Schwecke, & C. Bostrom (Eds.), *Psychiatric nursing* (3rd ed.). St. Louis: Mosby, pp. 270–297.

Laraia, M. (2001). Psychopharmacology. In G. Stuart & M. Laraia (Eds.), *Principles and practice of psychiatric nursing* (7th ed.) St. Louis: Mosby, pp. 572–607.

Lehne, R. (1998). *Pharmacology for nursing care* (3rd ed.). Philadelphia: W. B. Saunders, pp. 297–320.

Pesut, D. J. & Herman, J. (1999). *Clinical reasoning: The art and science of critical and creative thinking.* Albany, NY: Delmar, pp. 160–181.

Schultz, J. M. & Videbeck, S. D. (1998). *Lippincott's manual of psychiatric nursing care plans* (5th ed.). Philidelphia: Lippincott, pp. 179–208.

Scott, C. M. (2000). Mood disorders. In V. B. Carson (Ed.), *Mental health nursing: The nurse-patient journey* (2nd ed.). Philadelphia: W. B. Saunders, pp. 679–720.

Sherr, J. (2000). Psychopharmacology and other biologic therapies. In K. Fortinash & P. Holoday-Worret (Eds.), *Psychiatric mental health nursing* (2nd ed.). St. Louis: Mosby, pp. 536–572.

Stuart, G. W. (2001). Emotional responses and mood disorders. In G. Stuart & M. Laraia (Eds.), *Principles and practice of psychiatric nursing* (7th ed.) St. Louis: Mosby, pp. 345–380.

Stuart. G. W. & Laraia, M. T. (1998). *Pocket guide to psychiatric nursing* (4th ed.). St. Louis: Mosby, pp. 225–247.

Townsend, M. C. (2001). *Nursing diagnoses in psychiatric nursing: Care plans and psychotropic medications* (5th ed.). Philidelphia: F. A. Davis, pp. 168–203.

Warren, B. & Keltner, N. (1999). Mood disorders. In N. Keltner, L. Schwecke, & C. Bostrom (Eds.), *Psychiatric nursing* (3rd ed.). St. Louis: Mosby, pp. 382–421.

CHAPTER 5

Anxiety Disorders

Susan Bobek, RN, PhD

CHAPTER OUTLINE

OBJECTIVES

- Discuss at least three theories commonly cited to explain the origin of anxiety disorders.
- Explain six characteristics of anxiety disorders.
- Describe at least two physiological, behavioral, cognitive, and affective responses to anxiety disorders.
- Identify three specific treatment modalities used in the treatment of anxiety disorders.

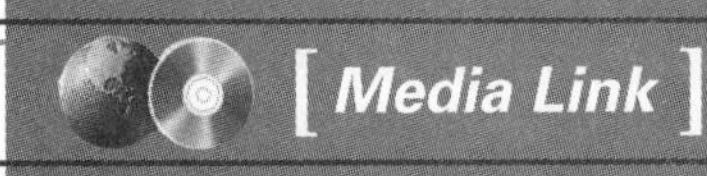

Use the CD-ROM enclosed with this text, or log onto the address given to access the free, interactive Companion Website created for this series. The CD-ROM and Companion Website accompanying this book offer additional practice opportunities and information—NCLEX Review, Case Studies, Glossary, In Depth with NCLEX, and more.

www.prenhall.com/hogan

Review at a Glance

agoraphobia *the fear of being incapacitated by being forced into or trapped in an unbearable situation from which there is no escape*

anxiety *a state of apprehension, dread, uneasiness, or uncertainty generated by a real or perceived threat whose actual source is unidentifiable*

burnout *a state of mental and/or physical exhaustion*

compulsion *unwanted behavioral pattern or act*

coping *efforts to manage specific demands that are appraised as threatening*

defense mechanism *unconscious psychological response designed to diminish or delay anxiety and protect the person*

fear *a reaction to a specific danger*

fight-or-flight reaction *an automatic psychological state of high anxiety mediated by the sympathetic nervous system*

general adaptation syndrome *an automatic physical reaction to stress mediated by the sympathetic nervous system*

obsession *unwanted, persistent, intrusive thoughts, impulses, or images related to anxiety*

panic attack *a sudden episode of symptoms such as dizziness, dyspnea, tachycardia, palpitations, and feelings of impending doom and death*

phobia *an irrational fear of a specific activity, object, or condition that leads to a compelling desire to avoid the feared stimulus*

stress *a state of imbalance between the demands placed on an individual and the individual's ability to deal with the demands*

stressor *an internal or external event or situation that leads to feelings of anxiety*

Pretest

1 During an assessment of a client the nurse finds that the client is trembling and restless, the client's blood pressure and pulse are elevated and the client is complaining of dry mouth, shortness of breath, inability to relax, lose of appetite, and an upset stomach. What is the client's level of anxiety?

(1) Mild
(2) Moderate
(3) Severe
(4) Panic

2 During an assessment interview the client tells the nurse, "I can't stop worrying about my makeup. I can't go anywhere or do anything unless my makeup is fresh and perfect. I wash my face and put on fresh makeup at least once and sometimes twice an hour." This behavior is *most* likely a sign of a(n):

(1) Acute stress disorder.
(2) Generalized anxiety disorder.
(3) Obsessive-compulsive disorder.
(4) Panic disorder.

3 When assessing an apparently anxious client, questions about anxiety should be:

(1) Abstract and nonthreatening.
(2) Avoided until the anxiety disappears.
(3) Avoided until the client brings up the subject.
(4) Specific and direct.

4 Which of the following nursing diagnoses has the *highest* priority for an anxious client?

(1) Defensive coping
(2) Ineffective denial
(3) Risk for loneliness
(4) Risk for self-directed violence

5 The *best* goal for a client learning a relaxation technique is that the client will:

(1) Confront the source of the anxiety.
(2) Experience anxiety without feeling overwhelmed.
(3) Keep a journal as a self-monitoring technique.
(4) Suppress anxious feelings.

6 The long-term goal, "The client will learn new ways of coping with anxiety," is *most* appropriate at which level of anxiety?

(1) Mild
(2) Moderate
(3) Severe
(4) Panic

7 Which of the following would be the *best* nursing action for a client who is having a panic attack?

(1) Remain with the client.
(2) Teach the client to recognize signs of a panic attack.
(3) Instruct the client to remain alone until the symptoms subside.
(4) Involve the client in a physical activity.

8 A client asks why a beta blocker has been prescribed for anxiety. When answering this question the nurse should explain that beta blockers are effective for treatment of which symptoms associated with anxiety?

(1) Cognitive dissonance and confusion
(2) Depression and suicidal ideations
(3) Insomnia and nightmares
(4) Palpitations and rapid heart rate

9 A client who has refused to take the regular prescribed dose of clonazepam (Klonopin) complains of irritability, insomnia, tremors, and sweating. It is likely the client is experiencing symptoms associated with:

(1) Addiction.
(2) Manipulation.
(3) Overdose.
(4) Withdrawal.

10 Which of the following statements by a client with post-traumatic stress disorder would indicate the most improvement?

(1) "I am responsible for what happened to me."
(2) "I enjoy being back at work with my friends."
(3) "I have forgotten some of the things that happened to me."
(4) "I stay alert all the time."

See page 117 for Answers and Rationales.

I. Overview/Theories

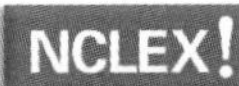

A. ***Anxiety:*** a state of apprehension, dread, uneasiness, or uncertainty generated by a real or perceived threat whose actual source is unidentifiable

1. Anxiety is an emotional, subjective response
   - **a.** Anxiety is commonly experienced by all human beings
   - **b.** Anxiety involves feelings of apprehension, worry, uneasiness, or dread
   - **c.** Acute anxiety is also known as state anxiety
   - **d.** Chronic anxiety is also known as trait anxiety
   - **e.** Primary anxiety is related to psychological factors
   - **f.** Secondary anxiety results as a reaction to a physical health problem
2. **Fear:** a reaction to a specific danger
3. **Stress:** a state of imbalance between demands placed on an individual and the individual's ability to deal with the demands
4. **Stressor:** an internal or external event or situation that leads to feelings of anxiety
   - **a.** Stressors are precipitating events that originate from the individual's internal or external environment
   - **b.** Physical illness, hospitalizations, and medical treatment can be stressors
   - **c.** It is not the stressor that causes anxiety, it is the person's perception of the stressor that leads to anxious feelings

   d. Individuals appraise stressors based on their past experiences, peer group practices, social circumstances, and current resources

5. **Burnout:** a state of mental and/or physical exhaustion; may be caused by excessive, prolonged stress

B. **Anxiety can be a healthy adaptive reaction** when it alerts the person to impending threats

C. **Anxiety is considered pathological** when it is disproportionate to the risk, continues after the threat no longer exists, and/or interferes with functioning

NCLEX!

D. **Anxiety exists on a continuum**

1. Mild
   a. Associated with the tension of everyday life
   b. The person is alert, the perceptual field is increased, and learning is facilitated
   c. Physiological responses are within normal limits
   d. The affect is positive
2. Moderate
   a. Focus is on immediate concerns
   b. The perceptual field is narrowed
   c. Low-level sympathetic arousal occurs
   d. Tension and fear are experienced
3. Severe
   a. Focus is on specific details and behavior is directed toward relieving anxiety
   b. The perceptual field is significantly reduced, and learning cannot occur
   c. The sympathetic nervous system is aroused
   d. Severe emotional distress is experienced
4. Panic
   a. Associated with dread and terror
   b. Details are blown out of proportion, the personality is disorganized, and the person is unable to function
   c. Physiological arousal interferes with motor activities
   d. Overwhelming emotions cause regression to primitive or childish behaviors

NCLEX!

E. ***General adaptation syndrome:*** an automatic physical reaction to stress mediated by the sympathetic nervous system; has three distinct stages—alarm, resistance, and exhaustion

1. Stress is viewed as a nonspecific body response to any demand
2. Alarm is the initial response to a stressor
   a. As a result of hormonal activity, generalized physical arousal develops and physical and psychological defenses are mobilized

b. The **"fight-or-flight" reaction,** an automatic psychological state of high anxiety mediated by the sympathetic nervous system, occurs

c. Increased alertness is focused on the immediate task or threat

d. The level of anxiety is mild to moderate

3. Resistance occurs when the body mobilizes resources to combat stress

a. The body stabilizes and adapts to stress, but functions below optimal level

b. **Coping,** efforts to manage specific demands that are appraised as threatening, and **defense mechanisms**, unconscious psychological responses designed to diminish or delay anxiety and protect the person, are used

c. Psychosomatic symptoms begin to develop

d. The level of anxiety is moderate to severe

4. Exhaustion occurs when adaptational resources are depleted

a. Results from inability to cope with overwhelming or long-lasting stress

b. Thinking becomes disorganized and illogical

c. The person may experience sensory misperceptions, delusions, hallucinations, and/or reduced orientation to reality

d. The level of anxiety is severe to panic

e. Physical illness and even death can occur if the period of exhaustion is prolonged

F. Anxiety is related to how a person appraises stressors

1. Events may be appraised as beneficial, benign, or stressful

2. Primary appraisal is used to evaluate personal and environmental factors or events

3. Secondary appraisal is used to determine how to cope with the anxiety generated by a stressful event

II. Etiology

A. Several theories have been postulated to account for a predisposition to anxiety

B. One's theoretical viewpoint affects the selection of treatment modalities

C. Biological factors

1. Anxiety results from improper functioning of the body systems involved in the normal stress response

2. Predisposition to the development of anxiety appears to be partially related to genetic factors

3. Hyperactivity of the autonomic nervous system is associated with anxiety

4. Several neurotransmitters have been associated with anxiety

a. A low level of gamma-aminobutyric acid (GABA), a neurotransmitter that inhibits the reactivity of neurons, is associated with anxiety

b. Norepinephrine is associated with the "fight-or-flight" reaction

c. **Panic attacks**, sudden episodes of symptoms such as dizziness, dyspnea, tachycardia, palpitations, and feelings of impending doom and death, have been related to high levels of norepinephrine

d. Obsessive-compulsive disorder is associated with high levels of serotonin

e. Cholecystokinin, a neuropeptide that functions as a neurotransmitter, may be related to the etiology of panic disorders

5. Changes in the structure and function of the brain are associated with anxiety

a. Anxiety appears to have its origin in the limbic system or the midline brainstem

b. Heightened activity in the cortex has been associated with obsessive thinking

c. PET scanning indicates that in some individuals anxiety leads to increased blood flow in the limbic system and certain areas of the midline brainstem

D. Psychodynamic factors

1. Anxiety is a warning of danger

a. Primary anxiety begins in response to the stimulation and trauma of birth

b. Subsequent anxiety represents a conflict between the instinctual drives (id) and the conscience (superego)

2. Anxiety and the personality are closely related

3. Symptoms of anxiety are a result of threatening unconscious mental content

4. Fear of punishment and pain may lead to anxiety

5. Unconscious repression of instinctual sexual drives may cause anxiety

6. Three types of anxiety have been identified

a. Reality anxiety is a painful affective experience related to the perception of danger in the external environment

b. Moral anxiety is related to feeling of guilt and/or shame

c. Neurotic anxiety is related to threats to instincts

E. Interpersonal factors

1. All human behavior is directed toward the attainment of satisfaction and security; anxiety occurs when individuals' needs are not met

2. Anxiety is a response to external environment factors arising out of contact with other human beings

a. Anxiety is first conveyed from the mother to the infant

b. Subsequent anxiety arises from fear of rejection, separation from significant others, and from feelings of inferiority

3. Symptoms of anxiety are a result of conflicts between individuals and their families, coworkers, and friends

4. Mild or moderate levels of anxiety may be expressed as anger

5. Severe anxiety produces confusion, forgetfulness, and decreased learning

6. Individuals with poor self-esteem are more susceptible to anxiety than are individuals with good self-esteem
   a. Individuals strive for security and relief from anxiety to protect the self
   b. The sense of self is based on how others evaluate the individual
   c. Individuals with low self-esteem have difficulty adapting to everyday events

F. Behavioral factors

1. Responses to stressors are often the result of learned or conditioned behavior
2. Anxiety may result from the inability to achieve desired goals
   a. Experimental psychologists believe anxiety begins with the attachment of pain to a specific stimulus
   b. Learning theorists believe individuals who have experienced intense fear early in life are likely to be anxious later in life
3. Anxiety may be generalized from specific stressors to similar objects and situations
4. When individuals experience too many life changes over a short period of time they may be unable to adjust and may display dysfunctional or maladaptive behavior

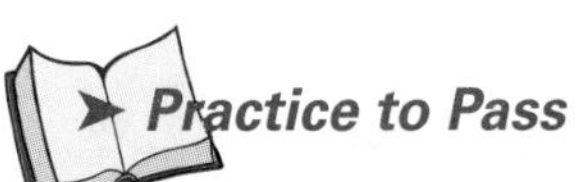

An anxious client states, "I can't help how I feel. Everyone in my family has this same problem. It's genetic. I inherited being worried all the time and there is nothing I can do about it, right?" How should you answer the client's question?

G. Other theories

1. Social theorists emphasize the role of social condition, such as socioeconomic status and racial inequalities, in the development of anxiety
2. Intrapersonal theorists believe an external locus of control and fear of future dangers contribute to the development of anxiety
3. Cognitive theorists believe unrealistic ideas and thoughts lead to anxiety
4. Feminist theorists believe women are likely to develop anxiety because they are taught to be dependent, passive, and submissive

III. Assessment

A. **Because stress affects each individual differently,** the signs and symptoms of anxiety are varied and numerous

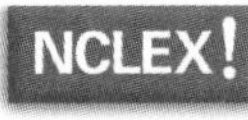

B. **Assessment should include data** to determine the level and stage of anxiety

C. **Several rating scales and diagnostic tools** are available to assess anxiety (e.g., Hamilton Anxiety Scale)

D. **Anxiety disorders are seen in all health settings**

1. Often individuals associate the symptoms of anxiety with physical disorders and seek treatment in medical-surgical healthcare settings
2. Shame and fear may prevent individuals from disclosing anxious feelings
3. All clients in all healthcare settings should be assessed for signs and symptoms of anxiety
   a. Anxiety should be assessed using direct, specific questions

b. The person's cognitive ability, level of education, and language ability should be considered when formulating individualized assessment questions

4. Because anxiety can contribute to organic illness, and organic illness can lead to anxiety, physical assessment must be included in the assessment of anxious individuals

E. **Assessment should include internal and external stressors** and the individual's specific and objective reactions to the stressors

F. **Biological, psychological, and social factors** should be assessed

1. Biological assessment should include appearance, substance use, sleep patterns, nutrition, physical activity, sexual function, and menstrual cycle

2. Psychological assessment should include thought and behavioral patterns, mood and affect, self-esteem, coping patterns, defense mechanisms, orientation to time, place and person, memory, insight, and suicide potential

3. Social assessment should include interpersonal relationships, support systems, diversional activities, ethnicity, and cultural factors

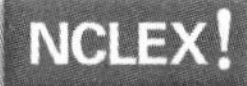

G. **Assessment should focus on the physical, affective, cognitive, social and spiritual symptoms of stress**

1. The physical signs of anxiety including increased blood pressure, respiration and heart rate, sweaty palms, diaphoresis, dilated pupils, dyspnea or hyperventilation, vertigo or light-headedness, blurred vision, urinary frequency, headache, sleep disturbance, muscle weakness or tension, anorexia, nausea, and vomiting

a. Physiologic symptoms of anxiety often mimic the symptoms of physical illness

b. Abnormal laboratory findings, including elevated adrenocorticotropic hormones, cortisol, catecholamine levels and hyperglycemia, may be evidence of anxiety

c. Individuals may not associate the physical signs of anxiety with stress and may believe they have physical health problems

A client being admitted to a medical-surgical unit asks why many of the assessment questions are related to anxiety. How should you respond to the client's concern?

2. Affective symptoms include depression, irritability, apathy, crying, hypercriticism, and feelings of guilt, grief, anger, worthlessness, apprehension, and helplessness

3. Cognitive symptoms include an inability to concentrate, indecisiveness, inability to learn and reason, lack of interest, and forgetfulness

4. Social symptoms include changes in the quality and quantity of communications, fear of social interactions, and social withdrawal

5. Spiritual symptoms include feelings of hopelessness and despair, fear of death, and inability to find life meaningful

IV. Nursing Diagnoses/Analysis

A. **Several nursing diagnoses are appropriate for anxious clients**

B. **Anxiety (panic)** related to situational and maturational crisis, real or perceived threat to self-concept or of death, unmet needs, and being exposed to a phobic stimulus

Box 5-1

Common Nursing Diagnoses for Anxious Clients

Altered family processes	Ineffective individual coping
Altered role performance	Post-traumatic stress response
Decisional conflict	Powerlessness
Hopelessness	Risk for self-harm
Dysfunctional grieving	Self-esteem disturbance
Impaired adjustment	Sleep pattern disturbance
Impaired social interaction	Social isolation
Ineffective family coping	Spiritual distress

C. Fear related to phobic stimulus or phobia, being in place or situation from which escape might be difficult or implausible and causing embarrassment to self in front of others

D. Ineffective individual coping related to ritualistic behaviors, obsessive thoughts, inability to meet basic needs, inability to meet role expectations, and inability to problem-solve effectively

E. Powerlessness related to lifestyle of helplessness, fear of disapproval from others, and unmet dependency needs

F. Social isolation related to panic level of anxiety, past experience of difficulty in interactions with others, and repressed fears

G. A more detailed list is found in Box 5-1

V. Planning and Implementation

A. Coping strategies

1. Coping is a process used by individuals to manage anxiety
2. The coping strategies selected by the individual are determined by the individual's intellectual ability, emotional state, physical health, beliefs, values, level of growth and development, and social status
3. Coping mechanisms may be effective or ineffective
4. NCLEX! Coping strategies to prevent and alleviate anxiety include such specific actions as: breathing exercises, guided imagery, meditation, listening to music, progressive muscle relaxation, recreational activities, crying, drinking, eating, exercising, laughing, sleeping, and swearing
5. NCLEX! General life management techniques related to diet, exercise, time management, and sleep can be used to prevent and alleviate stress
6. "Problem-focused coping" is task-oriented and designed to eliminate or change the source of the anxiety or deal with the consequences of the stressor
   a. Cognitive processes are used to reduce anxiety, solve problems, and resolve conflicts
   b. NCLEX! Problem-focused coping utilizes the steps in the problem solving process
      1) Assessment of the facts
      2) Development of goal
      3) Determination of alternatives for coping with the problem

Box 5-2

Common Defense Mechanisms Used by Anxious Individuals

Compensation	Rationalization
Denial	Reaction Formation
Displacement	Regression
Identification	Repression
Idealization	Splitting
Intellectualization	Sublimation
Introjection	Suppression
Isolation	Undoing
Projection	

4) Identification of the risks and benefits of each possible coping alternative

5) Selection of an alternative

6) Implementation of the selected alternative

7) Evaluation of the outcome

8) Modification of actions based on evaluation

7. "Emotional-focused coping" reinterprets the meaning of the situation

a. Defense mechanisms are automatic unconscious emotionally focused coping strategies

b. Defense mechanisms are often used to delay the onset of anxiety

c. Common defense mechanisms used by anxious individuals are listed in Box 5-2

B. Psychopharmacology

1. Common antianxiety agents (also known as anxiolytics or minor tranquilizers) used to treat anxiety are listed in Table 5-1

2. Benzodiazepines are the most commonly used and most effective medications for treatment of the symptoms of anxiety

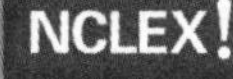

a. Prolonged use may lead to dependency and abuse

b. Benzodiazepines appear to increase the effectiveness of GABA and may also alter the brain's metabolism of serotonin and norepinephrine

c. All benzodiazepines are readily absorbed in the gastrointestinal tract after oral administration

d. The onset of action is very rapid and peak levels are often reached within an hour or less

e. The doses of specific benzodiazepines vary

f. Few drugs interact with benzodiazepines

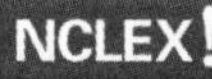

g. Common side effects include, ataxia, drowsiness, and impaired cognition, memory, and coordination

1) Long-acting benzodiazepines tend to cause early morning drowsiness

Table 5-1

Medications Commonly Used to Treat Anxiety

Generic Name	Trade Name	Clinical Use
Benzodiazepines		
Alprazolam	Xanax	Antianxiety
Chlordiazepoxide	Librium	Antianxiety
Clonazepam	Klonopin	Antianxiety and anticonvulsant
Diazepam	Valium	Antianxiety
Flurazepam	Dalmane	Hypnotic
Lorazepam	Ativan	Antianxiety and hypnotic
Oxazepam	Serax	Antianxiety and hypnotic
Temazepam	Restoril	Hypnotic
Triazolam	Halcion	Hypnotic
Nonbenzodiazepines		
Zolpidem	Ambien	Hypnotic
Zaleplon	Sonata	Hypnotic
Serotonin and dopamine agonist		
Buspirone	Buspar	Antianxiety
Barbiturates		
Amobarbital	Amytal	Hypnotic
Pentobarbital	Nembutal	Hypnotic
Phenobarbital	Luminal	Hypnotic
Secobarbital	Seconal	Hypnotic
Beta blocker		
Propranolol	Inderal	Antianxiety
Antihistamine		
Diphenhydramine	Benadryl	Hypnotic

2) Short-acting benzodiazepines may lose their effectives during the night, leading to nocturnal wakefulness and fatigue during the day

3) Benzodiazepines reduce rapid-eye-movement (REM) sleep

NCLEX!

h. Severe side effects are rare, however sedation and death may occur when alcohol and benzodiazepines are used together

i. Benzodiazepines should be tapered to minimize symptoms of withdrawal and rebound

NCLEX!

j. Withdrawal symptoms include difficulty concentrating, fatigue, irritability, insomnia, muscle aches, sweating, and tremors

3. Nonbenzodiazepine sedative-hypnotics are a new class of drugs used for short-term treatment of insomnia associated with anxiety

a. Zolpidem (Ambien) acts on the benzodiazepine receptors

1) Zolpidem has a short half-life

2) Zolpidem has fewer side effects than the benzodiazepines and does not cause rebound drowsiness, nor does it reduce REM sleep

3) There is little potential for dependency and abuse of zolpidem

b. Zaleplon (Sonata) is similar to zolpidem

1) Zaleplon is a schedule IV controlled substance

2) Because of its rapid onset of action and short half-life, zaleplon can be taken up to 4 hours before the client must awaken

4. Buspirone (Buspar) is a serotonin and dopamine agnosist used in the short-term treatment of anxiety

a. Buspirone is well-absorbed orally

NCLEX!

b. It generally takes 2 to 3 weeks for the antianxiety effects to become apparent and 4 to 6 weeks or longer for the drug to become fully effective

c. Side effects of buspirone rarely occur

1) Common side effects include dizziness, drowsiness, headache, nausea, nervousness, lightheadedness, and excitement

2) Side effects generally decrease over time as the body adapts to the medication

NCLEX!

d. Buspirone is not habit forming and does not potentiate the depressant effects of alcohol, barbiturates, and other central nervous system (CNS) depressants

e. Due to its short half-life, buspirone must be administered three times daily

f. Because buspirone does not induce an immediate calming effect it should not be used as a prn medication for anxiety

g. Withdrawal symptoms do not occur when the drug is discontinued

h. Because of its high cost and slow onset of action, buspirone is not widely prescribed

5. Barbiturates and sedative-hypnotic drugs were commonly used to treat anxiety before the development of the benzodiazepines

a. These drugs are very addictive and dangerous in overdose

b. Tolerance to their antianxiety and sedative effects develop with prolonged use

c. Because of their high potential for abuse and their tendency to depress the respiratory system and the CNS, barbiturates are not widely used to treat anxiety

6. Beta blockers have a calming effect on the CNS

a. Propranolol (Inderal) is a beta blocker sometimes used to treat anxiety

NCLEX!

b. Beta blockers are effective in treatment of physical symptoms of anxiety, such as tremors and tachycardia

An anxious client reports using over-the-counter Benadryl at bedtime to promote sleep and control "uncomfortable feelings." The client believes that because this medication is available without a prescription it is safe to use for an extended period of time. What information should you convey to the client?

7. The antihistamine diphenhydramine (Benadryl) is occasionally used to treat sleep disorders associated with anxiety
   a. Diphenhydramine may be purchased without a prescription
   b. Diphenhydramine shortens the time of sleep onset, but does not improve the quality of sleep
   c. Anticholinergic side effects, such as blurred vision and urinary hesitancy, may cause significant problems for elderly clients
8. Antidepressants may be used to treat coexisting depression and insomnia associated with anxiety (refer back to Chapter 4)
9. Highly sedating antipsychotics are sometimes used to treat sleep disorders associated with anxiety in elderly clients (see also Chapter 9)

C. Individual and group therapy

1. Most anxious individuals experience a marked decrease in their symptoms when they have the opportunity to discuss their feelings and problems with empathetic listeners
2. Individual and group therapy can be used to help anxious individuals develop insight into the reasons for their anxious feelings
   a. Insight therapy is most effective for highly motivated individuals who are not severely disabled by their symptoms
   b. Psychoanalysis is a form of insight therapy used by specially trained health care providers
3. Group therapy is an effective treatment modality for anxiety

NCLEX!

   a. Group therapy provides multiple sources of feedback and an interpersonal testing ground for practicing new behaviors
   b. Group experiences increase security, satisfaction, self-esteem, and commitment
   c. Nurses can serve as group leaders and can facilitate group therapy by referring clients to groups, preparing clients for group meetings, and debriefing clients following group meetings
   d. There are several different types of groups
      1) Growth groups are designed to increase an individual's sensitivity and problem-solving ability
      2) Support groups assist individuals to deal with normal life changes and crises
      3) Task groups use problem-solving strategies to achieve an outcome
      4) Self-help groups are autonomous from mental health professionals and are designed to assist individuals who have common problems

NCLEX!

      5) Education groups are designed to provide information and teach new skills

Box 5-3

Guidelines for Therapeutic Nursing Interventions to Assist Anxious Individuals

- Be aware of own level of anxiety.
- Remain calm.
- Establish a trusting relationship.
- Protect and reassure the client.
- Structure the environment to eliminate stressors.
- Assessment of client's anxiety should be ongoing.
- Assess the client's use of caffeine, nicotine, and other stimulants.
- Asses the client for signs of depression and suicidal ideations.
- Assist the client to identify stressors.
- Encourage the client to express feelings and explore sources of feelings.
- Help the client to examine cognitive processes and encourage positive self-talk.
- Assist the client to maintain hope and find meaning in life.
- Support the client's use of effective coping mechanisms.
- Teach the client new coping behaviors.
- Provide opportunities for the client to practice new coping behaviors.
- Teach the client relaxation techniques.
- Encourage appropriate grooming, sleep, diet, recreational activity, and exercise.
- Facilitate the client's interactions with supportive significant others.
- Use role-playing to assist the client to rehearse appropriate reactions to stressors.
- Stay with clients who display high levels of anxiety.
- Refer the client to community resources.

NCLEX!

4. Guidelines for therapeutic nursing interventions to assist anxious clients are listed in Box 5-3
   - **a.** An effective therapeutic relationship is based on trust
   - **b.** The goal of nursing interventions is not to totally eliminate anxiety, but to assist the client to tolerate mild anxiety and use constructive coping mechanisms to deal with stressors and anxious feelings
   - **c.** Client dependence on the nurse should be avoided
   - **d.** The client should actively participate in planning goals and interventions and in evaluating outcomes
   - **e.** When the client is hospitalized the environment should be structured to protect the client and provide activities and therapeutic interactions to reduce anxiety
   - **f.** Termination should occur when the client has gained optimal benefit

NCLEX!

5. Teaching is an important intervention for anxious clients
   - **a.** Anxious clients should be taught to reduce their intake of caffeine, nicotine, and other stimulants

b. Information pertaining to diet, exercise, and general health maintenance should be included in the teaching plan

c. Relaxation techniques such as deep rhythmic breathing, progressive muscle relaxation, visualization, and meditation should be taught

d. Social skill training and assertiveness training may also be useful

D. Behavior modification

1. Cognitive-behavior therapy can assist individuals to learn to identify stressors and plan responses to stressors

   a. To discourage dependency, cognitive therapy is brief and time-limited

   b. Cognitive therapy is structured and orderly

   c. Clients are encouraged to realistically appraise stressors

   d. Questions, rather than suggestions and advice, are used to encourage the clients to use and develop their own coping strategies

   e. "Homework" assignments are used to develop coping strategies

NCLEX!

2. In cognitive restructuring, clients are encouraged to examine involuntary negative thoughts and to replace negative self-talk with more positive thoughts

3. Response prevention is a form of behavior modification used to teach obsessive-compulsive clients how to prevent compulsive behaviors associated with obsessive thoughts

NCLEX!

4. Systematic desensitization is a form of behavior modification used to treat anxiety

   a. The client is first taught to relax

   b. While in a state of relaxation the client is exposed to a progressive hierarchy of stress-provoking stimuli

   c. The client helps to develop the hierarchy used during the desensitization process

5. Flooding, also known as implosion therapy, is a form of behavior modification used to treat anxiety

   a. Relaxation training is not used

   b. The client is exposed to imaginary or real-life stress provoking stimuli for an extended period of time

   c. The session is terminated when the client's anxiety decreases

6. Thought-stopping involves such techniques as instructing the client to shout "Stop!" or snap a rubber band placed on the wrist when unwelcome thoughts occur

7. Other behavior modification techniques used to treat anxiety include modeling, shaping, token economy, role-playing, social skill training, aversion therapy, response prevention, and contingency contracting

An agoraphobic client verbalizes some interest in attending a support group designed to help people learn how to cope with stress. What specific action should you take to refer this client to the group?

VI. Evaluation/Outcomes

A. **The client's progress** toward the identified outcomes should be evaluated during each nurse–client interaction

B. **Complete remission of symptoms** and total avoidance of stress producing stimuli is generally not an obtainable outcome

NCLEX!

C. **Evaluation should focus on changes** in lifestyle, behavior, feelings, interpersonal relationships, level of anxiety, perception of stressors, ability to recognize signs and symptoms of anxiety, thought processes, coping skills, use of medications, utilization of community resources, client's understanding of the disorder, and view of the future

D. **Standardized rating scales** can be used to evaluate the client's level of anxiety

E. **Clients may be encouraged to keep logs of daily experiences,** which can be used to evaluate such factors as severity, frequency, and duration of panic attacks, ritualistic behaviors, feelings, and relaxation strategies

VII. Specific Disorders

A. Phobic disorders

1. Individuals with phobic disorders recognize that their **phobias** (fears of specific objects, activities and situations) are irrational
2. Contact with the feared stimuli, or mere thought of the stimuli, causes immediate, severe anxiety

NCLEX!

3. Individuals with phobic disorders attempt to manage their anxiety by avoiding the feared stimuli
4. Avoidance of the feared stimuli may drastically interfere with routine activities
5. There are three types of phobia
   a. **Agoraphobia** (the fear of being incapacitated by being forced into or trapped in an unbearable situation from which there is no escape) without panic attacks involves fear of places or situations such as crowds, standing in line, being on a bridge, and traveling in a plane, bus, train, or car
   b. Social phobia is excessive fear of embarrassment and humiliation in public settings
      1) A social phobia may be related to a specific situation or generalized to several similar situations
      2) Social phobias strain interpersonal relationships and the phobic individual may become more anxious when significant others attempt to provide support and assistance
      3) Treatment with alprazolam and exposure therapy has been effective in reducing the anxiety associated with social phobias
   c. Specific phobia involves unrealistic fear of a particular object or situation
      1) The feared stimuli may be an object or a concern
      2) Panic level anxiety may be experienced
      3) The ethnic or cultural background of the client should be considered during assessment

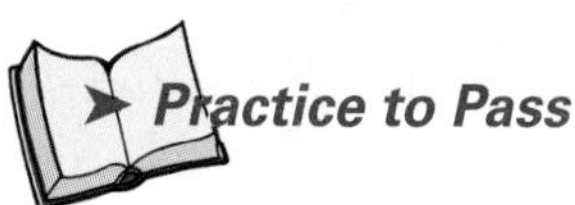

A client being admitted to the hospital verbalizes fear of "shots and blood." The client reports, "My heart pounds and I can hardly breathe just thinking about shots and blood. I don't know how I am going to survive being in the hospital." How can you assist this client?

6. Cognitive therapy and graduated exposure or desensitization are generally used to treat phobias

7. Antianxiety medications may provide short-term relief of phobic anxiety

NCLEX!

8. Nursing care should include accepting but not supporting the phobia, exploring the client's perceptions of threats, discussing feelings that may contribute to irrational fears, and identifying strategies for change

B. Generalized anxiety disorder

1. Individuals with generalized anxiety disorder have a great deal of difficulty controlling unrealistic, excessive anxiety associated with common daily experiences

2. The continued high level of anxiety causes symptoms such as restlessness, irritability, fatigue, depression, difficulty concentrating, muscle tension, sleep disturbance, and feeling of helplessness

3. Symptoms interfere with normal daily activities

4. In an attempt to control the symptoms of generalized anxiety disorder, individuals sometimes become dependent on alcohol or other substances

5. Generalized anxiety disorder has been successfully treated by a combination of cognitive therapy and relaxation training

NCLEX!

6. Nurses should encourage clients with generalized anxiety disorder to rethink their perceptions of the stressor, recognize that some anxiety is a normal part of life, and learn new coping mechanisms

7. Benzodiazepines and buspirone are sometimes used to treat generalized anxiety disorders

C. Panic disorder

1. Individuals who have panic disorder have recurrent panic attacks

2. Between panic attacks, the individual may have little or no debilitating anxiety or may suffer from chronic worry about future panic attacks

3. The onset of a panic attack is sudden and the source of the anxiety may not be identifiable

4. The symptoms of panic attacks include a desire to escape, chest pain, chills or hot flashes, choking sensations, depersonalization, dizziness, nausea, palpitations, shortness of breath, sweating, trembling, and fear of loss of control and mental illness

5. Individuals with panic attacks frequently associate their symptoms with physical illness and are concerned about death

6. Feelings of hopelessness, helplessness, and despair may lead to suicidal ideations

7. Agoraphobia is frequently associated with panic disorder

NCLEX!

8. During panic attacks the nurse should remain calm, stay with the client, offer reassurance, use short clear sentences, and reduce environmental stimuli

NCLEX!

9. When the level of anxiety is mild or moderate, the nurse should encourage the client to assume as much responsibility for self as possible, explore the possible causes of panic attacks, teach the signs and symptoms of escalating anxiety, reinforce appropriate coping and teach new coping strategies
10. Benzodiazepines and antidepressants are used to treat panic disorders

D. Obsessive-compulsive disorder

1. Individuals with obsessive-compulsive disorder (OCD) recognize that their recurrent obsessive thoughts and uncontrollable compulsive behaviors are irrational
2. Control of self, others, and the environment is an important issue for obsessive-compulsive individuals
3. Common **obsessions** (unwanted, persistent, intrusive thoughts, impulses or images related to anxiety) include thoughts about specific objects, contamination, questions, order, sex, aggressive feelings, and unacceptable impulses
4. Common **compulsions** (unwanted behavioral patterns or acts) include counting, praying, hand washing, repeating words, checking, and seeking assurance
5. In OCD, the obsessions and compulsions are either not realistically associated with preventing feared occurrences or are obviously excessive
6. Anxiety will increase if obsessive thoughts and compulsive behaviors are interrupted
7. Depression and/or substance abuse may occur as a complication of OCD
8. Relaxation and cognitive-behavioral techniques such as flooding and thought-stopping are used to treat OCD

NCLEX!

9. Nurses should assist clients with OCD to identify situations that increase anxiety and lead to unwanted thoughts and ritualistic behaviors
   a. The client should be assisted to explore the meaning and purpose of the thoughts and behavior
   b. Client's attempts to decrease obsessions and compulsions should be supported
      1) Initially, time should be structured to allow the client to complete rituals
      2) Limits should gradually be applied to the time allowed for rituals
      3) The nurse and client should mutually agree on limitations of rituals

NCLEX!

   c. Teaching should be conducted immediately following the completion of a ritual when the client's level of anxiety is at it lowest
10. Selective serotonin reuptake inhibitor (SSRI) antidepressant agents are the most effective somatic treatment for OCD
11. Electroconvulsive therapy has been used to treat depressive symptoms associated with OCD

E. Post-traumatic stress disorder (PTSD)

1. PTSD is associated with exposure to an extremely traumatic, menacing event such as military combat, rape, assault, kidnapping, torture, incarceration, disasters, and life-threatening illnesses

2. Symptoms of PTSD include, blunted affect, inability to show affection, lack of trust, lack of responsiveness, social withdrawal, loss of interest in activities, hopelessness, restlessness, irritability, intrusive and unwanted memories of the traumatic event, amnesia for certain aspects of the trauma, depression, nightmares, flashbacks, and occasional outburst of anger and rage
3. Individuals with PTSD use denial, repression, and suppression to cope with anxious feelings
4. Nurses should obtain an accurate account of the traumatic event, assess and acknowledge feelings of guilt, grief, and shame, provide a nonthreatening environment, encourage the client to discuss the traumatic event and feelings about the event, reinforce appropriate coping strategies, teach new coping strategies and assist the client to resume regular activities
5. Beta-blockers seem to be somewhat effective in the treatment of PTSD

NCLEX!

Case Study

An anxious client hospitalized on a psychiatric unit indicates her goal is to "feel more comfortable around other people." The client states, "I get so tense around other people my muscles hurt. I just don't know how to talk to other people. I am afraid I will do something wrong and offend someone. So I just stay home where it is safe. I don't have any friends here on the unit. I know I should go to the activities, but I just can't make myself do it. I wish I could relax more around others."

❶ What would be the most important nursing diagnosis for this client?

❷ What additional information would you need to obtain from this client?

❸ How could you get this client involved in activities on the unit?

❹ Which relaxation exercise would it be best for you to teach this client?

❺ How would you determine that the client had attained her goal?

For suggested responses, see page 306.

Posttest

1 Before an anxious client begins treatment with benzodiazepines it is *most* important to assess the client's:

(1) Level of motivation for treatment.
(2) Situational and social support.
(3) Stressors and use of coping mechanisms.
(4) Use of alcohol or other central nervous system depressant agents.

2 A physician has just told a client that surgery will be required to treat a health problem. After the physician leaves, the client reports feeling angry, tense, and shaky. The nurse notes that the client's palms are sweaty and the pupils are dilated. The nurse should assess the client's stage of anxiety as:

(1) Alarm.
(2) Exhaustion.
(3) Generalized anxiety.
(4) Resistance.

3 The nursing assessment indicates a client is experiencing a panic attack. The client is unable to understand directions and is preoccupied with thoughts of danger. Which of the following would be the *most* appropriate nursing diagnosis?

(1) Altered health maintenance
(2) Altered thought processes
(3) Ineffective individual coping
(4) Impaired communication

4 Which of the following would be the *most* appropriate goal for a client who has been diagnosed as having generalized anxiety disorder?

(1) The client will describe dissociative ideations.
(2) The client will display the ability to cope with mild anxiety.
(3) The client will relive the traumatic event.
(4) The client will verbalize a sense of control over ritualistic behaviors.

5 A client who is receiving an anxiolytic medication is reluctant to participate in group therapy. The client states, "The pills I am taking will take care of my stress. I don't need to talk about my problems." In response to the client's statement the nurse should explain that:

(1) Group therapy is the treatment of choice for anxiety.
(2) Medications relieve symptoms, but do not change the source of the anxiety.
(3) The client will need to attend group therapy only until the medication becomes effective.
(4) The medications will not work unless the client participates in group therapy.

6 A client states, "I am always late for everything because I can't leave my house without checking every door and window to make sure it is locked. If I don't make sure everything is locked I get so worried and I have to go back home. I can't seem to stop my behavior." The nurse should encourage this client to:

(1) Adjust the personal schedule to allow time for the ritual.
(2) Explore childhood experiences that may have led to the behavior.
(3) Remain at home until the symptoms subside.
(4) Stop worrying about the locks.

7 The *most* appropriate nursing action for a client experiencing a panic attack is to:

(1) Allow the client to determine the amount of stress that can be tolerated.
(2) Change the client's coping mechanisms.
(3) Explain the irrational nature of the situation.
(4) Expose the client to the source of the stress.

8 Which of the following statements made by a client with obsessive-compulsive disorder (OCD) would be the *best* indicator of improvement?

(1) "I have more control over my thoughts and behaviors."
(2) "I know that my thoughts and behaviors are not normal."
(3) "I only do my ritual to reward myself when I have been good."
(4) "My friends don't know about my disorder."

9 Which of the following statements by a client taking triazolam (Halcion) for anxiety indicates that teaching has not been effective?

(1) "The doctor wants me to take this drug at bedtime because it will help me sleep better."
(2) "I should not abruptly stop taking this medication."
(3) "I might not be able to drive while I am taking this medication."
(4) "I will probably have to take this medication for the rest of my life."

10 A client with generalized anxiety disorder states, "I now know the best thing for me to do is just to try to forget my worries." How should the nurse evaluate this statement?

(1) The client is developing insight.
(2) The client's coping skills are improving.
(3) The client needs to be encouraged to verbalize feelings.
(4) The nurse–client relationship should be terminated.

See pages 117–118 for Answers and Rationales.

Answers and Rationales

Pretest

1 **Answer: 3** ***Rationale:*** These are signs of the "fight-or-flight" response that occur at the severe level of anxiety. Mild anxiety is associated with the tension of everyday life; the person is alert, the perceptual field is increased, and learning is facilitated. In moderate anxiety, the perceptual field is narrowed, and low-level sympathetic arousal occurs. Panic anxiety is associated with dread and terror, and physiological arousal interferes with motor activities.
Cognitive Level: Application
Nursing Process: Assessment; ***Test Plan:*** PSYC

2 **Answer: 3** ***Rationale:*** Frequent and repetitive worries and behaviors are signs of an obsessive-compulsive disorder. Acute stress disorder and generalized anxiety disorders are characterized by a great deal of difficulty controlling unrealistic, excessive anxiety associated with common daily experiences or activities. Panic disorders are characterized by recurrent panic attacks and the source of the anxiety may not be identifiable.
Cognitive Level: Application
Nursing Process: Assessment; ***Test Plan:*** PSYC

3 **Answer: 4** ***Rationale:*** Because of shame, clients may be reluctant to talk about anxiety. Questions should be specific, direct, and individualized to the client. Option 1 is incorrect because when a client is experiencing anxiety abstract thinking and questions should be avoided. Options 2 and 3 are incorrect because the nurse should ask direct questions about the client's anxiety.
Cognitive Level: Comprehension
Nursing Process: Assessment; ***Test Plan:*** PSYC

4 **Answer: 4** ***Rationale:*** Safety needs generally have a higher priority than psychosocial needs. Options 1, 2, and 3 are applicable nursing diagnoses for anxious clients, but safety has the highest priority.
Cognitive Level: Application
Nursing Process: Planning; ***Test Plan:*** PSYC

5 **Answer: 2** ***Rationale:*** The goal of teaching calming techniques is to assist the client to learn to experience anxiety without feeling threatened and overwhelmed. Relaxation therapy does not assist a client to confront sources of anxiety. Likewise, keeping a journal is a self-monitoring technique but is not used to measure the outcome of relaxation. The goal is not to suppress anxious feelings but to make them more manageable.
Cognitive Level: Application
Nursing Process: Planning; ***Test Plan:*** PSYC

6 **Answer: 2** ***Rationale:*** Long-term goals for moderate anxiety should focus on assisting the client to understand the causes of anxiety and learn new coping strategies. These goals cannot be accomplished when the anxiety level is high because the client cannot focus on learning at this anxiety level.
Cognitive Level: Application
Nursing Process: Planning; ***Test Plan:*** PSYC

7 **Answer: 1** ***Rationale:*** To promote safety, nurses should stay with extremely anxious clients. During a panic attack a client is unable to focus on teaching. Physical activity should be avoided during a panic attack.
Cognitive Level: Application
Nursing Process: Implementation; ***Test Plan:*** PSYC

8 **Answer: 4** ***Rationale:*** Beta blockers are effective for the cardiovascular symptoms associated with anxiety. Options 1, 2, and 3 are not cardiovascular symptoms and reflect symptoms that beta blockers will not relieve.
Cognitive Level: Application
Nursing Process: Implementation; ***Test Plan:*** PSYC

9 **Answer: 4** ***Rationale:*** Abrupt withdrawal from a benzodiazepine may lead to symptoms associated with hyperarousal. There is not enough data to support addiction or manipulation. Signs of benzodiazepine overdose include severe drowsiness, ataxia, and impaired coordination.
Cognitive Level: Application
Nursing Process: Evaluation; ***Test Plan:*** PSYC

10 **Answer: 2** ***Rationale:*** People with post-traumatic stress disorder (PTSD) often avoid interactions and develop an isolated lifestyle that prevents them from working and socializing with others. Option 1 is an incorrect statement; clients are generally not responsible for the traumatic event. Options 3 and 4 reflect symptoms of PTSD, indicating the client is not yet showing improvement.
Cognitive Level: Application
Nursing Process: Evaluation; ***Test Plan:*** PSYC

Posttest

1 **Answer: 4** ***Rationale:*** Combined use of benzodiazepines and other central nervous system

depressants can lead to death from respiratory failure. Options 1, 2, and 3 are not the most important items to assess at this time.
Cognitive Level: Application
Nursing Process: Assessment; *Test Plan:* PSYC

2 **Answer: 1** *Rationale:* The symptoms displayed by the client reflect the "fight-or-flight" response, which occurs during the alarm stage of the general adaptation syndrome. Exhaustion and resistance consist of different symptoms within the general adaptation syndrome. General anxiety is characterized by a great deal of difficulty controlling unrealistic, excessive anxiety associated with common daily experiences.
Cognitive Level: Application
Nursing Process: Assessment; *Test Plan:* PSYC

3 **Answer: 2** *Rationale:* Altered thought processes related to understanding directions and/or obsessive thoughts is an appropriate nursing diagnosis for clients with severe or panic-level anxiety. The nursing diagnoses listed in options 1 and 4 do not reflect the cognitive state of the client. Option 2 is correct but is not the *most* appropriate diagnosis, since the question requires priority setting.
Cognitive Level: Application
Nursing Process: Analysis; *Test Plan:* PSYC

4 **Answer: 2** *Rationale:* Clients with generalized anxiety disorder should be able to demonstrate effective coping with mild anxiety. Clients with generalized anxiety disorder do not generally have dissociative ideations or ritualistic behaviors. Anxiety related to traumatic events is associated with posttraumatic stress disorder.
Cognitive Level: Application
Nursing Process: Planning; *Test Plan:* PSYC

5 **Answer: 2** *Rationale:* Anxiolytics relief symptoms, thus allowing the client to benefit from individual and group therapy. Anxiolytics cannot change the source of the anxiety.
Cognitive Level: Application
Nursing Process: Implementation; *Test Plan:* PSYC

6 **Answer: 1** *Rationale:* Clients who display compulsive behaviors need support and encouragement to manage their daily lives by modifying the environment and allowing time for the behaviors. Attempting to interfere with the ritualistic behaviors will only increase anxiety and ritualistic behaviors.
Cognitive Level: Application
Nursing Process: Implementation; *Test Plan:* PSYC

7 **Answer: 1** *Rationale:* Allowing the client to determine the amount of stress that can be tolerated will facilitate the client's feelings of safety. During a panic attack a client is unable to learn new coping mechanisms and is unable to identify the irrational nature of the situation (options 2 and 3). Removing the source of the stress can assist the client in coping with panic attacks, but exposing the client to the source of the stressor will worsen anxiety (option 4).
Cognitive Level: Application
Nursing Process: Implementation; *Test Plan:* PSYC

8 **Answer: 1** *Rationale:* Loss of control is a major concern for clients who have OCD. Goals related to control of unwanted thoughts and behaviors are appropriate for these clients. Options 2 and 4 do not indicate control over behavior. Option 3 is incorrect because the behaviors are utilized to reduce anxiety, not to reward self for good behavior.
Cognitive Level: Application
Nursing Process: Evaluation; *Test Plan:* PSYC

9 **Answer: 4** *Rationale:* Hypnotic and anxiolytic agents should be taken for as short a period of time as possible. Options 1, 2, and 3 are correct statements for clients taking triazolam, and as such are incorrect options. The question targets an incorrect statement to indicate ineffective teaching.
Cognitive Level: Application
Nursing Process: Evaluation; *Test Plan:* PSYC

10 **Answer: 3** *Rationale:* Suppression of feelings requires energy and will lead to increased anxiety. Clients need to talk about their feelings. The client's statement does not suggest insight nor is this an effective way to cope with generalized anxiety. The nurse–client relationship should be maintained because the client continues to require guidance and support.
Cognitive Level: Application
Nursing Process: Assessment; *Test Plan:* PSYC

References

American Psychiatric Association (2000). *Diagnostic and statistical manual of mental disorders, text revision* (4th ed.). Washington, DC: American Psychiatric Association.

Charron, H. S. (1998). Anxiety disorders. In E. M. Varcarolis (Ed.). *Foundations of psychiatric mental health nursing* (3rd ed.). Philadelphia: Saunders, pp. 443–477.

Frisch, L. E. & Wilson, W. (1998). Pharmacology in psychiatric care. In N. C. Frisch, & L. E. Frisch (Eds.), *Psychiatric mental health nursing: Understanding the client as well as the condition*. Albany, NY: Delmar, pp. 609–641.

Frisch, N. C. & Frisch, L. E. (1998). The client experiencing anxiety. In N. C. Frisch & L. E. Frisch (Eds.), *Psychiatric mental health nursing: Understanding the client as well as the condition.* Albany, NY: Delmar, pp. 174–207.

Fontaine, K. L. & Fletcher, J. S. (1999). *Mental health nursing* (4th ed.). Menlo Park, CA: Addison-Wesley, pp. 29, 169–204, 516.

Fortinash, K. M. & Holoday-Worret, P. A. (2000). *Psychiatric mental health nursing* (2nd ed.). St. Louis: Mosby, pp. 234, 249, 563, 565.

Johnston, C. J. (2000). *Psychotropic drugs.* In V. B. Carson (Ed.), *Mental health nursing: The nurse-patient journey* (2nd ed.). Philadelphia: Saunders, pp. 406–461.

Keltner, N. L. (1999). Antianxiety drugs. In N. L. Keltner, L. H. Schwecke, & C. E. Bostrom (Eds.), *Psychiatric nursing* (3rd ed.). St. Louis: Mosby, pp. 298–308.

Laraia, M. T. (2001). Psychopharmacology. In G. W. Stuart & M. T. Laraia (Eds.), *Principles and practice of psychiatric nursing* (7th ed.). St. Louis: Mosby, pp. 572–607.

LaSalle, P. C. & LaSalle, A. J. (2001). Therapeutic groups. In G. W. Stuart & M. T. Laraia (Eds.), *Principles and practice of psychiatric nursing* (7th ed.). St. Louis: Mosby, pp. 673–686.

Lee, K. (1998). Anxiety and related disorders. In M. A. Boyd & M. A. Nihart (Eds.), *Psychiatric nursing contemporary practice.* Philadelphia: Lippincott, pp. 476–529.

Molloy, M. (2000). Anxiety and related disorders. In K. M. Fortinash & P. A. Holoday-Worret (Eds.), *Psychiatric mental health nursing* (2nd ed.). St. Louis: Mosby, pp. 232–256.

Rittenmeyer, L. & Fontaine, K. L. (1999). Treatment modalities. In K. L. Fontaine & J. S. Fletcher (Eds.), *Mental health nursing* (4th ed.). Menlo Park, CA: Addison-Wesley, pp. 127–143.

Schwecke, L. H. (1999). Anxiety, coping, and crisis. In N. L. Keltner, L. H. Schwecke, & C. E. Bostrom (Eds.), *Psychiatric nursing* (3rd ed.). St. Louis: Mosby, pp. 147–156.

Sheer, J. (2000). Psychopharmacology and other biologic therapies. In K. M. Fortinash & P. A. Holoday-Worret (Eds.), *Psychiatric mental health nursing* (2nd ed.). St. Louis: Mosby, pp. 536–571.

Shives, L. R. (1998). *Basic concepts of psychiatric-mental health nursing* (4th ed.). Philadelphia: Lippincott, pp. 281–334.

Shoemaker, N. (2000). Stress and anxiety disorders. In V. B. Carson (Ed.), *Mental health nursing: The nurse-patient journey* (2nd ed.). Philadelphia: Saunders, pp. 608–634.

Stuart, G. W. (2001). Anxiety responses and anxiety disorders. In G. W. Stuart & M. T. Laraia (Eds.), *Principles and practice of psychiatric nursing* (7th ed.). St. Louis: Mosby, pp. 274–298.

Stuart, G. W. (2001). Cognive behavioral therapy. In G. W. Stuart & M. T. Laraia (Eds.), *Principles and practice of psychiatric nursing* (7th ed.). St. Louis: Mosby, pp. 658–672.

Stuart, G. W. & Laraia, M. T. (2001). *Principles and practice of psychiatric nursing* (7th ed.). St. Louis: Mosby, pp. 290, 291.

Townsend, M. C. (1999). *Essentials of psychiatric/mental health nursing.* Philadelphia: Davis, pp. 167–184, 199–235, 419–460.

Townsend, M. C. (2000). *Psychiatric mental health nursing concepts of care* (3rd ed.). Philadelphia: Davis, pp. 177–186, 225–281, 481–501.

Townsend, M. C. (2001). *Nursing diagnoses in psychiatric nursing: Care plans and psychotropic medications* (5th ed.). Philadelphia: F. A. Davis, pp. 209–218.

Varcarolis, E. (1998). Reducing stress and anxiety. In E. M. Varcarolis (Ed.), *Foundations of psychiatric mental health nursing* (3rd ed.). Philadelphia: Saunders, pp. 333–363.

Varcarolis, E. M. (1998). *Foundations of psychiatric mental health nursing* (3rd ed.). Philadelphia: Saunders, p. 454.

Videbeck, S. L. (2001). *Psychiatric mental health nursing.* Philadelphia: Lippincott, pp. 260–295.

Vincent-Pounds, K. G. (1999). Psychopharmacology. In K. L. Fontaine & J. S. Fletcher (Eds.), *Mental health nursing* (4th ed.). Menlo Park, CA: Addison-Wesley, pp. 145–166.

CHAPTER 6

Somatoform Disorders

Karma Castleberry, PhD, RN, APRN, BC

CHAPTER OUTLINE

OBJECTIVES

- Discuss five characteristics associated with somatoform disorders.
- State examples of at least four nursing diagnoses frequently used in the management of clients experiencing somatoform disorders.
- Formulate three intervention strategies for clients with somatoform disorders.

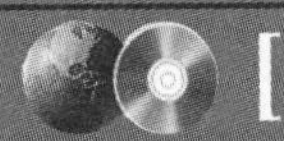

[Media Link]

Use the CD-ROM enclosed with this text, or log onto the address given to access the free, interactive Companion Website created for this series. The CD-ROM and Companion Website accompanying this book offer additional practice opportunities and information—NCLEX Review, Case Studies, Glossary, In Depth with NCLEX, and more.

www.prenhall.com/hogan

Review at a Glance

body dysmorphic disorder *a somatoform disorder characterized by preoccupation with a defect in appearance, either as an imagined defect or excessive concern about a minor anomaly*

conversion disorder *a somatoform disorder in which motor, sensory, or visceral function is lost and about which the client is usually indifferent*

hypochondriasis *a somatoform disorder in which a physical symptom is interpreted as severe or life-threatening, resulting in exaggerated worry*

la belle indifference *a calm, indifferent attitude toward symptoms or situations about which most persons would be concerned*

organic basis *an understanding of physical symptoms that are based upon structural and/or functional changes revealed by objective, diagnostic tests*

pain disorder *a somatoform disorder characterized by pain as the dominant physical symptom*

primary gain *symbolic resolution of unconscious conflict that decreases anxiety and keeps the conflict from awareness*

secondary gain *receipt of extra support and caring when experiencing an illness*

somatoform disorder *a psychiatric disorder in which there is no organic basis for the physical symptoms that are the chief complaints*

somatization disorder *a somatoform disorder characterized by multiple complaints in multiple body systems*

Pretest

1 A client with chronic low back pain receives cooking and cleaning help from her extended family. This is best described as:

(1) Primary gain.
(2) Secondary gain.
(3) Attention-seeking.
(4) Malingering.

2 The spouse of a woman diagnosed with somatization disorder asks the nurse if his wife has so many health problems on purpose. The *best* response is:

(1) "Have you tried asking her? I think she'd tell you the truth."
(2) "Your wife is trying to gain your attention."
(3) "She doesn't have the problem on purpose; however, this is probably difficult for both of you."
(4) "She has some significant emotional problems that she cannot admit."

3 The nurse would know that the plan of care for a client with a pain disorder was successful if the client states:

(1) "I realize that my pain can be influenced by stress."
(2) "I should avoid most physical activity."
(3) "Relaxation techniques only help when I am anxious about my pain."
(4) "I should keep myself pain-free by increasing my pain medications as I need."

4 The *most* appropriate nursing diagnosis for a client with a conversion disorder manifested by a stocking anesthesia is:

(1) High risk for impaired tissue integrity.
(2) Altered thought processes.
(3) Sensory-perceptual alteration.
(4) Ineffective individual coping.

5 What would the nurse expect the client with a somatization disorder to reveal in the nursing history?

(1) Abrupt onset of physical symptoms at menopause
(2) Exaggeration of the importance of a minor symptom
(3) Ignoring physical symptoms until role performance was altered
(4) Numerous physical symptoms in many organ systems

6 A goal of care for a client with hypochondriasis is:

(1) The nurse will respond matter-of-factly to the client's complaints.
(2) The client will seek second opinions about the symptom from health care providers.
(3) The client will state the relationships between life events and physical symptoms.
(4) The spouse will encourage the client to talk more about the symptoms.

7 The nurse would anticipate that health assessment of a client with a conversion disorder is likely to reveal which of the following?

(1) Elevated serum calcium levels
(2) Sensory loss along affected nerve tracks
(3) No significant physical or laboratory findings
(4) Motor loss to body parts along the nerve tracks

8 The *most* appropriate nursing diagnosis for a client with a somatoform disorder is:

(1) Altered role performance.
(2) Knowledge deficit: medication.
(3) High risk for violence, self-directed.
(4) Acute trauma reaction.

9 A hospitalized client diagnosed as having a somatization disorder asks for her "PRN" for stomach pain. The nurse's *best* response is to:

(1) Matter-of-factly assess the pain and administer PRN medication.
(2) Confront her with the negative gastroscopy findings.
(3) Ask her to take slow, deep breaths.
(4) Delay fulfilling her request to see if the pain subsides first.

10 A client treated for hypochondriasis would demonstrate understanding of his disorder by which statement?

(1) "I realize that tests and lab results cannot pick up on the seriousness of my illness."
(2) "Once my family realizes how severely ill I am, they will be more understanding."
(3) "I know that I don't have a serious illness even though I still worry a little about the symptoms."
(4) "I realize that exposure to toxins can cause significant organ damage."

See pages 134–135 for Answers and Rationales.

I. Overview/Theories

A. Psychophysiological responses

1. Amplified awareness of somatic stimuli caused by impaired CNS inhibitory function

2. Deficient communication between hemispheres of brain that impairs the ability to express emotions directly

B. Defense against anxiety

1. A person may express conflict and resultant anxiety through physical symptoms

a. Being physically ill is socially acceptable

b. Receives help and nurturance, as well as having dependency needs met

2. Conflict does not have to be acknowledged
    a. May consciously seek relief from physical symptoms
    b. May unconsciously not want to give up the symptoms because they decrease anxiety

C. Family dynamics

1. Family rules may prevent direct expression of conflict
2. Family may view physical illness as an acceptable way to avoid meeting otherwise required developmental tasks and role demands
3. Family may provide secondary gain
4. Symptoms may serve to control others or to stabilize relationships

II. Etiology

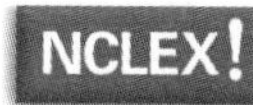

A. **Physical symptoms have no *organic basis;*** i.e., objective diagnostics tests do not reveal structural or functional changes

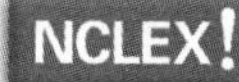

B. **Physical symptoms for which there is no organic basis** allow clients to meet dependency needs without admitting such needs exist

C. **Clients may be admonished to be mentally "strong"** and to not express emotional needs or problems

D. ***Somatoform disorders,*** in which there is no organic basis for the physical symptoms, may or may not begin after a physical illness or injury

E. Culture influences physical expressions

1. Cultures may expect distress to be manifested in bodily symptoms, with psychological distress viewed as unacceptable
2. Somatization is defined as a disorder in primarily Western societies
3. Some symptoms may be culture-bound, appearing only in some groups, such as the feeling of worms in the head being found only in some parts of Africa and South Asia
4. Many culture-bound illnesses have little influence on role performance

F. ***Somatization disorders,*** characterized by multiple complaints in multiple body systems, are more prevalent in women than in men

III. Assessment

A. History

1. Onset is variable, depending upon the disorder
2. Has seen multiple care providers without relief of symptoms
3. Sees the problem as "physical," and denies psychological influences on symptoms
4. **Primary gain:** illness allows reprieve from responsibilities
5. **Secondary gain:** sick role allows for dependency needs to be met
6. Over time, client is increasingly socially isolated and physically inactive
7. Family may insist on client seeking assistance due to altered role performance

B. Mental status variations

1. Depends upon type of disorder
2. Appearance: ranges from deeply anguished to indifferent; may assume antalgic position
3. Mood: may be depressed, anxious, or unaffected; mood may be labile
4. Thought: usually preoccupied with symptoms
5. NCLEX! Insight: highly impaired, usually denying any stressors or minimizing reactions to stressful events; not "psychologically-minded"

C. Physical symptoms

1. Respectfully and thoroughly evaluate physical symptoms
2. Common organ system responses; see Table 6-1 for specific symptoms
   a. Cardiovascular
   b. Musculoskeletal
   c. Respiratory
   d. Gastrointestinal
   e. Integumentary
   f. Genitourinary
3. NCLEX! Thorough health assessment including laboratory studies necessary to rule out physical illnesses with organic basis or other mental disorders

Table 6-1

Specific Symptoms of Common Organ System Responses

Organ System	Specific Symptom
Cardiovascular	Fainting Hypertension Migraine headache Tachycardia
Musculoskeletal	Back pain Fatigue Tension headache Tremor
Respiratory	Bronchospasm Dyspnea Hyperventilation
Integumentary	Pruritis
Genitourinary	Difficulties in micturation Menstrual disturbances Sexual dysfunction

IV. Nursing Diagnoses/Analysis

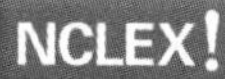

A. **Coping, ineffective individual** related to severe level of anxiety, low self-esteem, regression to earlier level of development and inadequate coping skills

B. **Family processes, altered** related to detachment and inability to express feelings or to struggle for power and control

C. **Denial, ineffective** related to threat to self-concept

D. **Social interaction, impaired** related to fear of leaving neighborhood or home or to physical symptoms and disability

E. **Body image disturbance** related to low self-esteem and unmet dependency needs

F. **Self-care deficit** related to paralysis of body part; inability to see, hear, or speak; and pain or discomfort

G. **Pain, chronic** related to severe level of anxiety and secondary gains from the sick role

V. Planning and Implementation

A. Specific strategies

1. Establish trusting, therapeutic relationship
   - **a.** Avoid describing the physical symptoms as "in the client's head"
   - **b.** Note that the symptoms are not an attempt to get attention
   - **c.** Recall that the client does not create symptoms consciously, or on purpose
   - **d.** Accept the reality of the symptoms as client presents them, avoiding dispute

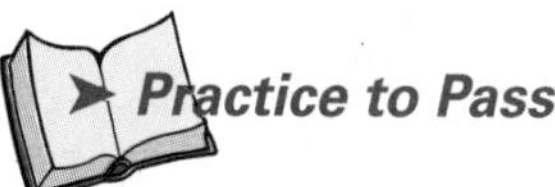

How could you explain symptoms from the stress response perspective for a person who presents with headache and low back pain?

2. Client education
   - **a.** Explain symptoms on a tissue level, using understandable and acceptable language
   - **b.** Present current knowledge of mind-body interaction, emphasizing how stress and anxiety affect physiological functioning
   - **c.** Teach methods to reduce physiological arousal, including relaxation techniques, visual imagery, self-talk strategies, and physical exercise (see Box 6-1)

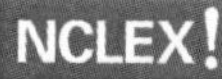

3. Encourage verbalization of thoughts and feelings, life events, and stressors

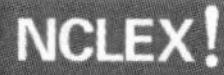

4. Assist in problem-solving specific conflicts or situations

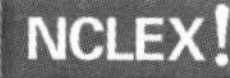

5. Self-care strategies
   - **a.** Modify exercise/activity plan to fit client's physical status
   - **b.** Employ nursing measures to promote sleep and rest
   - **c.** Promote healthy nutritional practices
   - **d.** Teach day-to-day client management of symptoms
6. Encourage gradual assumption of expected work, family, and community roles, commensurate with physical capabilities

Box 6-1

Tips for Teaching Relaxation Training

- Emphasize the relationship between stress and physiological arousal/symptoms
- Note that relaxation techniques work by:
  - Focusing attention to relaxation task, thus interrupting the preoccupation with symptoms
  - Decreasing physiological arousal, which negates physical symptoms of anxiety
- Remind the client that *s/he* effects the change (not the technique) to increase a sense of control
- Promote a daily return to physiological and psychological baseline to calm the mind and body through relaxation techniques, thus keeping general arousal low
- Note that daily practice builds skill level, not episodic use
- Suggest additional use of techniques when anticipating a stressful situation, or when client finds himself or herself becoming anxious
- Explain and teach a variety of techniques so that client can choose a technique that is acceptable and can be used in specific client environments

B. Pharmacological treatment

1. No specific psychotropic medications for somatoform disorders
2. Some evidence for use of antidepressants with pain and somatization disorders
3. Co-morbid anxiety or depression treated symptomatically with anxiolytics and antidepressants

NCLEX!

4. Medication for physical symptoms
   - **a.** Assess requests for medication and effectiveness of medication matter-of-factly
   - **b.** Encourage client to express thoughts and feelings experienced at the time of discomfort
   - **c.** Thorough client education regarding medication use, emphasizing provider-client collaboration to reduce self-adjustment of dosages

C. Individual/group treatment

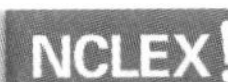

1. Cognitive-behavioral approaches
   - **a.** Identify self-statements and assumptions about stress, anxiety, and sick role
   - **b.** Challenge irrational beliefs and self-statements regarding seriousness of illness, inability to cope, and/or mind–body relationships
   - **c.** Provide accurate data to counter misinformation
   - **d.** Encourage positive, self-coping statements

Explain why a gradual assumption of responsibilities is indicated, especially since there is no organic basis for the disorder.

2. Groups for clients and families
   - **a.** Discussion of mind-body relationships
   - **b.** Forum for discussion and encouragement to "talk" out problems as a deterrent to physical symptoms
   - **c.** Correct misinformation about origin of somatoform disorders
   - **d.** Support for families and/or clients as roles shift during recovery

3. Supportive approaches
   a. Convey empathy: "This must be very trying for you"
   b. Convey respect: "I am impressed by how you have been able to do as much as you have, given how you feel"
   c. Explore with client ways to decrease isolation, improve role performance, and enhance self-esteem

NCLEX!

   d. Focus on verbally expressing feelings and coping techniques rather than symptoms
   e. Keep discussion of symptoms brief and matter-of-fact, but without dismissal

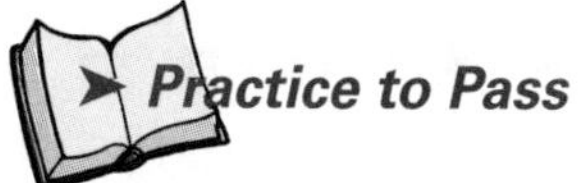

How might you teach family members to reinforce verbal expressions rather than symptoms?

4. Behavior modification
   a. In addition to cognitive behavioral approaches, engage client in self-modification to reward for engagement in treatment plan
   b. Teach family members to reinforce verbalization of stressors and life difficulties rather than symptoms

VI. Evaluation/Outcomes

A. Identifies the interaction of mind and body and the effects of stress

B. Increases ability to verbalize thoughts and feelings

C. Identifies conflicts and/or problems in situations and relationships

D. Seeks to actively solve problems through talking and concrete actions

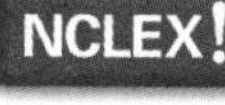

E. Assumes appropriate roles in work, family, and community

F. Employs self-help strategies

1. Challenges irrational thoughts
2. Corrects own misinformation
3. Uses positive coping statements
4. Engages in physical activity on regular basis
5. Employs relaxation techniques or visual imagery
6. Demonstrates sound nutritional practices

G. Diminished or less incapacitating physical symptoms

VII. Specific Disorders

A. Somatization disorder

1. Onset prior to age 30 with symptoms of several years duration

NCLEX!

2. Multiple physical complaints in multiple body systems
   a. Must include four pain symptoms
   b. Must include two gastrointestinal symptoms
   c. Must include sexual symptoms
   d. Must include symptoms suggesting neurological disorders
   e. Many clients complain of fatigue

3. New symptoms often arise with increased emotional distress
4. Tends to run in families
5. Lifestyle changes evoked by physical illness, affecting occupational, family and community relationships, and self-care
    a. Client is often disabled
    b. Client may be unable to work and economic hardships result
6. Seeks treatment for physical symptoms, only occasionally for problems in psychosocial functioning

NCLEX!

    a. Frequently goes from provider to provider, seeking relief (see Figure 6-1)
    b. Often a history of multiple surgeries
7. Special interventions
    a. Client requires long-term management, often in a medical setting

NCLEX!

    b. Treat physical symptoms conservatively, matter-of-factly
    c. Antidepressants may be prescribed if depressive symptoms present
    d. If anxiety present, focus should be on nonpharmacological treatments

B. ***Conversion disorder***

1. A somatoform disorder in which a motor, sensory, or visceral function is lost and about which the client is usually indifferent
2. Symptoms do not have an underlying organic cause
    a. Motor symptoms: mutism, paralysis, tremors (Figure 6-2)
    b. Sensory symptoms: blindness, deafness, numbness
    c. Visceral symptoms: urinary retention, breathing difficulties, headaches

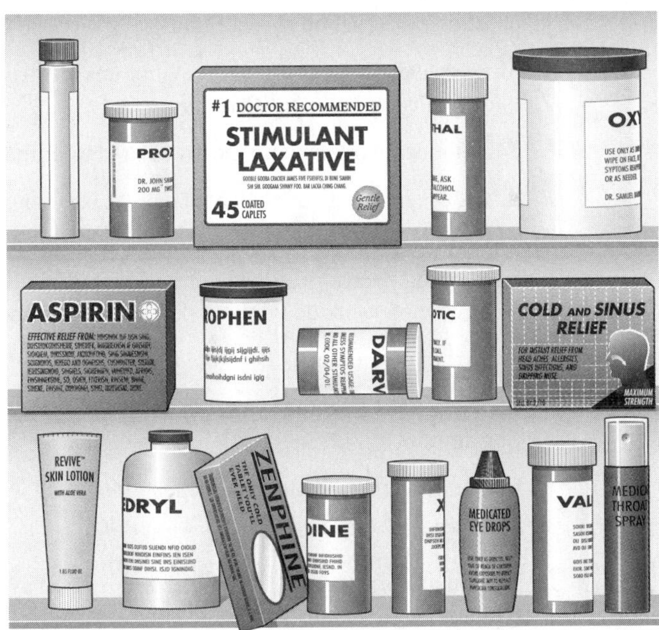

Figure 6-1

Clients with somatization disorder seek relief for a multitude of symptoms.

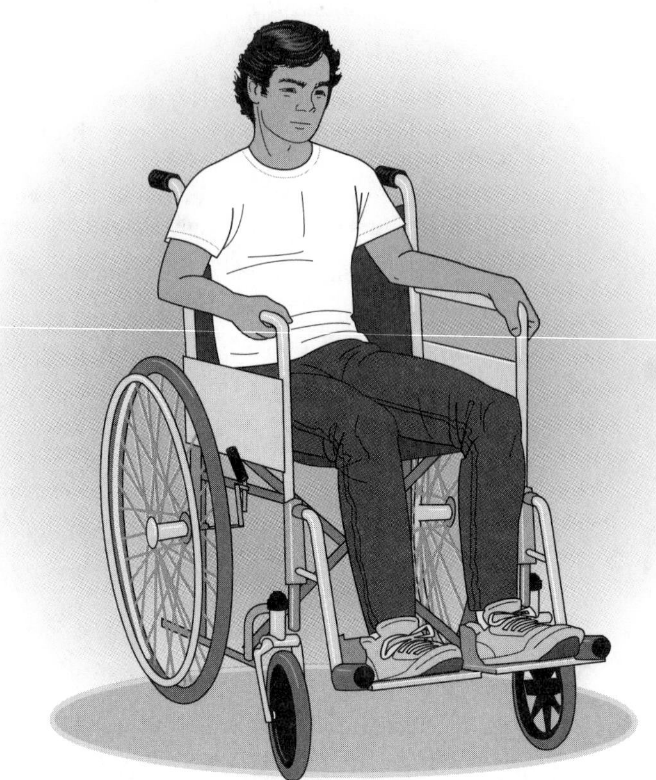

Figure 6-2

The client's symptoms reveal his needs.

3. The more medically naïve the client, the more implausible the symptoms
   a. Symptoms correspond to the client's ideas of the problem
   b. Symptoms do not follow neurological pathways
4. Clear, identifiable psychological factors (stress, conflict) are related to the onset or exacerbation of symptoms

NCLEX!

5. Mood may be inappropriate for symptoms, displaying little concern for symptoms (called ***la belle indifference***)
6. Symptoms are often symbolically related to primary gain
   a. Glove anesthesia of student about to take comprehensive examination so that answers cannot be written and he does not have to graduate
   b. Bilateral paralysis of lower extremities of man about to get married, so that he cannot "walk down the aisle" when he is uncertain of his decision
7. Special interventions

NCLEX!

   a. Nurse must treat the symptom as "real," as the client experiences the symptom
   b. Use problem-solving approaches for dealing with conflicts and stressors

C. ***Pain disorder***

1. Is a somatoform disorder characterized by pain as the dominant physical symptom

2. Client seeks medical attention for severe, prolonged pain with no organic basis for pain or the pain intensity
3. Preoccupation with pain that is not helped significantly by analgesics
4. Manifestations vary: low back pain, headache, chronic pelvic pain

NCLEX!

5. Historical relationship between stress, conflict, and initiation or exacerbation of pain
   a. Often follows physical trauma or injury
   b. Usually refuses to consider psychological origin
6. Diagnosis difficult because of personal and cultural differences in definition and expression of pain
7. Commonly accompanied by depression
   a. Hopelessness, helplessness
   b. Anger, irritability

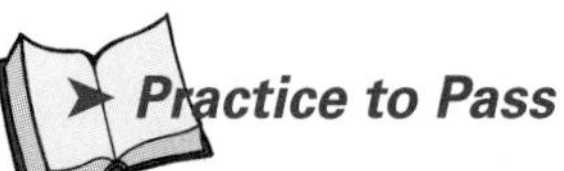

Explain how medications for pain and anxiety might be used most effectively for a client with pain disorder.

8. Special interventions
   a. Teach client how stress increases muscle tension, which creates increased pain (stress-tension-pain cycle)
   b. Acupuncture, biofeedback training, transcutaneous nerve stimulation
   c. Specific exercise programs, physical therapy
   d. Visualization, and relaxation training
   e. Education about pain management techniques

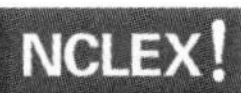

   f. *Note:* analgesics and antianxiety agents may be ineffective for pain, and addiction is possible

D. ***Hypochondriasis***

1. A disorder in which a physical symptom is interpreted as severe or life-threatening, resulting in exaggerated worry
2. Physical symptoms may begin with sensitivity to vague physical sensations or mild physical symptoms that most people would not notice

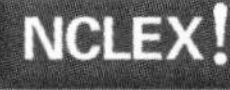

3. Exaggerated worry and preoccupation with physical symptoms and sensations occur
   a. Client interprets symptom as severe or life-threatening when it is not
   b. Symptom may be related to particular body function such as constipation, or to organ system such as coronary artery disease
   c. Often seeks information from clinicians or data sources to substantiate concerns
4. History of multiple visits to multiple practitioners
   a. May begin with physical illness in childhood
   b. May originate after severe medical problems as an adult
   c. Concern persists in spite of negative findings and clinician reassurances

5. Accompanied by significant anxiety
6. Special interventions
   a. Teach rational interpretation of body sensations
   b. Assist resolution of family conflict over medical treatment and client distress
   c. Non-pharmacological treatment of anxiety

E. ***Body dysmorphic disorder***

1. Is a somatoform disorder characterized by preoccupation with a defect in appearance, either an imagined defect or excessive concern over a minor anomaly
   a. Causes significant distress or impairment in role function
   b. Varies from flaws of face or head (complexion, hair thinning, asymmetry) to abdomen, extremities, or body shape/size
   c. Embarrassed about defects so may express them vaguely ("ugly," for example)
2. May frequently check defects, avoid reminders (removing mirrors), seek reassurances from others, or attempt to improve the defect (exercise, surgery, cosmetics)
3. Often leads to social isolation
4. Disorder is persistent; client has repeated surgeries, dental work, or dermatological treatment for defects

NCLEX!

5. Emotional distress may be severe enough to lead to depression and suicidal ideation
6. Special interventions
   a. Respect preoccupation; avoid challenging the validity of client perceptions
   b. Focus on coping techniques
   c. Contract with client to increase social activities and relationships

Case Study

G. A., a middle-aged man diagnosed with pain disorder, has been unable to work for the past year. Usually affable and gregarious, G. A. has become increasingly irritable with friends and family and prefers to spend time alone. An infrequent drinker (several beers a month) in the past, he now easily finishes a 6-pack of beer every evening. G. A. is now hospitalized on a psychiatric inpatient unit.

❶ G. A. requests a PRN pain medication that has been ordered. What principles would guide the nurse in handling his request?

❷ In a meeting with G. A. and his wife, she asks why he is so irritable. How could the nurse explain his mood change?

❸ G. A. questions going to group therapy. "I need my pain meds, not this jabbering about so-called problems." What is the best response?

❹ One of the staff members comments that he just thinks G. A. is trying to get out of working. Explain what is known about the origin of somatoform disorders, and the roles of primary and secondary gain.

❺ What are possible pain management strategies that could be included in a teaching plan for G. A.?

For suggested responses, see pages 306–307.

Posttest

1 Which of the following is the *most* appropriate nursing diagnosis for a client with pain disorder who is homebound and unable to work for the past 5 years?

(1) Impaired role performance
(2) Anxiety
(3) High risk for injury
(4) Sensory/perceptual alteration

2 A client who developed a glove anesthesia of the right (dominant) hand was unable to play in the piano competition yesterday. The consequence of the symptom, not having to perform, is best described as:

(1) Phobia.
(2) Primary gain.
(3) Carpal tunnel dysmorphia.
(4) Secondary gain.

3 Which of the following would be an outcome criterion for a client with body dysmorphic disorder, who is preoccupied with the size of her ears?

(1) Client will seek a second opinion for plastic surgery.
(2) Client will list three benefits of plastic surgery.
(3) Client will devise a plan for healthy eating and exercise.
(4) Client will explore possible explanations for dissatisfaction with body image.

4 A female client with a 15-year history of somatization disorder is to be discharged from her first psychiatric hospitalization. Which statement would indicate that nursing care has been effective?

(1) "I need to make sure that all of my medications are sent home with me."
(2) "I see now that when I get stressed, my 'body' speaks for me."
(3) "My family is so good to me when I am sick like this."
(4) "There are so many illnesses that you nurses simply do not know about."

5 A client treated for hypochondriasis has an upsetting phone conversation with her husband and subsequently requests an analgesic. "My head is killing me, and I know there is a tumor in there somewhere or it wouldn't hurt like this." The nurse's *best* response is:

(1) "You have no brain tumor. It is just your anger towards your husband."
(2) "I'll get your vital signs and then call your doctor if they are abnormal."
(3) "You must try not to rely on the pain pills so much since they are addictive."
(4) "I'll get your medication and then let's talk about what just happened."

6 While taking the nursing history, a client with body dysmorphic disorder complains that his jaw line "still isn't right" after three surgeries. He adds that it took five surgeons to finally fix his nose. The *most* appropriate nursing diagnosis is:

(1) Health-seeking behaviors.
(2) Body image disturbance.
(3) Personal identity disturbance.
(4) Risk for self-mutilation.

7 A client with pain disorder is likely to reveal in the nursing history:

(1) Good responses to pharmacological treatment.
(2) Indifference to the discomfort.
(3) Pain originated after physical trauma.
(4) Insight into stress-pain relationship.

8 A client is assessed as having bilateral stocking anesthesia. The *most* important goal of care is that the client will:

(1) Explore how his life is affected by being unable to walk.
(2) List the side effects of prescribed medication.
(3) Be referred for outpatient physical therapy.
(4) Demonstrate crutch-walking techniques.

9 A client is convinced that her pelvic pain is from an advanced malignancy, and that she is likely to die. Extensive testing has revealed no abnormalities. "You think this is in my head, don't you?" she asks. The nurse's *best* response is:

(1) "Sometimes doctors miss a diagnosis."
(2) "Yes, I think you think you have pain."
(3) "It must be hard for you to hear the testing results."
(4) "How about resting now and asking your doctor later?"

10 A client with a somatization disorder has been attending group therapy. Which statement indicates that the care has been effective?

(1) "I think I'd better get some pain pills. My back hurts from sitting in group."
(2) "The other women in the group have *mental* problems!"
(3) "I haven't said much, but I get a lot out of listening."
(4) " I feel better physically just from getting a chance to talk."

See pages 135–136 for Answers and Rationales.

Answers and Rationales

Pretest

1 Answer: 2 ***Rationale:*** Secondary gains are unintentionally sought "benefits" that result from an illness, such as support that otherwise might not be available. These benefits serve to reinforce illness behavior. Primary gains are symbolic resolutions of unconscious conflict that decrease anxiety and keep the conflict from awareness. Attention-seeking and malingering are deliberate behaviors.
Cognitive Level: Comprehension
Nursing Process: Analysis; ***Test Plan:*** PSYC

2 Answer: 3 ***Rationale:*** Family members must understand the mechanism of somatization disorder, and to have their own needs addressed. The chronic nature of the physical complaints are very frustrating and disrupting of family functioning.
Cognitive Level: Analysis
Nursing Process: Implementation; ***Test Plan:*** PSYC

3 Answer: 1 ***Rationale:*** Understanding the relationship between physical symptoms and stress helps the client to gain control of outcomes. Physical activity and limited use of pain medications are indicated.

Relaxation techniques are most effective when practiced on a regular, not episodic basis, although they can be employed when pain levels are just beginning to rise.
Cognitive Level: Application
Nursing Process: Evaluation; *Test Plan:* PSYC

4 **Answer: 4** ***Rationale:*** In a conversion disorder, symptoms assist the client to avoid anxiety about unconscious conflicts. Effective means of coping reduce the need to use physical symptoms.
Cognitive Level: Analysis
Nursing Process: Analysis; *Test Plan:* PSYC

5 **Answer: 4** ***Rationale:*** Somatization disorder is characterized by chronic, multiple vague physical symptoms in multiple body systems that impair role performance. The disorder usually begins before age 30, and symptoms are a major source of concern in the client's life.
Cognitive Level: Analysis
Nursing Process: Assessment; *Test Plan:* PSYC

6 **Answer: 3** ***Rationale:*** Discharge criteria for clients with somatoform disorders, which are associated with anxiety, include understanding the relationships between symptoms and anxiety-provoking events. Family members must also learn not to reinforce physical symptoms or illness behavior. The client with hypochondriasis usually has a number of care providers in succession, going from one to another, in a search for a cure.
Cognitive Level: Application
Nursing Process: Planning; *Test Plan:* PSYC

7 **Answer: 3** ***Rationale:*** Clients with a conversion disorder have no physiological basis for the symptoms. Options 1, 2, and 4 have a physiological basis.
Cognitive Level: Application
Nursing Process: Assessment; *Test Plan:* PSYC

8 **Answer: 1** ***Rationale:*** Somatoform disorders result in altered role performance because the illness interferes with the usual responsibilities in life. There is not enough data to support knowledge deficit or risk for self-directed violence. Acute trauma reaction does not exist.
Cognitive Level: Analysis
Nursing Process: Analysis; *Test Plan:* PSYC

9 **Answer: 1** ***Rationale:*** The nurse's response to requests for PRN medications for the client with a somatization disorder should be designed to accept the reality and intensity of the pain, and to not reinforce the client's using physical symptoms as communication.
Cognitive Level: Application
Nursing Process: Implementation; *Test Plan:* PSYC

10 **Answer: 3** ***Rationale:*** Education for a client with hypochondriasis is effective if the client is aware that the symptoms present no real danger. Giving up the preoccupation with the serious nature of the symptoms is a gradual process of cognitive restructuring.
Cognitive Level: Application
Nursing Process: Evaluation; *Test Plan:* PSYC

Posttest

1 **Answer: 1** ***Rationale:*** Chronic pain interferes with social and occupational functioning, prompting further stress and anxiety. The other nursing diagnoses do not address the long-term homebound status and unemployment.
Cognitive Level: Analysis
Nursing Process: Analysis; *Test Plan:* PSYC

2 **Answer: 2** ***Rationale:*** Unconscious avoidance of responsibilities or conflicts (competing in the recital) is primary gain. The client does not have to take personal responsibility for not playing; rather, he can "blame" his illness. Glove anesthesia does not have an organic basis for the symptom.
Cognitive Level: Comprehension
Nursing Process: Assessment; *Test Plan:* PSYC

3 **Answer: 4** ***Rationale:*** Cognitive-behavioral approaches such as identifying and challenging distorted perceptions of the client or interrupting self-critical thoughts are effective to deal with preoccupation with imagined physical defects. Options 1, 2, and 3 would support the client's poor body image.
Cognitive Level: Application
Nursing Process: Planning; *Test Plan:* PSYC

4 **Answer: 2** ***Rationale:*** The client's statement indicates accurate awareness of mind–body interaction. She does not suggest the symptoms are something to medicate, nor does she persist in identifying her illness as physical in origin, both of which are characteristic of somatization disorder.
Cognitive Level: Application
Nursing Process: Evaluation; *Test Plan:* PSYC

5 **Answer: 4** ***Rationale:*** The nurse should provide physical care for the client in a matter-of-fact manner and, at the same time, should help the client note how symptoms increase at the time of stress and can be a way of coping with stress.
Cognitive Level: Application
Nursing Process: Implementation; *Test Plan:* PSYC

6 **Answer: 2** ***Rationale:*** Body dysmorphic disorder is characterized by preoccupation with imagined

defects, usually on the face or head, that prompt the client to seek medical treatment.
Cognitive Level: Analysis
Nursing Process: Analysis; ***Test Plan:*** PSYC

7 **Answer: 3** ***Rationale:*** The client with pain disorder continues to express discomfort, does not respond well to medication, and exhibits no insight into his condition. Pain often begins after physical injury. The client usually shows no insight into the role of stress on pain perception.
Cognitive Level: Analysis
Nursing Process: Assessment; ***Test Plan:*** PSYC

8 **Answer: 1** ***Rationale:*** Focusing on the effects of the symptoms may help the client understand the relationship between symptoms and stressors. Options 2, 3, and 4 will only assist the client to manage bilateral stocking anesthesia.
Cognitive Level: Application
Nursing Process: Planning; ***Test Plan:*** PSYC

9 **Answer: 3** ***Rationale:*** Verbalizing feelings helps the client learn to express herself in other ways, especially about issues that are anxiety-producing, such as negative test results.
Cognitive Level: Application
Nursing Process: Implementation; ***Test Plan:*** PSYC

10 **Answer: 4** ***Rationale:*** Participating in group therapy offers a chance to talk and to gain support from others, both of which free up energy.
Cognitive Level: Application
Nursing Process: Evaluation; ***Test Plan:*** PSYC

References

American Psychiatric Association. (2000). *Diagnostic and statistical manual of mental disorders, text revision* (4th ed.). Washington, DC: American Psychiatric Association.

Boyd, M. (1998). Somatoform and related disorders. In M. Boyd & M. Nihart (Eds.), *Psychiatric nursing: Contemporary practice.* Philadelphia: Lippincott, pp. 582–610.

Doenges, M., Townsend, M., & Moorhouse, M. (1998). *Psychiatric care plans* (3rd ed.). Philadelphia: F. A. Davis, pp. 356, 360.

Fontaine, K. (1999). Anxiety disorders. In K. Fontaine & S. Fletcher (Eds.), *Mental health nursing* (4th ed.). Menlo Park, CA: Addison Wesley Longman, pp. 169–204.

Fontaine, K. (1999). Communicating and teaching. In K. Fontaine & S. Fletcher (Eds.), *Mental health nursing* (4th ed.) Menlo Park, CA: Addison Wesley Longman, pp. 89–113, 180.

Johnson, M., Bulechek, G., Dochterman, J., Maas, M., & Moorhead, S. (2000). *Nursing diagnoses, outcomes, and interventions: NANDA, NOC, and NIC linkages.* St. Louis: Mosby.

Kennedy, W. (1999). Somatoform disorders, factitious disorders, and malingering. In P. O'Brien, W. Kennedy, & K. Ballard (Eds.), *Psychiatric nursing: An integration of theory and practice.* New York: McGraw-Hill, pp. 331–350, 366.

Malloy, M. (2000). Anxiety and related disorders. In K. Fortinash & P. Holoday-Worret (Eds.), *Psychiatric mental health nursing* (2nd ed.). St. Louis: Mosby, pp. 231–256.

McDonald, S. (2000). Principles of communication. In K. Fortinash & P. Holoday-Worret (Eds.), *Psychiatric mental health nursing* (2nd ed.). St. Louis: Mosby, pp. 148–173.

Rittenmeyer, L., & Fontaine, K. (1999). Treatment modalities. In K. Fontaine & S. Fletcher (Eds.), *Mental health nursing* (4th ed.). Menlo Park, CA: Addison Wesley Longman, pp. 127–166.

Spelic, S. (1998). Somatoform disorders. In C. Glod (Ed.), *Contemporary psychiatric nursing: The brain-behavior connection.* Philadelphia: F. A. Davis, pp. 403–424.

Stewart. G. (2001). Anxiety responses and anxiety disorders. In G. Stewart & M. Laraia (Eds.), *Principles and practice of psychiatric nursing* (7th ed.). St. Louis: Mosby, pp. 274–316.

Stewart, G. (2001). Psychophysiological responses and somatoform and sleep disorders. In G. Stewart & M. Laraia (Eds.), *Principles and practice of psychiatric nursing* (7th ed.). St. Louis: Mosby, pp. 299–316.

Thomas, S. (2000). Psychophysiological disorders. In V. Carson (Ed.), *Mental health nursing: The nurse-patient journey* (2nd ed.). Philadelphia: W. B. Saunders, pp. 897–923.

Townsend, M. (2000). *Psychiatric mental health nursing: Concepts of care* (3rd ed.). Philadelphia: F. A. Davis, pp. 514, 517, 519.

Townsend, M. (2001). *Nursing diagnoses in psychiatric nursing* (5th ed.). Philadelphia: F. A. Davis, p. 228.

CHAPTER 7

Dissociative Disorders

Karma Castleberry, PhD, RN, APRN, BC

CHAPTER OUTLINE

Overview/Theories
Etiology
Assessment
Nursing Diagnoses/Analysis
Planning and Implementation
Evaluation/Outcomes
Specific Disorders

OBJECTIVES

- Discuss five characteristic behaviors associated with dissociative disorders.
- State examples of at least four nursing diagnoses frequently used in the management of clients experiencing dissociative disorders.
- Formulate three intervention strategies for clients with dissociative disorders.

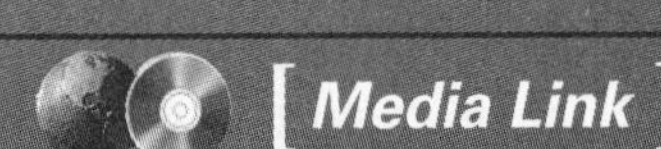

Use the CD-ROM enclosed with this text, or log onto the address given to access the free, interactive Companion Website created for this series. The CD-ROM and Companion Website accompanying this book offer additional practice opportunities and information—NCLEX Review, Case Studies, Glossary, In Depth with NCLEX, and more.

www.prenhall.com/hogan

Review at a Glance

alter *personality state or identity that recurrently takes over the behavior of a person with dissociative identity disorder*

continuous amnesia *inability to recall successive events as they occur*

depersonalization *feeling of detachment or separation from one's self, as if in a dream-like state*

derealization *feeling that the external world is unreal or strange*

dissociation *defense mechanism in which experiences are blocked off from consciousness, so that affect, behavior, identity, memories, and/or thoughts are not integrated*

dissociative amnesia *dissociative disorder in which there is an inability to remember important personal information that cannot be accounted for by ordinary forgetfulness*

dissociative fugue *dissociative disorder characterized by suddenly wandering or taking a trip away from one's usual place, accompanied by amnesia for some or all of the past*

dissociative identity disorder *dissociative disorder characterized by two or more distinct personalities or identities (alters) in an individual person*

generalized amnesia *inability to recall entire life*

host personality *primary identity that holds the person's name*

localized amnesia *inability to recall events in a circumscribed time period*

repression *defense mechanism in which thoughts and feelings are kept from consciousness*

selective amnesia *inability to recall some events within a circumscribed time*

Pretest

1 The client, although oriented to person, place, and time, cannot remember being extracted from his burning automobile the day before. His inability to remember events surrounding the accident is best described as:

(1) Denial.
(2) Localized amnesia.
(3) Confabulation.
(4) Continuous amnesia.

2 The *most* appropriate nursing diagnosis for a client experiencing a fugue state is:

(1) Anxiety.
(2) Self-esteem disturbance.
(3) Altered family processes.
(4) Relocation stress syndrome.

3 The nurse who assesses the client in a fugue state is *most* likely to note:

(1) A history of childhood trauma.
(2) Coexisting depression.
(3) Exposure to a major stressor.
(4) Selective amnesia.

4 A *priority* goal for a client who is unable to recollect events surrounding the tornado that demolished his farm is:

(1) The client will report decreased depression by day 2.
(2) The client will express anger about his loss by day 2.
(3) The client will apply for job retraining by day 2.
(4) The client will attend a support group for disaster survivors by day 2.

5 A nursing assistant asks for advice about talking with a client recently diagnosed with dissociative identity disorder: "Should I talk about her childhood abuse?" The nurse's *best* answer is:

(1) "If she brings up the abuse, listen to her and be supportive."
(2) "You will need to really push her to get it all out."
(3) "Ask her to discuss this only with her therapist."
(4) "Remind her that sometimes adults exaggerate about their childhood experiences."

6 The nurse realizes a dissociative client may best be able to recover memories through which of the following types of therapy?

(1) Electroconvulsive therapy
(2) Hypnosis
(3) Relaxation techniques
(4) Antianxiety agents

7 The nurse would determine that client education to manage dissociative episodes is effective if the client states, "Once I start to dissociate, I should:

(1) Immediately take my antianxiety medication."
(2) Focus on what I can see and hear externally."
(3) Begin my relaxation technique."
(4) Focus on my internal feelings."

8 A client with dissociative identity disorder, who is now 20 minutes late for group, is adamant that she was *never* told to go to the cognitive therapy group. The nurse's *best* response is:

(1) "You can't get out of group that easily."
(2) "People with dissociative identity disorder forget quite a bit."
(3) "Have you thought about just why you might be resisting treatment?"
(4) "It is possible that you were not aware of group time."

9 The wife of a client who has returned to his prefugue state asks if her husband will be able to remember what happened during the time of the fugue. The nurse's *best* response is:

(1) "He will have no memory for events during the fugue."
(2) "He will be able to tell you—if you can gently encourage him to talk."
(3) "Only his therapist should have him talk."
(4) "Avoid mentioning it, or he may start alternating old and new identities."

10 The nurse may note switching from one alter to another by observing for which of the following in a client?

(1) Orthostatic hypotension
(2) Blinking or rolling of the eyes
(3) Dystonic reactions
(4) None of these; there are no discernable features of switching

See page 148 for Answers and Rationales.

I. Overview/Theories

A. Usually consciousness, memory, identity, and perception are integrated functions

B. In dissociative disorders, there is a sudden disruption in client's consciousness, identity, or memory

C. Defense mechanisms of dissociation and repression are used

1. May experience considerable anxiety caused by expressed or fantasized forbidden wishes, often of sexual or aggressive nature
2. May have considerable anxiety related to stressors or traumatic events
3. Person does not consciously "decide" to dissociate

D. Anatomical/physiological origins of "trance states" or dissociation

1. Childhood trauma resulting in neurotransmitter and anatomical changes in the brain
2. Genetic predisposition to dissociate is hypothesized

II. Etiology

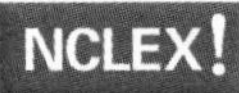

A. Traumatic experience (commonly accidents, natural disasters, assault)

1. Strong emotional response
2. Psychological conflict

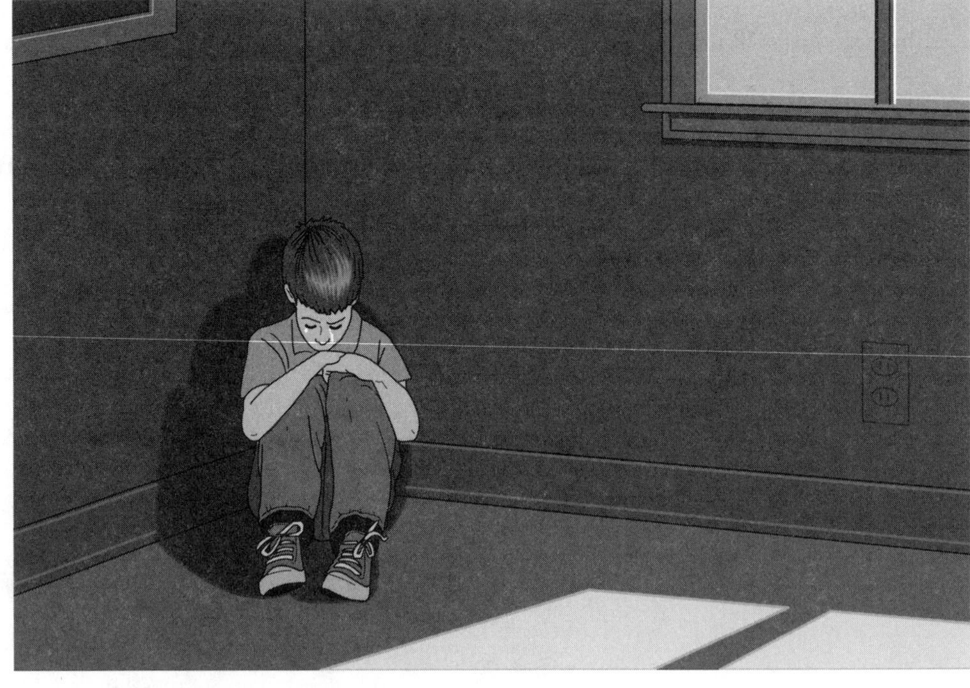

Figure 7-1

Children may learn to dissociate from intolerable situations such as severe abuse.

3. May be long-term, chronic stressors

B. **More easily induced if using psychoactive drugs** (hallucinogens or cannabis)

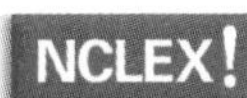

C. **Severe childhood physical, sexual, or emotional abuse**

1. Implicated in dissociative identity disorder (DID)
2. Child learns to detach or dissociate from intolerable situation (Figure 7-1)
3. Continues to dissociate when experiencing stressful (even non-abusive) events as an adult, which interferes with normal functioning

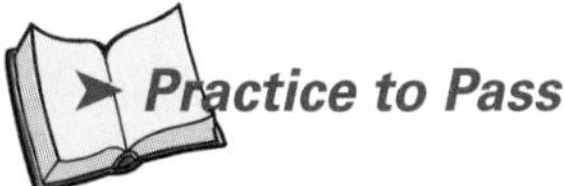

Practice to Pass

How would you explain the stress-anxiety-dissociation relationship to a client who is dissociative and is puzzled about her behavior?

III. Assessment

A. History

1. Recounts trauma and/or severe stress
   a. History of childhood abuse, but often does not recall trauma
   b. Symptoms appear in adulthood after stressful event(s)
   c. Symptoms appear immediately or may be delayed for years
2. Extent of dissociation or amnestic symptoms varies widely with different dissociative disorders
   a. **Dissociation** is a defense mechanism in which experiences are blocked off from consciousness, so that affect, behavior, identity, memories, and/or thoughts are not integrated
   b. **Repression** is a defense mechanism in which thoughts and feelings are kept from consciousness
3. May report symptoms of depression or anxiety

Practice to Pass

What questions could you routinely use in all assessments that might uncover a history of trauma?

B. Physical symptoms

1. Headaches common with DID
2. Other dissociative disorders have no associated physical symptoms

C. Mental status examination

1. Appearance: facial expressions and mannerisms may vary widely within one session or appearance may vary widely from day to day (DID)
2. Mood: anxious, depressed; some clients have little mood change
3. Memory: amnesia for events (variable extent)
4. Perception: feelings of detachment from self or environment, feeling of physical change in body
5. Insight: impaired, unaware of memory impairment

NCLEX!

NCLEX!

NCLEX!

NCLEX!

IV. Nursing Diagnoses/Analysis

A. **Anxiety** related to traumatic experience

B. **Ineffective individual coping** related to childhood trauma, childhood abuse, low self-esteem, and inadequate coping skills

C. **Personal identity disturbance** related to threat to physical integrity, threat to self-concept, and underdeveloped ego

D. **Sensory-perceptual alterations** related to severe level of anxiety, repressed and decreased perceptual field

E. **Altered thought processes** related to physical integrity and threat to self-concept

F. **Powerlessness** related to unmet dependency needs and fear of memory loss

G. **High risk for self-mutilation** related to response to increasing anxiety and inability to verbalize feelings

V. Planning and Implementation

A. Specific strategies

1. Create safe, calm environment
   a. Mutually develop plan of care
   b. Prevent stressors that could elicit dissociation
2. Teach stress management and coping techniques
   a. Progressive muscle relaxation
   b. Physical exercise
   c. "Grounding" or the focus on external environment (what client can see and hear) rather than on internal feelings, thoughts, or sensations that can lead to "spacing out" (a lay term indicating lack of awareness of the immediate environment)
   d. Problem-solving strategies to resolve conflicts and stressors
   e. Distraction

NCLEX!

NCLEX!

A client who is dissociative remarks that he has tried using visual imagery to reduce stress, but finds it anxiety producing and "spacey." How could you explain this phenomenon and what alternatives could the client use to reduce stress?

3. Discuss traumatic event and its meaning
4. Reconstruct memories through client's account and those of others
5. Educate about specific dissociative disorder
    a. Relationship between anxiety and dissociation
    b. Include family and significant others
6. Assist staff and other clients to understand the disorder (especially DID)
7. Plan for use of leisure time (anxiety often increases when alone without activities)

B. Pharmacology

Why are antianxiety agents recommended for short-term use?

1. Drug-facilitated interviews using thiopental sodium (Pentothal) or sodium amytal to recovery memory
2. Antianxiety agents for short-term symptomatic treatment
3. Antidepressants for depression and antipsychotics for extreme agitation (if those symptoms are present)

C. Individual/group

1. Hypnosis to recover memories
2. Focus on emotional responses to trauma or stressors
3. Work through unacceptable impulses or behavior verbally

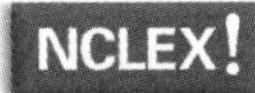

4. Refer to support groups
    a. Related to specific stressors such as parenting or occupational
    b. "Survivor" groups, particularly for natural disasters or abuse

D. Behavior modification

1. Teach cognitive techniques to promote positive self-statements about coping ability

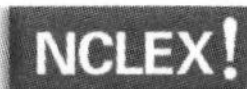

2. Reinforce client's use of stress management and coping strategies rather than dissociation

VI. Evaluation/Outcomes

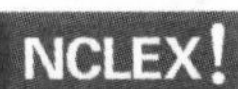

A. Client explains the relationship between trauma/stress, anxiety, and dissociation

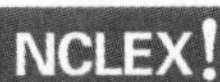

B. Client can prevent dissociative states by employing stress-management and positive coping behaviors

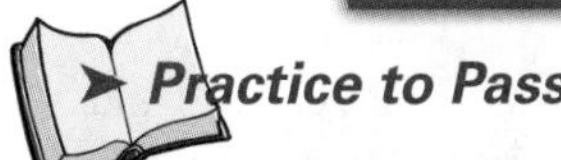

How could you determine that the client's traumatic events are remembered with appropriate affect?

C. Client can remember stressors and traumatic events with congruent affect

D. Client actively seeks to solve problems

E. Client assumes or resumes social and occupational roles

F. Client uses leisure time in constructive ways

VII. Specific Disorders

A. ***Dissociative amnesia:*** a dissociative disorder, in which the client cannot remember important personal information that cannot be accounted for by ordinary forgetfulness

NCLEX!

1. Suddenly unable to recall memories
   - **a. Localized amnesia:** short time period (hours) after a disturbing event
   - **b. Selective amnesia:** amnesia for some, but not all events
   - **c. Generalized amnesia:** amnesia for whole lifetime of experiences (very rare)
   - **d. Continuous amnesia:** forgets successive events as they occur
2. Not ordinary forgetfulness
3. Able to recall other information, learn, and function coherently
4. Most common during wars and natural disasters
5. Primary gain: symbolic resolution of unconscious conflict that decreases anxiety and keeps the conflict from awareness
6. Secondary gain: receipt of extra support and caring when experiencing an illness
7. Usually terminates abruptly
8. Special interventions
   - **a.** Survivor support groups
   - **b.** Gradual reconstruction of events through talking and listening/reading of others' accounts of the trauma

B. ***Dissociative fugue:*** a dissociative disorder characterized by suddenly wandering away or taking a trip away from one's usual place, accompanied by amnesia for some or all of the past (Figure 7-2)

NCLEX!

1. Travels from usual environment

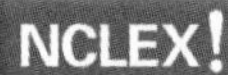

2. Unable to recall important aspects of identity and assumes new identity
   - **a.** Old and new identities do not alternate
   - **b.** Incomplete new identity
   - **c.** Does not know information is forgotten
3. Usually lasts from hours to days, rarely months; considerable confusion when returns to pre-fugue state
4. Often is a response to psychological stressors (war, family, marital)

NCLEX!

5. Once the client has returned to pre-fugue state, has no memory for events during the fugue
6. Special interventions: hypnosis, drug-facilitated interviews, support groups

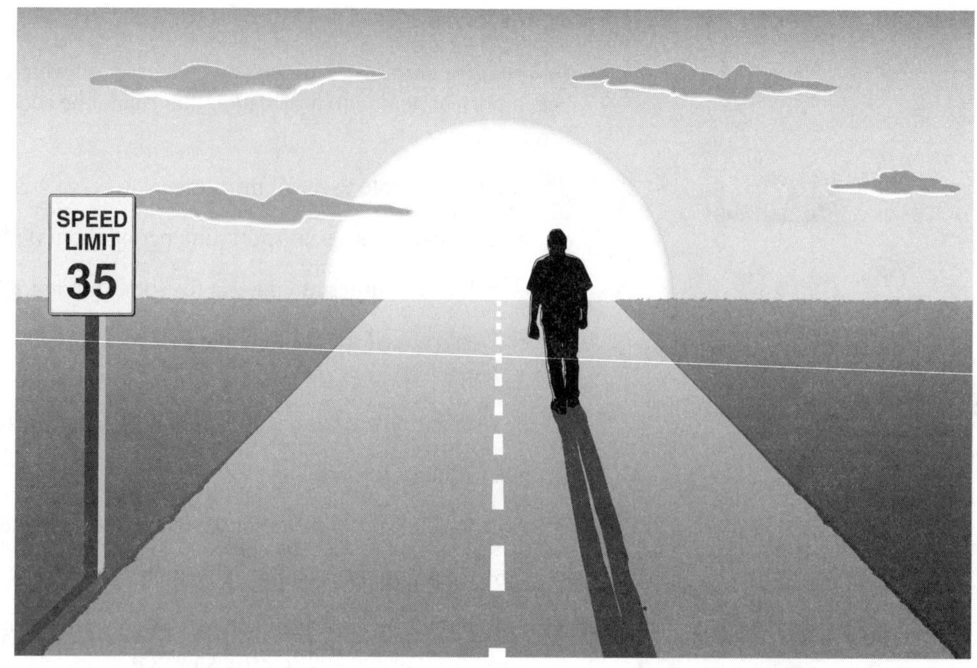

Figure 7-2

A dissociative fugue involves leaving one's usual environment and is accompanied by amnesia for all or part of the past.

C. ***Dissociative identity disorder* (DID):** a dissociative disorder characterized by two or more distinct personalities or identities (alters) in an individual person

NCLEX!

1. Client has two or more alters (separate, distinct identities or "personalities")
   a. An **alter** is a personality state or identity that recurrently takes over the behavior of a person with DID
   b. Each alter has relatively enduring pattern of perceiving, relating to, and thinking about oneself and the environment
   c. Formerly known as multiple personality disorder (MPD)
2. Personalities with different influences and power over one another
   a. May represent different ages, genders
   b. Alters each have different physiological responses and disorders (one alter may be myopic, while another is not)
   c. Communicate with one another through "executive" alter
   d. Some alters share "co-consciousness," aware of each other's experience and behavior; others only aware of own existence
   e. "Switching" occurs by dissociating from one alter to another
   f. Number of personalities range from 2 to over 100, with 50 percent of clients having more than 10 personalities
   g. **Host personality:** primary identity that holds the person's name
   h. The host personality is typically unaware of the alters (the anxiety-provoking aspects of personality), but the alters are typically aware of the host personality

NCLEX!

3. "Loses time" when alternate personality is present for a period of time
   a. Usually client is unable to give full account of childhood (few memories) because of dissociation
   b. May appear forgetful and is often accused of lying

NCLEX!

4. Mental status variations
   a. Marked variation in appearance from time to time
   b. Blinking, eye rolls, headaches, covering or hiding the face, and twitches may occur when "switching" from one alter to another
   c. Marked variation in speech in brief periods of time
   d. Impaired insight, usually unaware of alters
   e. May appear anxious or depressed

NCLEX!

5. Associated with severe physical or sexual abuse during childhood
   a. Many post-trauma symptoms (nightmares, flashbacks, hypervigilance)

NCLEX!

   b. Self-mutilation, suicidal, or aggressive behavior
6. Special interventions

NCLEX!

   a. No-harm contract and environmental safety if client is suicidal or is self-mutilating

NCLEX!

   b. Meeting and recognizing alters and their unique experiences and needs

NCLEX!

   c. "Mapping" personality system, noting characteristics of alters and co-consciousness
   d. Creation of emotionally safe environment for all alters
   e. Individual therapy with therapist skilled in working through trauma leading to integration (moving together of aspects of all identities)
   f. Development of new coping skills for integrated client and for clients who choose not to integrate so that dissociation is either not necessary or is under control

NCLEX!

   g. Family therapy with partners and children to help client avoid dissociation, deal with hostile personalities, understand therapy process, and to confirm experience with client's behavior
   h. Hypnosis or drug-facilitated interviews; use is controversial because of the possibility of remembering "too much, too soon" and being overwhelmed with anxiety
   i. Issue: the therapist's "creating" memories and alters by his or her verbal and nonverbal behavior in suggestible client

D. Depersonalization disorder

NCLEX!

1. Experiences recurrent alterations in self-perception
   a. **Depersonalization:** feeling of detachment or separation from one's self, as if in a dream-like state
   b. Client describes self as "detached from my body" or "being in a dream"

c. Feels strange or unreal

d. Able to function during the experience

NCLEX!

2. Client may report distress about experiences and become depressed and anxious
   a. Often fears being "crazy"
   b. May be accompanied by **derealization,** which is the feeling that the external world is unreal or strange
3. Precipitated by stress and anxiety
4. Most common in teenagers and young adults
5. Special interventions
   a. Problem-solving to reduce stress in general
   b. Stress-management techniques
   c. "Grounding" or focus on external environment

Case Study

C. J., a 35-year-old woman diagnosed with depression and dissociative identity disorder, is hospitalized when outpatient therapy proved insufficient to manage her mood. You are part of the interdisciplinary team working with C. J.

1. What are some of the safety issues might you anticipate?
2. You overhear one of the nursing assistants urging another to "go see C. J. and her eleven faces." How could you handle this situation?
3. What could you do to decrease confusion about which "personality" you are interacting with at a given point in time?
4. C. J.'s husband is concerned about involving their two school-age children in family therapy. How might you explain how children might benefit from family therapy?
5. One of the evening nurses comments that C. J. does this "multiple business" just to get attention, even though she has a lovely family—and a nice house. What is your best response?

For suggested responses, see page 307.

Posttest

1 The nurse working with a client who has a dissociative disorder understands that this disorder is likely to begin as a:

(1) Gradual loss of memory for names and phone numbers.
(2) Means to avoid adult responsibilities.
(3) Consequence of using hallucinogens.
(4) Protective defense against anxiety.

2 A *priority* nursing intervention for a person recently admitted to an inpatient unit with a dissociative disorder is:

(1) Creation of a calm, safe environment.
(2) Increasing sensory stimulation.
(3) Working through past trauma.
(4) Promoting social skills.

3 The nurse assessing a client with dissociative identity disorder (DID) is *most* likely to note:

(1) History of headaches.
(2) Elated mood.
(3) Intact memory for recent and remote events.
(4) Stocking anesthesia.

4 A client with DID is admitted after an overdose of alcohol and benzodiazepines, claiming that another alter "did it." The *priority* nursing diagnosis is:

(1) Post-trauma response.
(2) Risk for self-directed violence.
(3) Personal identity disturbance.
(4) Anxiety.

5 A client is brought to the emergency room after a brutal physical assault. Although oriented and coherent, she cannot remember the assault or events surrounding it. The *priority* intervention is to provide:

(1) Frequent reality orientation.
(2) Physical comfort and safety.
(3) Thoughtful questioning for the police report.
(4) Referral to a community support group.

6 A client with DID suddenly begins to speak with a child's vocabulary and voice. This is *best* understood as:

(1) An attempt to gain attention.
(2) Regression to a more comfortable state.
(3) Switching to a child alter.
(4) Resistance to therapeutic work.

7 A client with DID suddenly begins to speak with a child's vocabulary and voice. Which of the following is the most therapeutic response by the nurse?

(1) "You must be feeling very needy."
(2) "Here are some toys you might enjoy."
(3) "Can you tell me what is happening?"
(4) "This behavior keeps you from working on your problems."

8 A client is diagnosed with depersonalization disorder. Which of the following is the nurse most likely to find in the assessment?

(1) Two or more personalities
(2) Feelings like "being in a dream"
(3) Indifference to the symptoms
(4) Amnesia about the event

9 The *priority* nursing diagnosis for a client experiencing amnesia is:

(1) High risk for self-directed violence.
(2) Powerlessness.
(3) Ineffective individual coping.
(4) Sensory/perceptual alteration.

10 A client reports episodic depersonalization experiences. Which of the following is an appropriate goal of care?

(1) The client will describe three stress management techniques by day 2.
(2) The client will report no suicidal thoughts by week 1.
(3) The client will create a chart of all personalities by week 1.
(4) The client will state five personal strengths by day 2.

See pages 148–149 for Answers and Rationales.

Answers and Rationales

Pretest

1 **Answer: 2** ***Rationale:*** A localized amnesia is characterized by the inability to recall all events associated with a stressful event; whereas, continuous amnesia would include the present (and the client is oriented to person, place, or time). Denial is an unconscious defense mechanism in which emotional conflict and anxiety are avoided by refusing to acknowledge those thoughts, feelings, or desires. Confabulation is the replacement of gaps in memory with imaginary information.
Cognitive Level: Application
Nursing Process: Assessment; ***Test Plan:*** PSYC

2 **Answer: 1** ***Rationale:*** A fugue state is a result of dissociation, a defense against overwhelming anxiety. Without further data, it is impossible to determine that the stress and anxiety are related either to family difficulties, self-esteem, or relocation.
Cognitive Level: Analysis
Nursing Process: Analysis; ***Test Plan:*** PSYC

3 **Answer: 3** ***Rationale:*** Fugue states usually begin abruptly after a major stressor such as war or natural disaster, and end abruptly. The client may or may not have a history of childhood trauma or depression. The client who experiences a fugue will have no memory of that period of time.
Cognitive Level: Analysis
Nursing Process: Assessment; ***Test Plan:*** PSYC

4 **Answer: 4** ***Rationale:*** Support groups for disaster survivors assist persons who have gone through the traumatic event. These groups provide the opportunity to work through the event, talking about the event to decrease anxiety. Feelings of depression and anger may occur later than 2 days and will take more than a few days to resolve. It is too early to consider job retraining.
Cognitive Level: Application
Nursing Process: Planning; ***Test Plan:*** PSYC

5 **Answer: 1** ***Rationale:*** Trust is the basis of a therapeutic relationship, and the client should proceed at a self-determined rate, particularly if the subject is painful. Self-pacing avoids flooding the client with severe anxiety. This self-disclosure should be accepted nonjudgmentally by all persons with whom the client has contact.
Cognitive Level: Application
Nursing Process: Implementation; ***Test Plan:*** PSYC

6 **Answer: 2** ***Rationale:*** Hypnosis may be used to access memories or other personalities that have not yet emerged. The other options do not affect memory retrieval.
Cognitive Level: Comprehension
Nursing Process: Planning; ***Test Plan:*** PSYC

7 **Answer: 2** ***Rationale:*** Objects or surroundings can be used to reorient the client by promoting concentration and external focus. Internal focusing only augments dissociation. Trying to take an antianxiety medication at the time of dissociation is not only too late to be an effective deterrent, but is also unlikely to be carried out as dissociation disrupts the client's integrated functioning.
Cognitive Level: Analysis
Nursing Process: Evaluation; ***Test Plan:*** PSYC

8 **Answer: 4** ***Rationale:*** Many clients with dissociative identity disorder have lack of awareness of events because another personality was present when these events were discussed. Thus, the host personality has no knowledge of them. Although the client eventually must be accountable for all actions of the personalities to the greatest extent possible, this may not initially be under the client's control.
Cognitive Level: Application
Nursing Process: Implementation; ***Test Plan:*** PSYC

9 **Answer: 1** ***Rationale:*** The client who has experienced a fugue is unable to remember events occurring during the fugue state, despite encouragement. The client does not have the ability to alternate his own identity with the partial identity he assumed during the fugue state.
Cognitive Level: Application
Nursing Process: Implementation; ***Test Plan:*** PSYC

10 **Answer: 2** ***Rationale:*** Switching from one alter to another is manifested in a variety of ways including blinking, facial changes, and changes in voice and train of thought. Orthostatic hypotension and dystonic reactions are not usually associated with switching from one alter to another.
Cognitive Level: Application
Nursing Process: Assessment; ***Test Plan:*** PSYC

Posttest

1 **Answer: 4** ***Rationale:*** Dissociative disorders result from using the defense mechanism of dissociation, which prevents anxiety about traumatic events or stressors from conscious awareness. Dissociation is

not consciously employed and does not involve a gradual loss of memory. Hallucinogens can facilitate dissociation in persons who are prone to "trance states" or spacing out.
Cognitive Level: Comprehension
Nursing Process: Assessment; ***Test Plan:*** PSYC

2 **Answer: 1** ***Rationale:*** Dissociation occurs when anxiety is high; thus, a calm, safe, and supportive environment is essential to decrease emotional arousal. Even if a history of trauma is a causative factor, anxiety must be reduced to a level compatible with verbal exploration. Social skills may or may not be problematic; they are not a priority.
Cognitive Level: Application
Nursing Process: Implementation; ***Test Plan:*** PSYC

3 **Answer: 1** ***Rationale:*** Clients with DID often have particular physical problems including headache, irritable bowel syndrome, and asthma. Memory is discontinuous, and although bipolar illness (elated mood) could be co-morbid, it is not a usual accompaniment to DID. Stocking anesthesia does not generally accompany DID.
Cognitive Level: Analysis
Nursing Process: Assessment; ***Test Plan:*** PSYC

4 **Answer: 2** ***Rationale:*** The overdose of alcohol and benzodiazepines is particularly lethal which demonstrates that the client is potentially harmful to self. The presenting personality may not be depressed, or may not have enough power to prevent the alter that is self-destructive from acting again, so substantial risk remains. Physical safety is a priority over the other options.
Cognitive Level: Analysis
Nursing Process: Planning; ***Test Plan:*** PSYC

5 **Answer: 2** ***Rationale:*** The client needs to have critical physical needs met, including comfort, as the first priority. Creating a sense of safety after an assault is essential as anxiety may fluctuate. Although the other nursing interventions are relevant, they are not priorities and can be deferred to a later time.
Cognitive Level: Analysis
Nursing Process: Planning; ***Test Plan:*** PSYC

6 **Answer: 3** ***Rationale:*** The change in the client's voice indicates a switch to a child alter, the reason for which could be regression, resistance, needing sustenance, or wanting to be understood.
Cognitive Level: Application
Nursing Process: Assessment; ***Test Plan:*** PSYC

7 **Answer: 3** ***Rationale:*** Switching often occurs with increases in anxiety. Asking the client to explain more will help the nurse understand what is happening on a system level, and why the child alter was emergent. Options 1 and 4 will increase anxiety. Option 2, although helpful, may not provide therapeutic outcomes.
Cognitive Level: Analysis
Nursing Process: Implementation; ***Test Plan:*** PSYC

8 **Answer: 2** ***Rationale:*** Feeling detached, as if in a dream, is characteristic of depersonalization disorder. Multiple personalities or alters are not part of depersonalization disorder (option 1). Indifference to the symptoms (*la belle indifference*) and amnesia are usually related to conversion disorder (option 3). The client remembers the event and usually is distressed by the experience (option 4).
Cognitive Level: Analysis
Nursing Process: Assessment; ***Test Plan:*** PSYC

9 **Answer: 3** ***Rationale:*** Amnesia is a result of being unable to cope with high levels of anxiety. There is no data to suggest other nursing diagnoses.
Cognitive Level: Analysis
Nursing Process: Analysis; ***Test Plan:*** PSYC

10 **Answer: 1** ***Rationale:*** Reducing anxiety through the use of stress management techniques will prevent depersonalization that is a reaction to high levels of anxiety. There is no data to support suicidal thoughts or multiple identities. Improving self-concept is helpful, but is not a priority when anxiety leads to dissociation.
Cognitive Level: Application
Nursing Process: Analysis; ***Test Plan:*** PSYC

References

American Psychiatric Association. (2000). *Diagnostic and statistical manual of mental disorders text revision* (4th ed.). Washington, DC: American Psychiatric Association, pp. 257, 527.

Barringer, B. & Glod, C. (1998). Therapeutic relationship and effective communication. In C. Glod (Ed.), *Contemporary psychiatric nursing: The brain-behavior connection.* Philadelphia: F. A. Davis, pp. 46–61.

Benter, S. (1999). Crisis intervention. In G. Stewart & M. Laraia (Eds.), *Principles and practice of psychiatric nursing* (7th ed.). St. Louis: Mosby, pp. 227–245.

Bostrom, C. & Schwecke, L. (1999). Anxiety-related disorders. In N. Keltner, L. Schwecke, & C. Bostrom (Eds.), *Psychiatric nursing* (3rd ed.). St. Louis: Mosby, pp. 442–450.

Carson, V. (2000). Basic interventions. In V. Carson (Ed.), *Mental health nursing: The nurse-patient journey* (2nd ed.). Philadelphia: W. B. Saunders, pp. 281–335.

Charron, H. (1998). Somatoform and dissociative disorders. In E. Varcarolis (Ed.), *Foundations of psychiatric mental health nursing* (3rd ed.). Philadelphia: W. B. Saunders, pp. 479–506.

Doenges, M., Townsend, M., & Moorhouse, M. (1998). *Psychiatric care plans* (3rd ed.). Philadelphia: F. A. Davis, pp. 368, 372.

Fontaine, K. (1999). Anxiety disorders. In K. Fontaine & S. Fletcher (Eds.), *Mental health nursing* (4th ed.). Menlo Park, CA: Addison Wesley Longman, pp. 169–204.

Fontaine, K. (1999). Communicating and teaching. In K. Fontaine & S. Fletcher (Eds.), *Mental health nursing* (4th ed.). Menlo Park, CA: Addison Wesley Longman, pp. 89–113.

Glod, C. (1998). Posttraumatic stress and dissociative disorders. In C. Glod (Ed.), *Contemporary psychiatric nursing: the brain-behavior connection.* Philadelphia: F. A. Davis, pp. 427–437.

Johnson, M., Bulechek, G., Dochterman, J., Maas, M., & Moorhead, S. (2000). *Nursing diagnoses, outcomes, and interventions: NANDA, NOC, and NIC linkages.* St. Louis: Mosby, p. 490.

Malloy, M. (2000). Anxiety and related disorders. In K. Fortinash & P. Holoday-Worret (Eds.), *Psychiatric mental health nursing* (2nd ed.). St. Louis: Mosby, pp. 231–256.

Marcus, P. (2000). Dissociative disorders. In V. Carson (Ed.), *Mental health nursing: The nurse-patient journey* (2nd ed.). Philadelphia: W. B. Saunders, pp. 799–820.

O'Brien, P. (1999). Anxiety and dissociative disorders. In P. O'Brien, W. Kennedy, & K. Ballard (Eds.), *Psychiatric nursing: An integration of theory and practice.* New York: McGraw-Hill, pp. 317–330.

Stewart. G. (2001). Anxiety responses and anxiety disorders. In G. Stewart & M. Laraia (Eds.), *Principles & practice of psychiatric nursing* (7th ed.). St. Louis: Mosby, pp. 274–298.

Stewart, G. (2001). Self-concept response and dissociation. In G. Stewart & M. Laraia (Eds.), *Principles & practice of psychiatric nursing* (7th ed.). St. Louis: Mosby, pp. 317–344.

Townsend, M. (2000). *Psychiatric mental health nursing: Concepts of care* (3rd ed.). Philadelphia: F. A. Davis, pp. 537, 545, 553.

Townsend, M. (2001). *Nursing diagnoses in psychiatric nursing* (5th ed.). Philadelphia: F. A. Davis, p. 245.

CHAPTER 8

Personality Disorders

Carol Stubblefield, RN, PhD

CHAPTER OUTLINE

OBJECTIVES

- Identify four predisposing factors that contribute to personality disorders.
- Describe five characteristics associated with each personality disorder.
- State examples of at least four nursing diagnoses frequently used for clients experiencing personality disorders.
- Formulate four intervention strategies for clients with personality disorders.

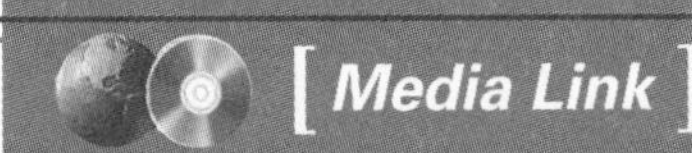

Use the CD-ROM enclosed with this text, or log onto the address given to access the free, interactive Companion Website created for this series. The CD-ROM and Companion Website accompanying this book offer additional practice opportunities and information—NCLEX Review, Case Studies, Glossary, In Depth with NCLEX, and more.

www.prenhall.com/hogan

Review at a Glance

antisocial personality disorder *a disorder characterized by a pattern of disregard for, and violation of, the rights of others unable to experience guilt related to inappropriate behavior; more commonly seen in prisons than in hospitals*

avoidant personality disorder *a disorder characterized by a pattern of social inhibition, feelings of inadequacy, and hypersensitivity to negative evaluation*

axis I disorders *clinical disorders such as mood and thought disorders are coded under this DSM-IV axis*

axis II disorders *personality disorders and mental retardation are coded under this DSM-IV axis; coding these disorders under a separate axis ensures they are not overlooked when clients are admitted with a more obvious axis I disorder*

borderline personality disorder *a disorder characterized by a pattern of instability in interpersonal relationships, self-image and affects, and marked impulsivity; carries a high risk for suicide and self-mutilation*

dependent personality disorder *a disorder characterized by a pattern of submissive and clinging behavior, including fear of abandonment and forcing others into making their decisions*

ego-dystonic *describes when patterns of personal behavior are perceived as uncomfortable, unnatural or foreign to the self; problems in living are perceived to an extent as internal; associated with a willingness to try to change behavior*

ego-syntonic *describes when patterns of personal behavior are perceived as comfortable, natural and a part of the self; problems in living are attributed to external causes; associated with an unwillingness to try to change behavior*

histrionic personality disorder *a disorder characterized by a pattern of excessive emotionality and attention seeking; suggestible*

narcissistic personality disorder *a disorder characterized by a pattern of grandiosity, need for admiration, and lack of empathy; exploits others to achieve personal goals*

obsessive-compulsive personality disorder *pattern of preoccupation with orderliness, perfectionism and control; includes focus on detail and difficulty with decision making related to a fear of making a mistake*

paranoid personality disorder *a disorder characterized by a pattern of distrust and suspiciousness such that others' motives are interpreted as malevolent*

personality *composed of enduring patterns or traits that determine how individuals perceive, relate to, and think about the environment and themselves*

personality disorder *a disorder characterized by personality patterns or traits that are inflexible, enduring, pervasive, maladaptive and cause significant functional impairment or subjective distress*

personality traits *reflected in how individuals cope with feelings and impulses, see themselves and others, respond to the surroundings, and find meaning in relationships*

schizoid personality disorder *a disorder characterized by a pattern of detachment from social relationships and a restricted range of emotions; not influenced by praise or criticism*

schizotypal personality disorder *a disorder characterized by a pattern of acute discomfort in close relationships, cognitive or perceptual distortions, and eccentricities of behavior; may be a mild form of schizophrenia*

Pretest

1 **The nurse would assess for which of the following characteristics in the behavior of any client diagnosed with a personality disorder?**

(1) Ability to charm and manipulate people
(2) Desire for interpersonal relationships
(3) Diminished need for approval
(4) Disruption in some aspect of his or her life

2 **A 27-year-old woman has been diagnosed with borderline personality disorder. She displays a labile affect, impulsivity, frequent angry outbursts, and difficulty tolerating her angry feelings without self-injury. A *priority* nursing diagnosis for this client is:**

(1) Anxiety.
(2) Risk for self-mutilation.
(3) Risk for violence towards others.
(4) Ineffective individual coping.

3 **The nurse assesses for the presence of which of the following etiologic factors that may explain the dichotomous thinking observed in an individual diagnosed with borderline personality disorder?**

(1) Gender stereotyping
(2) Family enmeshment
(3) Perfectionistic standards
(4) Physiological under-arousal

4 A client recently released from prison for embezzlement has a history of blaming others for his problems and becoming defensive and angry when criticized. He has expressed no remorse for his actions nor any response to his conviction. He claims his actions were justified since his employer did not treat him fairly. He is displaying characteristics of which personality disorder?

(1) Narcissistic
(2) Histrionic
(3) Antisocial
(4) Borderline

5 A 35-year-old client is being interviewed by the nurse. The client's history indicates that she has few friends, fears criticism and rejection from others, and withholds information about her thoughts and feelings because she anticipates a negative reaction. Based on the data, the nurse suspects that the client may have which of the following personality disorders?

(1) Schizotypal
(2) Paranoid
(3) Avoidant
(4) Schizoid

6 Which nursing diagnosis may be a priority of care at the time of admission for a client diagnosed with antisocial personality disorder?

(1) Personal identity disturbance
(2) Fear
(3) Risk for violence directed at others
(4) Social isolation

7 The nurse anticipates that which of the following intervention would be appropriately ordered for a client admitted with an axis I diagnosis of major depression and an axis II diagnosis of schizoid personality disorder?

(1) Group psychotherapy
(2) Individual psychotherapy
(3) Family therapy
(4) Participation in a support group

8 The nurse would look for signs of which of the following as a prominent behavioral characteristic of an individual diagnosed with narcissistic personality disorder?

(1) Splitting
(2) Hypersensitivity
(3) Suspiciousness
(4) Entitlement

9 An intervention strategy routinely included in the nursing care plan for a client diagnosed with antisocial personality disorder is:

(1) Establishing clear and enforceable limits.
(2) Varying unit rules based on client demands.
(3) Varying unit rules based on staff needs.
(4) Letting the client have a voice in when unit rules should apply.

10 Which of the following interventions would be appropriate for the nurse to implement when caring for the client with obsessive-compulsive personality disorder?

(1) Assertiveness training
(2) Decision-making skills
(3) Anxiety management
(4) Values clarification

See pages 167–168 for Answers and Rationales.

I. Overview

A. Personality

1. Composed of enduring patterns or traits that determine how individuals perceive, relate to, and think about the environment and themselves

2. Develops as individuals adjust to their physical, emotional, social, and spiritual environments

3. **Personality traits** or patterns are reflected in how individuals cope with feelings and impulses, see themselves and others, respond to their surroundings, and find meaning in relationships

B. Personality disorders

NCLEX!

1. **Personality disorders** are diagnosed when personality patterns or traits are inflexible, enduring, pervasive, maladaptive, and cause significant functional impairment or subjective distress

NCLEX!

2. Reflect patterns of inner experience and behavior that differ from cultural expectations

NCLEX!

3. Result in problems in living rather than in clinical symptoms

NCLEX!

4. Clients frequently experience their personality patterns as natural or comfortable (**ego-syntonic**) rather than painful or uncomfortable (**ego-dystonic**)

NCLEX!

5. If personality patterns are experienced as egosyntonic, clients rarely seek treatment as they tend to externalize the cause of any functional impairment or subjective distress

6. If personality patterns are experienced as egodystonic, clients are more likely to seek treatment to ease their distress

7. Are coded under **axis II disorders** (personality disorders or mental retardation) using the American Psychiatric Association's *Diagnostic and Statistical Manual of Mental Disorders, fourth edition* (DSM-IV) diagnostic criteria

8. Frequently overlap: individuals may exhibit patterns or traits associated with more than one personality disorder

9. Develop before or during adolescence and persist throughout life; symptoms may become less obvious by middle or old age

10. Occur in 6 to 13 percent of the general population

11. May coexist with clinical disorders coded as **axis I disorders** (mood and thought disorders) using DSM-IV

12. Are organized into three diagnostic clusters

NCLEX!

a. *Cluster A disorders:* individuals with these disorders appear odd and eccentric

NCLEX!

b. *Cluster B disorders:* individuals with these disorders appear dramatic and erratic

NCLEX!

c. *Cluster C disorders:* individuals with these disorders appear anxious and fearful

13. Characteristics of personality disorders are manifested in four areas

a. Behavioral manifestations: include patterns of day-to-day behavior and impulse control

b. Affective manifestations: include the range, intensity, lability, and appropriateness of emotional response

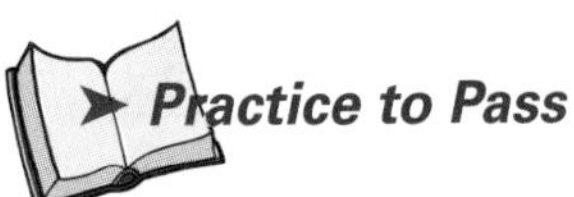

What qualities must personality patterns reflect for an individual to be diagnosed with a personality disorder?

c. Cognitive manifestations: reflect how the self, others, and events are interpreted

d. Sociocultural manifestations: reflect interpersonal functioning

II. Etiology

A. Neurobiological theories

1. Limbic system dysregulation and central nervous system (CNS) irritability may result in decreased impulse control
2. Decreased levels of serotonin (5-HT) have been associated with a tendency to self-mutilate, experience intense rage, and behave aggressively toward others
3. Elevated levels of norepinephrine (NE) have been associated with hypersensitivity to the environment
4. Abnormal levels of dopamine (DA) may explain the psychotic episodes associated with borderline and schizotypal personality disorders
5. Physiological underarousal to stimulation may contribute to the risk taking associated with some disorders
6. Schizotypal personality disorder may be a milder form of schizophrenia
7. Genetic factors may play a role
    a. In individuals with certain personality disorders, there is an increased prevalence of the disorder in relatives
    b. A familial relationship exists between certain personality disorders and some axis I disorders
    c. Certain personality disorders are diagnosed more frequently in men than in women and vice versa

B. Intrapersonal theories

1. Hostility toward the self may be projected onto others resulting in fear, mistrust, and defensive withdrawal to avoid being hurt
2. Individuals may try to live up to perfectionistic standards imposed on them by their parents or others during childhood
3. An underdeveloped superego may result in a failure to both internalize authority and cultural morals and to experience guilt when violating rules
4. Inadequate parenting and unsatisfied basic needs may lead to hostility toward caregivers, fear of both own anger and of abandonment resulting in a fear of intimacy, and an acting out of rage including self-destructive behavior to manage feelings of guilt
5. Anxiety may manifest itself as a personality disorder

C. Social theories

1. Social oppression may have a negative effect on the development of self-esteem and a healthy identity

2. A changing societal value system, with personal needs being viewed as more important than group needs, may be reflected in the behavior associated with Cluster B disorders

D. Family theories

1. Inability to manage conflict, inconsistent parenting resulting in emotional deprivation, inadequate supervision and discipline, and role modeling of inappropriate behavior may affect personality development in some individuals

NCLEX!

2. Growing up in a multigenerational enmeshed family system and failure to individuate the self may be associated with the dichotomous thinking or splitting observed in some individuals diagnosed with borderline personality disorder

3. A chaotic and abusive environment may be associated with the development of borderline personality disorder in some individuals

E. Feminist theory: the diagnosis of a personality disorder reflects the influence of rigid gender-role stereotyping rather than that of genetic factors

III. Assessment

A. General guidelines

NCLEX!

1. Since the client probably does not perceive that a problem exists or believes that any problem is related to the behavior of others, maintain sensitivity in the interview process so the client does not become guarded or defensive

2. If it is necessary to interview family members to obtain accurate assessment data, exercise professional judgment to protect client rights and to maintain confidentiality

B. Specific guidelines: assess client's level of function in the areas of affect, cognition, behavior (including impulse control), and sociocultural adaptation (interpersonal relationships)

IV. Nursing Diagnoses/Analysis

A. Cluster A disorders (paranoid personality, schizoid personality, and schizotypal personality)

NCLEX!

1. Ineffective individual coping related to inability to trust

NCLEX!

2. Fear related to perceived threats from others or the environment

NCLEX!

3. Social isolation related to craving of solitude

4. Spiritual distress related to lack of connectedness to others

B. Cluster B disorders (antisocial personality, borderline personality, histrionic personality, and narcissistic personality)

NCLEX!

1. Impaired social interaction related to manipulation of others, unstable mood, poor impulse control, extreme emotional reactions including overidealization and devaluation of the self and others, extreme self-centeredness, and seductive behavior

NCLEX!

2. High risk for violence self-directed (suicide or self-mutilation) related to intense emotional pain including rage and a sense of emptiness, and poor impulse control

NCLEX!

3. High risk for violence directed at others or objects related to intense rage, poor impulse control

NCLEX!

4. Personal identity disturbance related to lack of a sense of self, changes in perceptions of body image, dissociation

NCLEX!

5. Fear related to feelings of abandonment

C. Cluster C disorders (avoidant personality, dependent personality, and obsessive-compulsive personality)

NCLEX!

1. Ineffective individual coping related to high dependency needs, rigid behavior and thoughts, fear of rejection, high need for approval from others, or inability to make independent decisions

NCLEX!

2. Fear related to feelings of abandonment, disapproval, or losing control

V. Planning and Implementation

NCLEX!

A. Basic principles of nursing intervention

1. Recognize that clients have the right to change or not to change; if patterns of behavior are egosyntonic, clients may lack the motivation required to effect change
2. Help clients to see how behavior affects their lives to motivate them to develop a more adaptive lifestyle
3. Remember that personality traits are too ingrained to expect radical, long-term behavioral change; interventions should be based on short-term goals and focus on small steps designed to improve role functioning and decrease distress
4. Maintain hope for each client's improvement; all clients have the potential for change
5. Identify your own emotional responses when caring for clients diagnosed with a personality disorder as power struggles between staff members related to the best treatment approach create staff divisiveness and a chaotic rather than a structured milieu

What basic understanding of the nature of personality patterns must undergird the treatment and nursing care of individuals diagnosed with personality disorders?

B. Specific strategies: cluster-specific nursing interventions can be individualized for each client

NCLEX!

1. Cluster A disorders (paranoid personality, schizoid personality, and schizotypal personality)
   a. Approach people in a gentle, interested, but nonintrusive manner
   b. Respect client's needs for distance and privacy
   c. Be mindful of own nonverbal communication as a client may perceive others as threatening
   d. Gradually encourage interaction with others, if appropriate

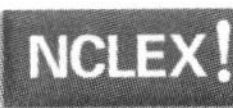

2. Cluster B disorders (antisocial personality, borderline personality, histrionic personality, and narcissistic personality)
   a. Be patient as clients display emotional and erratic behavior
   b. Provide a consistent and structured milieu to avoid manipulation and power struggles

Why are interventions focused on limit setting so important in the nursing management of clients diagnosed with antisocial personality disorder?

NCLEX!

Why are interventions focused on diminishing the tendency toward dichotomous thinking so important in the nursing management of clients diagnosed with borderline personality disorder?

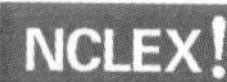

c. Safety is always the first priority of care—protect clients from suicide and self-mutilation until they can protect themselves

d. Set limits as necessary to help clients maintain impulse control in order to protect themselves and others from injury

e. Engage in frequent staff conferences to counteract client's ability to play one staff member against the other

f. Help clients recognize and discuss their fear of abandonment

g. Help clients recognize the presence of dichotomous thinking or splitting, in which self and others are perceived as all good or all bad

h. Encourage direct communication to minimize attention seeking through the use of dramatic, seductive behavior

i. Help clients who display a sense of entitlement to acknowledge the needs of others

3. Cluster C disorders (avoidant personality, dependent personality, and obsessive-compulsive personality)

a. Point out avoidance behaviors and related losses and secondary gains

b. Provide problem solving and assertiveness training to increase self-confidence and independence

c. Encourage expression of feelings to decrease rigidity and need for control

d. Help clients recognize any impairment or distress related to their need for perfection and control

e. Help clients acknowledge and discuss their sense of inadequacy and fear of rejection

C. Psychopharmacology

1. Antipsychotic agents may be prescribed on a short-term basis to alleviate psychotic symptoms associated with schizotypal or borderline personality disorders

2. Selective serotonin reuptake inhibitors (SSRIs) may be prescribed to diminish the rapid mood swings, impulsive, aggressive, and self-destructive behavior associated with borderline personality disorder

3. SSRIs may be prescribed to treat the obsessive rumination associated with certain personality disorders

D. Individual and group therapy

1. A decision for participation in individual or group therapy or both is based on a client's level of function and specific needs

2. Self-help groups may increase clients' self-awareness and assist them in coping with problems in living

E. Behavioral therapy

1. Impulse-control training is designed to support client safety by decreasing the risk of suicide or self-mutilation through the use of anti-harm contracts, staff and client (self) monitoring, identifying triggers and patterns related to self-destructive behavior, and identifying alternative coping strategies

NCLEX!

2. Limit setting is designed to discourage the tendency to test and manipulate others

a. Involves establishing a structured environment with clear ground rules

Why is impulse-control training crucial to the effective nursing management of some individuals diagnosed with a personality disorder?

b. Limit setting reflects three principles: limits must be clearly stated, necessary, and enforceable

c. Clearly stating limits and seeking clarification from clients of their understanding of limits decreases attempts at manipulation based on "not understanding what was expected"

d. Establishing necessary limits establishes staff members as business-like authority figures rather than as individuals who are perceived as harsh, judgmental, or punitive; this diminishes a client's tendency to try to engage in a power struggle

e. Limits must be enforceable or they encourage rather than discourage the tendency to manipulation

3. Behavioral modification: social skills

NCLEX!

a. For clients who are helpless and dependent, the goal is to increase coping skills and independent functioning

1) They need to acknowledge their feelings of helplessness and fear of becoming more independent

What are the basic principles supporting the intervention of limit setting?

2) Explore clients' dichotomous thinking or the tendency to see themselves as totally dependent or totally independent

3) Help clients identify what they would gain and lose by becoming less helpless

4) Engage clients in problem-solving exercises to increase their self-confidence

5) Provide assertiveness training

6) Take care not to be seen as a rescuer

NCLEX!

b. For clients who are socially isolative related to a fear of rejection, the goal is to increase self-confidence

1) They need to acknowledge their fear of criticism and rejection

2) Help clients identify what they would gain and lose by risking criticism and rejection

3) Help clients identify the interpersonal effects of social isolation and the feelings associated with them

4) Engage clients in problem solving exercises to increase their self-confidence

5) Provide assertiveness training

NCLEX!

c. For clients who are socially isolated related to suspiciousness and mistrust of others, respect their need to be isolative while gradually encouraging interaction with others; if appropriate, help clients identify the interpersonal effects of social isolation and the feelings associated with them

NCLEX!

d. For clients who seek out relationships with others through behavior that is attention seeking (dramatic, seductive) but superficial, help them to interact in a more direct fashion; help clients identify what they would gain and lose by communicating more directly

NCLEX!

e. For clients whose relationships are based on manipulation, call attention to their attempts at manipulation and help them to identify ways to interact that are more collaborative and less power-based; help clients identify what they would gain and lose by becoming less manipulative

F. Psychological comfort promotion—anxiety reduction

NCLEX!

1. Some clients avoid decisions to avoid the anxiety of failure; encourage decision making to support a sense of competence and an internal locus of control; point out that an imperfect decision may be better than no decision and that many decisions can be remade

NCLEX!

2. Some clients become perfectionistic to guard against the anxiety of feeling inferior; explore why they fear the evaluation of others

NCLEX!

3. Anxiety prevents some clients from asking for help as they fear rejection; help clients identify what they would gain and lose by asking for help

VI. Evaluation/Outcomes

A. **Based on assessment** of behavioral, affective, cognitive and sociocultural manifestations, identify realistic, specific and measurable short-term goals for nursing interventions

B. **Be aware that realistic goals** must reflect small steps to improving function and decreasing subjective distress; personality traits are too ingrained to expect immediate, radical, long-term change

C. **Evaluate the effectiveness** of the nursing interventions in relationship to stated outcomes

VII. Specific Disorders

A. Cluster A disorders (using DSM-IV diagnostic criteria)

NCLEX!

1. **Paranoid personality disorder:** pattern of distrust and suspiciousness such that others' motives are interpreted as malevolent (APA, 2000)

   a. Behavioral manifestations

      1) Secretive

      2) Hyperalert to danger

      3) Argumentative to maintain a safe distance between themselves and others

   b. Affective manifestations

      1) Avoid sharing feelings except for quick expressions of anger, bear grudges

      2) Rarely forgive perceived slights

      3) Fear losing power or control to others

c. Cognitive manifestations

1) Pervasive distrust and suspicious

2) Expect to be used or harassed

3) Tendency to look for hidden, demeaning, or threatening meanings and to respond by criticizing others

d. Sociocultural manifestations

1) Interact in a cold and aloof manner to avoid intimacy

2) Expect to be harmed or exploited by others and question the loyalty or trustworthiness of family and friends

3) Often pathologically jealous of a significant other

NCLEX!

2. Schizoid personality disorder: pattern of detachment from social relationships and a restricted range of emotions (APA, 2000)

a. Behavioral manifestations

1) Neither desire nor enjoy relationships with others

2) Have little interest in activities or sexual relationships

b. Affective manifestations

1) Mood stable but restricted range of expression of emotions

2) May become anxious if forced into a close interaction

3) Affect is bland, blunted, or flat

c. Cognitive manifestations

1) Appear to have poverty of thought

2) Expressed thoughts are often vague

3) Indifferent to the attitudes and feeling of others

4) Not influenced by praise or criticism

d. Sociocultural manifestations

1) Interact with others in a cold, aloof manner

2) Desire no close friends

NCLEX!

3. Schizotypal personality disorder: pattern of acute discomfort in close relationships, cognitive or perceptual distortions, and eccentricities of behavior (APA, 2000)

a. Behavioral manifestations

1) Exhibit odd/eccentric behavior and speech that is coherent but often tangential, vague, or overelaborate

2) May be a mild form of schizophrenia

3) May display transient psychotic symptoms under periods of extreme stress and anxiety

b. Affective manifestations

1) Emotionally constricted

2) Affect may be inappropriate

What are the underlying differences in attitudes toward interpersonal relationships of individuals diagnosed with Cluster A personality disorders?

c. Cognitive manifestations

1) Paranoid ideation may be present

2) Ideas of reference may be present

3) Illusions may be present

4) Magical thinking may be present

d. Sociocultural manifestations

1) Are uncomfortable with intimacy and avoid relationships with others

2) Are usually avoided by others because of their odd/eccentric behavior

B. Cluster B disorders

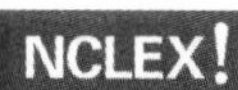

1. **Antisocial personality disorder:** pattern of disregard for and violation of the rights of others (APA, 2000)

   a. Behavioral manifestations: childhood manifestations are lying, stealing, truancy, vandalism, fighting and running away from home; adults fail to conform to social norms such as functioning within the law; lie pathologically and "con" others for personal profit; consistent irresponsibility related to financial obligations and work behavior; impulsive and reckless in regard to own safety and that of others

   b. Affective manifestations: superficial expression of emotion; lack of guilt or remorse related to inappropriate behavior; irritable and aggressive

   c. Cognitive manifestations: egocentric and grandiose; perceive themselves as more clever than others

   d. Sociocultural manifestations: consistently violate the rights of others as well as the values of society; unable to sustain personal relationships; may be abusive

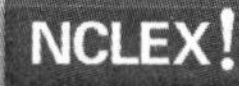

2. **Borderline personality disorder:** pattern of instability in interpersonal relationships, self-image, and affect, and marked impulsivity (APA, 2000)

   a. Behavioral manifestations

   1) Unpredictable

   2) Fear of real or imagined abandonment

   3) Engage in self-destructive behaviors such as reckless driving, substance abuse, and binge-eating

   4) High risk for suicide and self-mutilation because of feelings of emptiness or rage

   5) Behavior may vary from one moment to the next

   b. Affective manifestations

   1) Moods are intense and unstable

   2) Difficulty in moderating anger, which may escalate rapidly

c. Cognitive manifestations

1) Identity disturbance because of a feeling of emptiness and a lack of sense of self

2) Splitting or dichotomous thinking present—tend to see self and others as all good or all bad

3) Paranoid ideation or dissociation may be present

d. Sociocultural manifestations: intense, unstable interpersonal relationships alternating between extremes of idealization and devaluation of others

NCLEX!

3. Histrionic personality disorder: pattern of excessive emotionality and attention seeking (APA, 2000)

a. Behavioral manifestations

1) Uncomfortable unless the center of attention

2) Display seductive and other attention-seeking behavior when interacting with others

3) Conversation is superficial

b. Affective manifestations

1) Overly dramatic

2) Rapidly shifting

3) Shallow expression of emotion

c. Cognitive manifestations: guided by feelings rather than logic; suggestible

d. Sociocultural manifestations

1) Assume role of victim or prince/princess in relationships

2) Consider relationships to be more intimate than they are

NCLEX!

4. Narcissistic personality disorder: pattern of grandiosity, need for admiration, and lack of empathy (APA, 2000)

a. Behavioral manifestations

1) Preoccupied with fantasies of power, success

2) Extremely grandiose and exploit others to achieve personal goals

3) Seek constant admiration

4) Sense of entitlement

b. Affective manifestations: labile moods varying from anger to anxiety

c. Cognitive manifestations

1) Arrogant, egotistical, sees self as more important/special than others

2) Lack empathy

3) May think others are envious or may be envious of others

d. Sociocultural manifestations

1) Disturbed relationships as a result of using others to meet own goals

2) Own needs are perceived as more important than the needs of others

What are the underlying differences in attitudes toward interpersonal relationships of individuals diagnosed with Cluster B personality disorders?

C. **Cluster C disorders**

1. **Avoidant personality disorder:** pattern of social inhibition, feelings of inadequacy, and hypersensitivity to negative evaluation (APA, 2000)
   a. Behavioral manifestations
      1) Avoid interpersonal contact and new situations related to fear of rejection and embarrassment
      2) Lack self-confidence and are extremely sensitive to rejection
   b. Affective manifestations: fearful, shy, hurt by criticism
   c. Cognitive manifestations
      1) View self as inadequate and inferior
      2) Are fearful of shame, criticism, and ridicule
   d. Sociocultural manifestations
      1) Desire relationships but reluctant to enter into them without a guarantee of unconditional acceptance
      2) Few close friends

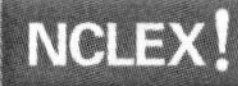

2. **Dependent personality disorder:** pattern of submissive and clinging behavior related to a need to be taken care of (APA, 2000)
   a. Behavioral manifestations
      1) Desire help with everyday decisions, and want others to take care of them
      2) Difficulty in disagreeing with others related to fear of rejection and abandonment
   b. Affective manifestations: anxious when left alone because of fear of being unable to do things for themselves
   c. Cognitive manifestations
      1) Lack self-confidence
      2) Preoccupied with fear of being abandoned
   d. Sociocultural manifestations
      1) Constantly strive to obtain support from others
      2) Uncomfortable unless involved in a supportive relationship

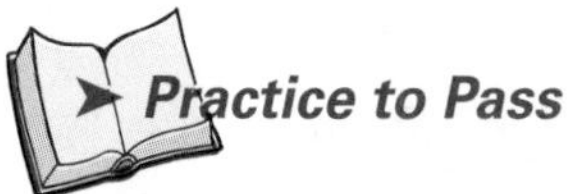

What are the underlying differences in attitudes toward interpersonal relationships of individuals diagnosed with Cluster C personality disorders?

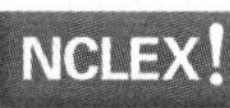

3. **Obsessive-compulsive personality disorder:** pattern of preoccupation with orderliness, perfectionism, and control (APA, 2000)
   a. Behavioral manifestations
      1) High need for routine
      2) Decreased ability to focus on the major goal of any activity as becomes overly involved in details
      3) Difficulty with task completion related to a need for perfection
      4) Inflexibility related to moral and ethical issues

Why is it important to recognize differences in individual's attitudes toward interpersonal relationships?

5) Unable to discard worthless objects

6) Unable to delegate for fear that others will not perform tasks correctly

b. Affective manifestations: rigid, stubborn, and emotionally constricted

c. Cognitive manifestations

1) Believe in a correct solution for every problem

2) Procrastinate because fearful of making mistakes

d. Sociocultural manifestations: impaired interpersonal relationships and absence of leisure activities due to devotion to work and productivity

D. Concomitant disorders: there is a correlation between certain personality disorders and some axis I disorders such as substance abuse, mood disorders, anxiety disorders, and psychotic disorders

Case Study

A client admitted with a diagnosis of borderline personality disorder describes dissatisfaction with her interpersonal relationships, stating, "My friends seem so wonderful at first and then they always let me down." When asked how she responds to this disappointment, she states, "Sometimes I'm filled with a sense of overwhelming rage and other times I just feel so empty." When asked to describe how she copes with these feelings, she states, "I try not to, but sometimes I cut myself. I know I shouldn't but I can't always stop myself."

❶ What are the priority nursing diagnoses for this client?

❷ What are your short-term goals for this client?

❸ What input will the client have in the development of the goals?

❹ What nursing interventions will you implement based on your goals?

❺ On what basis will you evaluate the effectiveness of your nursing interventions?

For suggested responses, see pages 307–308.

Posttest

1 **The nurse would look for which of the following characteristics that reflect the attitude toward treatment of most individuals diagnosed with personality disorders? These individuals usually:**

(1) Actively seek treatment related to subjective distress.
(2) Avoid treatment related to the tendency to externalize the cause of problems in living.
(3) Actively seek treatment related to impaired functioning.
(4) Avoid treatment related to the stigma associated with mental illness.

2 **Which nursing outcome would indicate that a client with a nursing diagnosis of Risk for self-mutilation due to feelings of abandonment related to the ending of a close relationship has improved?**

(1) Client verbalizes fear of abandonment in a realistic way.
(2) Client vows never to get involved in a relationship again.
(3) Client expresses rage over the ending of this relationship.
(4) Client suppresses feelings of abandonment.

3 **During your interaction with a client diagnosed with antisocial personality disorder, the client keeps asking where you live, whom you date, and other personal information. The client states the reason for this is, "I just want to get to know you better. You're the only one I can really talk to." The most effective nursing response is:**

(1) "You're getting too involved with me. Maybe another nurse would be more appropriate for you."
(2) "Let's talk about my purpose in working with you and your feelings about it."
(3) "Why are you focusing on me all the time?"
(4) "Stop trying to avoid talking about yourself and your problems."

4 **A client comes in for her psychiatric appointment wearing a cocktail dress and theatrical makeup. She announces dramatically and flirtatiously that she needs to be seen immediately as she is experiencing overwhelming psychological distress. The most likely axis II diagnosis would be:**

(1) Borderline personality disorder.
(2) Narcissistic personality disorder.
(3) Histrionic personality disorder.
(4) Antisocial personality disorder.

5 **A client diagnosed with antisocial personality disorder tells Nurse A, "You're a much better nurse than Nurse B said you were." The client then tells Nurse B, "Nurse A is upset with you for some reason." To Nurse C, the client states, "I think you're great, but Nurse A said she saw you make three mistakes this morning." This interaction can best be described as an attempt to:**

(1) Gain acceptance.
(2) Gain attention.
(3) Create guilt in the staff.
(4) Manipulate the staff.

6 **The nurse assigned to care for a client interviews him about his reportedly abusive relationship with his wife. Which statement would be characteristic of the thinking of an individual diagnosed with antisocial personality disorder?**

(1) "I've done a stupid thing, but I've learned my lesson."
(2) "I'm feeling awful about the way I've hurt my wife."
(3) "I have a quick temper, but I can usually keep it under control."
(4) "I hit her because she nags at me."

7 **The client diagnosed with borderline personality disorder tends to label certain persons on the staff as being good or bad. This behavior is an example of:**

(1) Secondary gain.
(2) Acting out.
(3) Passive aggression.
(4) Dichotomous thinking.

8 **The most important short-term goal for the client who consistently tries to manipulate others is to:**

(1) Stop initiating arguments.
(2) Sustain lasting relationships.
(3) Explore childhood experiences.
(4) Acknowledge own behavior.

9 **In evaluating the progress of the client whose interpersonal relationships are based on manipulation, the most important criteria are the client's:**

(1) Plans.
(2) Promises.
(3) Actions.
(4) Words.

10 **The nurse determines that a client who is described as a loner and who does not express a desire for close interpersonal relationship reflects a behavioral pattern associated with which type of personality disorder?**

(1) Antisocial
(2) Schizotypal
(3) Paranoid
(4) Schizoid

See page 168 for Answers and Rationales.

Answers and Rationales

Pretest

1 **Answer: 4** ***Rationale:*** To meet DSM-IV diagnostic criteria for a personality disorder, behavioral patterns must be pervasive and maladaptive, resulting in functional impairment or subjective distress. The other behavioral patterns (options 1, 2, and 3) are associated with some but not all personality disorders.
Cognitive Level: Application
Nursing Process: Assessment; ***Test Plan:*** PSYC

2 **Answer: 2** ***Rationale:*** The priority of care is always client safety. Intervening to minimize a client's risk of self-harm maintains a safe environment. The nursing diagnoses of Anxiety and Ineffective individual coping are of secondary importance to maintaining the client's safety. Although the client is impulsive and exhibits angry outbursts, more assessment data are required to determine if she is a risk for violence directed toward others.
Cognitive Level: Analysis
Nursing Process: Analysis; ***Test Plan:*** PSYC

3 **Answer: 2** ***Rationale:*** Growing up in a multigenerational enmeshed family system and failure to separate/individuate the self is associated with the development of borderline personality disorder. Conflict in the area of separation/individuation can result in splitting or dichotomous thinking—perceiving the self and others as all good or all bad. The other etiologic factors (options 1, 2, 3) are not associated with the development of dichotomous thinking.
Cognitive Level: Analysis
Nursing Process: Assessment; ***Test Plan:*** PSYC

4 **Answer: 3** ***Rationale:*** The described behavior reflects DSM-IV diagnostic criteria for antisocial personality disorder. His behavior is not characteristic of individuals diagnosed with narcissistic, histrionic, or borderline personality disorder.
Cognitive Level: Application
Nursing Process: Assessment; ***Test Plan:*** PSYC

5 **Answer: 3** ***Rationale:*** The described behavior reflects the DSM-IV diagnostic criteria for avoidant personality disorder. Her behavior is not characteristic of individuals diagnosed with schizotypal, paranoid, or schizoid personality disorder.
Cognitive Level: Application
Nursing Process: Analysis; ***Test Plan:*** PSYC

6 **Answer: 3** ***Rationale:*** Individuals diagnosed with antisocial personality disorder display decreased impulse control, can be irritable and aggressive, and lack remorse for their actions. Recognizing the potential risk for violence and maintaining client safety is the first priority of nursing care. The other nursing diagnoses do not reflect the behavioral patterns associated with individuals diagnosed with antisocial personality disorder.
Cognitive Level: Analysis
Nursing Process: Analysis; ***Test Plan:*** PSYC

7 **Answer: 2** ***Rationale:*** Since individuals diagnosed with schizoid personality disorder have no desire for interpersonal relationships and are indifferent to the opinions of others, individual rather than group therapy would be the treatment of choice.
Cognitive Level: Analysis
Nursing Process: Planning; ***Test Plan:*** PSYC

8 **Answer: 4** ***Rationale:*** A sense of entitlement is reflected in the DSM-IV diagnostic criteria for narcissistic personality disorder. Splitting, hypersensitivity, and suspiciousness are not behavioral patterns associated with individuals diagnosed with narcissistic personality disorder.
Cognitive Level: Application
Nursing Process: Assessment; ***Test Plan:*** PSYC

9 **Answer: 1** ***Rationale:*** As the behavioral patterns of individuals diagnosed with antisocial personality reflect a tendency to test and manipulate others, it is important to establish the parameters of acceptable behavior upon admission through limit setting. The other interventions would result in an unstructured environment with no consistent limits on behavior. This would increase rather than decrease an individual's tendency to test and try to manipulate others in the environment.
Cognitive Level: Application
Nursing Process: Implementation; ***Test Plan:*** PSYC

10 **Answer: 2** ***Rationale:*** Because they need perfection and control, individuals diagnosed with obsessive-compulsive personality disorder usually have trouble making decisions. This difficulty frequently negatively affects their occupational functioning. Learning that decisions do not always have to be perfect and that they can be changed may be a first small step toward improvement. Individuals with obsessive-compulsive personality disorder tend to be assertive in stressing the importance or rules and regulations and in arguing in support of their own value system. Anxiety may occur when their attempts to control the

environment fail, but it has less impact on functioning than does the difficulty in making decisions.
Cognitive Level: Application
Nursing Process: Implementation; *Test Plan:* PSYC

Posttest

1 **Answer: 2** *Rationale:* Clients diagnosed with a personality disorder usually avoid rather than seek treatment as their personality patterns are perceived as ego-syntonic or natural. They tend to externalize the cause of any problem in living they encounter. The stigma associated with mental illness would not be a factor in avoiding treatment; to be concerned with stigma is to recognize that one has a problem.
Cognitive Level: Analysis
Nursing Process: Assessment; *Test Plan:* PSYC

2 **Answer: 1** *Rationale:* Verbalizing rather than suppressing one's fear of abandonment is the first step in recognizing its effect on the self and on interpersonal relationships. A fear of abandonment often drives significant others away as it may be reflected in extremes of emotion or extremes of idealization or devaluation of the other. It can be associated with a heightened risk of self-mutilation. Vowing never to get involved in another relationship reveals a lack of insight into the desire for a relationship and the related fear of abandonment. Expressing rage reflects both an emotional extreme and, perhaps, a devaluation of the self and the other. It may be associated with a heightened risk of self-mutilation.
Cognitive Level: Analysis
Nursing Process: Evaluation; *Test Plan:* PSYC

3 **Answer: 2** *Rationale:* In returning the focus of the conversation to the client, the nurse intervenes in his/her attempt at manipulation in a manner that is business-like without appearing uncomfortable (options 1 and 3) or defensive (option 4).
Cognitive Level: Analysis
Nursing Process: Implementation; *Test Plan:* PSYC

4 **Answer: 3** *Rationale:* The client's pattern of attention seeking behavior reflects DSM-IV diagnostic criteria for histrionic personality disorder. This behavioral pattern is not associated with a diagnosis of borderline, narcissistic, or antisocial personality disorder.
Cognitive Level: Analysis
Nursing Process: Analysis; *Test Plan:* PSYC

5 **Answer: 4** *Rationale:* Individuals diagnosed with antisocial personality disorder frequently attempt to play one staff member against another. Their goal is not to gain acceptance or attention but to manipulate or control their environment. Creating guilt is just one manifestation of their attempt to control others.
Cognitive Level: Analysis
Nursing Process: Assessment; *Test Plan:* PSYC

6 **Answer: 4** *Rationale:* Individuals diagnosed with antisocial personality disorder rarely take responsibility (options 1 and 3) or express remorse (option 2) for their actions. They can be irritable and aggressive.
Cognitive Level: Analysis
Nursing Process: Assessment; *Test Plan:* PSYC

7 **Answer: 4** *Rationale:* Individuals diagnosed with borderline personality disorder frequently display a tendency to dichotomous thinking or splitting. They perceive the self and others as all good or all bad. The secondary gain that may be associated with illness, acting out, and passive aggressive behavior do not involve a tendency to perceive the self and others as all good or all bad.
Cognitive Level: Application
Nursing Process: Assessment; *Test Plan:* PSYC

8 **Answer: 4** *Rationale:* Being encouraged to acknowledge attempts at manipulation is a small step in recognizing maladaptive communication patterns and their effect on relationships. Sustaining lasting relationships is a long-term goal. Neither decreasing the tendency to initiate arguments or exploring childhood experiences are relevant goals in relationship to the behavioral pattern of manipulation.
Cognitive Level: Analysis
Nursing Process: Planning; *Test Plan:* PSYC

9 **Answer: 3** *Rationale:* Plans, promises and words do not reflect actual behavioral change. Change is reflected in action.
Cognitive Level: Comprehension
Nursing Process: Evaluation; *Test Plan:* PSYC

10 **Answer: 4** *Rationale:* Individuals with schizoid personality disorder are aloof when interacting with others as they have no desire for close relationships. This behavior pattern is described in DSM-IV diagnostic criteria for schizoid personality disorder. Individuals diagnosed with antisocial personality disorder tend to develop relationships that meet their own needs. Individuals diagnosed with schizotypal personality disorder are uncomfortable in relationships with others; individuals diagnosed with paranoid personality disorder mistrust others.
Cognitive Level: Application
Nursing Process: Assessment; *Test Plan:* PSYC

References

American Psychiatric Association (2000). *Diagnostic and statistical manual of mental disorders* (4th ed. text revision). Washington, DC: American Psychiatric Association.

Burgess, A. W. (1997). *Psychiatric nursing: Promoting mental health.* Stamford, CT: Appleton-Lange.

Carpenito, L. J. (2000). *Nursing Diagnosis: Application to clinical practice* (8th ed.). Philadelphia: Lippincott.

Doenges, M. E., Townsend, M. C., & Moorhouse, M. F. (1998). *Psychiatric care plans: Guidelines for individualizing care* (3rd ed.). Philadelphia: F. A. Davis.

Fontaine, K. L. & Fletcher, J. S. (1999). *Mental health nursing* (4th ed.). Menlo Park, CA: Addison-Wesley, pp. 354–369.

Fortinash, K. M. & Holoday-Worret, P. A. (1999). *Psychiatric nursing care plans.* (3rd ed.). St. Louis: Mosby.

Fortinash, K. & Holoday-Worret, P. (2000). *Psychiatric mental health nursing.* (2nd ed.). St. Louis: Mosby.

Frisch, N. & Frisch, L. (1998). *Psychiatric mental health nursing.* Albany, NY: Delmar.

Glod, C. (1998). *Contemporary psychiatric-mental health nursing: The brain-body connection.* Philadelphia: F. A. Davis.

Perlin, C. (2001). Social responses and personality disorders. In G. Stuart & M. Laraia (Eds.), *Principles and practice of psychiatric nursing* (7th ed.) St. Louis: Mosby, pp. 438–439.

Townsend, M. C. (2001). *Nursing diagnoses in psychiatric nursing: Care plans and psychotropic medications.* (5th ed.). Philadelphia: F. A. Davis.

CHAPTER 9

Schizophrenia and Other Psychotic Disorders

Linda Manfrin-Ledet, APRN, MN, CS

CHAPTER OUTLINE

OBJECTIVES

- Describe at least three factors regarding the development of schizophrenia.
- Differentiate between positive and negative symptoms of schizophrenia.
- Describe four treatment modalities for clients with schizophrenia.
- Differentiate between schizophrenia and other psychotic disorders.

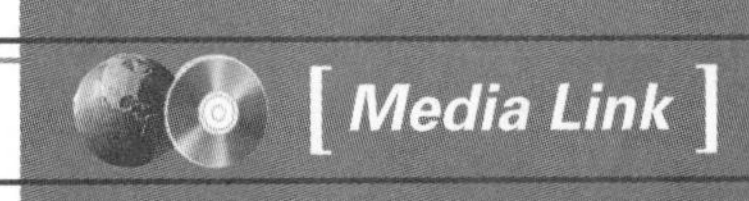

Use the CD-ROM enclosed with this text, or log onto the address given to access the free, interactive Companion Website created for this series. The CD-ROM and Companion Website accompanying this book offer additional practice opportunities and information—NCLEX Review, Case Studies, Glossary, In Depth with NCLEX, and more.

www.prenhall.com/hogan

Review at a Glance

catatonic *position of the body in a fixed, wax-like state*

clang association *rhyming of words in a sentence that make no sense*

delusional ideation *a false belief brought about without appropriate external stimulation and inconsistent with the individual's own knowledge and experience*

echolalia *an involuntary parrot-like repetition of words spoken by others*

echopraxia *a meaningless imitation of motions made by others*

hallucination *a false sensory perception that may involve any of the five senses (auditory, visual, tactile, olfactory, and gustatory)*

illusion *an inaccurate perception or misinterpretation of sensory impressions*

milieu therapy *a method of psychotherapy that controls the environment of the client to provide interpersonal contacts in order to develop trust, assurance, and personal autonomy*

neologisms *new words that are invented by and have meaning to only one person*

psychosis *a disorderly mental state in which a client has difficulty distinguishing reality from his or her own internal perceptions*

thought broadcasting *the delusional belief that others can hear one's thoughts*

thought control *the delusional belief that others can control a person's thoughts against one's will*

thought insertion *the delusional belief that others have the ability to put thoughts in a person's mind against one's will*

word salad *the combining of words in a sentence that have no connection and make no sense*

Pretest

1 A client with a diagnosis of schizophrenia, paranoid type, is admitted to an acute-care psychiatric hospital unit. In anticipation of the client's needs, what nursing diagnosis would be given the highest priority?

(1) Altered thought processes
(2) Social isolation
(3) Impaired verbal communication
(4) Risk for violence directed at self or at others

2 While working with a client who is having delusions, what nursing intervention would be *most* helpful?

(1) Avoid challenging the content of the client's delusion.
(2) Promise the client that antipsychotic meds will improve thought processes.
(3) Challenge the content of the client's delusion.
(4) Seclude the client in his room to decrease stimulation.

3 A male client diagnosed with schizophrenia is having negative symptoms associated with his illness. Which of the following is classified as a negative symptom?

(1) Abnormal thoughts
(2) Ideas of reference
(3) Blunted affect
(4) Hallucinations

4 A female home health client in your care was recently started on a typical antipsychotic medication. While assessing the client, you notice that the client's hands are trembling and she complains of muscle stiffness. Her vital signs indicate hyperthermia and tachycardia. Based on this information, what should you do next?

(1) Administer the prn acetaminophen (Tylenol) ordered for the client.
(2) Tell the client to rest today and increase her fluid intake.
(3) Transport client to the hospital ER for further evaluation.
(4) Schedule an appointment with the client's physician for further evaluation.

5 While meeting with a schizophrenic client's family, you are asked the question, "What causes schizophrenia?" The *best* response to this question is:

(1) "Research indicates that schizophrenia is caused by a genetic predisposition."
(2) "The exact cause of schizophrenia is unclear at this time."
(3) "Poor parenting skills most likely caused schizophrenia to occur."
(4) "An early-age trauma most likely caused schizophrenia to occur."

6 While working with a client who is withdrawn and disconnected, which of the following is an appropriate short-term goal?

(1) The client will attend one group meeting accompanied by a staff member within 1 week.
(2) The client will voluntarily lead the unit community meeting by discharge from the hospital.
(3) The client will be more connected to the unit in 3 days.
(4) The client will attend many of the unit group meetings by discharge from the hospital.

7 A client presents in the intake assessment office of the mental health clinic with mutism and wax-like flexibility of the extremities. What type of schizophrenia is characteristic of these findings?

(1) Disorganized type
(2) Undifferentiated type
(3) Residual type
(4) Catatonic type

8 A client with a diagnosis of schizophrenia is speaking in a group by putting rhyming words that have no meaning together. This speech pattern is known as:

(1) Echopraxia.
(2) Echolalia.
(3) Clang associations.
(4) Neologisms.

9 The nurse administering atypical antipsychotic medications is aware that they have been defined as having which of the following characteristics?

(1) High risk for tardive dyskinesia
(2) Minimal to no risk for extrapyramidal effects
(3) Effective in treating only positive symptoms of schizophrenia
(4) Effective in treating only negative symptoms of schizophrenia

10 A male client with a diagnosis of schizophrenia tells you that his roommate is putting thoughts in his mind against his will. This is an example of:

(1) Thought broadcasting.
(2) Thought blocking.
(3) Thought insertion.
(4) Thought control.

See pages 184–185 for Answers and Rationales.

I. Overview/Classification

NCLEX!

A. Schizophrenia is one of a cluster of related psychotic brain disorders of unknown etiology

B. Schizophrenia is a combination of disordered thinking, perceptual disturbances, behavioral abnormalities, affective disruptions, and impaired social competency

C. Symptoms of schizophrenia typically include the following

NCLEX!

1. **Delusional ideation:** a false belief brought about without appropriate external stimulation and inconsistent with the individual's own knowledge and experience

NCLEX!

2. **Hallucinations:** false sensory perceptions that may involve any of the five senses (auditory, visual, tactile, olfactory, and gustatory)
3. Disorganized speech patterns
4. Bizarre behaviors

D. At least two of these symptoms must be present for a significant portion of the time during a 1-month period

E. Other manifestations include social impairment and cognitive impairment: the subtypes of schizophrenia have similar features, but differ in their clinical presentations

F. Critical essential features of each subtype of schizophrenia

1. Paranoid type

NCLEX!

   a. Auditory hallucinations
   b. Preoccupation with one or more delusions usually of a persecutory nature
   c. May appear hostile or angry
   d. None of the following are present: flat or inappropriate affect, disorganized speech or behavior, or **catatonic** behavior; in catatonic behavior the body remains in a fixed position, wax-like state

2. Catatonic type

   a. Stupor (state of daze or unconsciousness) or extreme motor agitation
   b. Excessive negativism

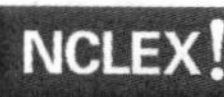

   c. Inappropriate or bizarre body postures
   d. **Echolalia** (an involuntary parrot-like repetition of words spoken by others) or **echopraxia** (a meaningless imitation of motions made by others)

3. Residual type

   a. Absence of prominent psychotic symptoms
   b. Social withdrawal and inappropriate affect
   c. Eccentric behavior
   d. Past history of at least one episode of schizophrenia

4. Disorganized type

   a. Disorganized speech
   b. Disorganized behavior
   c. Inappropriate or flat affect

5. Undifferentiated type

   a. Disorganized behaviors
   b. Psychotic symptoms (including delusions and hallucinations)

II. Etiology

A. Approximately 1 percent of the population has schizophrenia; schizophrenia is the most common psychotic disorder and often results in a chronic illness

B. Schizophrenia is a disorder of the brain like epilepsy or multiple sclerosis

NCLEX!

C. Generally the individual is fairly normal early in life, experiences subtle changes after puberty, and undergoes severe symptoms in the late teens to early adulthood

D. The vast majority of individuals develop the disorder in adolescence or young adulthood, with only 10 percent of cases first diagnosed in people over the age of 45

E. The current knowledge base on the cause of schizophrenia is uncertain

F. Several factors have been identified as having a high correlation or association with the development of schizophrenia; they include:

1. Brain structure and functioning
    - **a.** An overactive basal ganglia
    - **b.** Enlarged ventricles, cerebral atrophy, decreased cerebral blood flow, decreased brain volume, and reduced glucose metabolism in the frontal and temporal lobes as seen on imaging studies (CT, MRI, and PET scans)
    - NCLEX! **c.** Imbalance between dopamine and serotonin neurotransmitter systems, usually with an excess of dopamine
    - **d.** Low levels of the neurotransmitter GABA (gamma-aminobutyric acid)
2. Genetic factors
    - NCLEX! **a.** Multiple studies have shown that there is increased risk for the development of schizophrenia with a positive family history of schizophrenia
    - **b.** The risk for the development of schizophrenia increases for those with first-degree relatives diagnosed with schizophrenia
    - **c.** There has been no specific genetic defect identified that causes schizophrenia

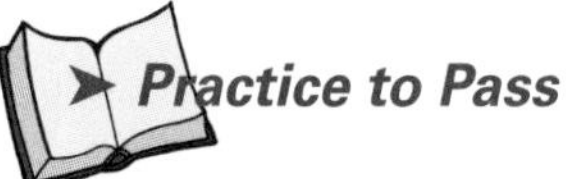

How would knowledge about a genetic predisposition to schizophrenia be helpful?

3. Psychological factors
    - **a.** There are no specific studies that indicate that stress causes schizophrenia, but studies have shown that stress does affect relapse and exacerbation of schizophrenic manifestations
    - **b.** The existence of several factors together such as genetic predisposition to schizophrenia along with the presence of stressful events may contribute to the development of schizophrenia
4. Environmental factors
    - **a.** Observations have suggested that exposure to infectious agents such as viruses in early infancy may contribute to the development of schizophrenia
    - **b.** Research studies have indicated an association between schizophrenia and complications during pregnancy or labor such as oxygen deprivation, short gestation periods, and low birthweights

III. Assessment for Symptomatology (Subjective/Objective)

NCLEX! **A. Positive symptoms** indicate a distortion or excess of normal functioning: they often occur as the initial symptoms of schizophrenia and precipitate the need for hospitalization; they include:

1. Delusions—fixed false beliefs or ideas
    - **a.** Paranoid type: the individual believes others are out to get him or her; the client may be hostile, suspicious, and aggressive
    - **b.** Grandiose type: the individual has excessive feelings of importance and power over others

c. Religious type: the individual has delusions that focus on a religious context

d. Somatic type: the individual has delusions that are fixed on an irrational belief about his or her body

e. Nihilistic: the client has delusions of nonexistence

f. Persecutory: the client has delusions that others are out to get or are plotting against him or her

NCLEX!

g. **Thought broadcasting:** the individual has the delusional belief that others can hear his or her thoughts

NCLEX!

h. **Thought insertion:** the individual has the delusional belief that others have the ability to put thoughts in a person's mind against that person's will

i. **Thought control:** the individual has the delusional belief that others can control a person's thoughts against one's will

NCLEX!

2. Hallucinations, usually auditory
3. **Psychosis** is a disorderly mental state in which a client has difficulty distinguishing reality from his or her own internal perceptions

NCLEX!

4. **Illusions:** inaccurate perception or misinterpretation of sensory impressions
5. Agitation
6. Hostility
7. Bizarre behaviors (catatonic, etc.)
8. Association disturbances

a. Echolalia: repeating the words of another person for no logical reason

b. Echopraxia: purposeless imitation of movements exhibited by others

NCLEX!

c. **Clang associations:** rhyming words in a sentence that make no sense

d. Illogical thinking patterns

NCLEX!

e. **Neologisms:** inventing new words, which are meaningful only to that person

NCLEX!

f. **Word salad:** combining words in a sentence that have no connection and make no sense

NCLEX!

B. **Negative symptoms** indicate a loss or lack of normal functioning; they develop over time and hinder the person's ability to endure life tasks; they include:

1. Anhedonia: diminished ability to experience pleasure or imtimacy
2. Alogia: poverty of speech
3. Anergia: lack of energy
4. Avolition: lack of motivation and goals
5. Ambivalence: inability to make a decision because of conflicting emotions
6. Affect disturbances

a. Blunted

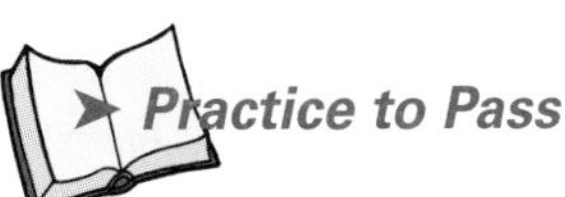

Practice to Pass

What are considered nursing priorities when a client is experiencing psychosis?

b. Flat

c. Inappropriate

7. Restricted emotion

8. Social withdrawal

9. Dependency

10. Lack of ego boundaries

11. Concrete thought processes

12. Lack of self-care

13. Sleep disturbance

IV. Nursing Diagnoses/Analysis

NCLEX!

A. **Impaired thought processes** related to possible hereditary factors, delusional thinking, hallucinations, or inaccurate interpretation of the environment

B. **Anxiety** related to inaccurate interpretation of the environment, unfamiliar environment, repressed fear, or panic level of stress

C. **Individual ineffective coping** related to inability to trust, low self-esteem, or inadequate support systems

NCLEX!

D. **Social isolation** related to lack of trust, regression to earlier level of function, delusional thinking, or past experiences of difficulty in interactions with others

NCLEX!

E. **Risk for violence, self-directed or directed toward others** related to lack of trust, panic-level anxiety, command hallucinations, delusional thinking, or perception of the environment as threatening

F. **Sensory-perceptual alterations: auditory/visual** related to hallucinations, delusional thinking, withdrawal into self, or perception of the environment as threatening

G. **Impaired verbal communication** related to inability to trust, regression to earlier level of development, or disordered and unrealistic thinking

H. **Self-care deficit (specify)** related to withdrawal into self, regression to earlier level of development, or perceptual or cognitive impairment

I. **Sleep pattern disturbance** related to repressed fears, hallucinations, or delusional thinking

J. **Chronic low self-esteem** related to withdrawal into self, lack of trust, poor socialization skills, or chronic illness

V. Planning and Implementation of Specific Treatment Modalities

NCLEX!

A. **Psychopharmacology** (see Table 9-1 for nursing considerations for clients on antipsychotic medications)

1. Typical antipsychotics (traditional)

a. Initially introduced in the 1950s

b. Also referred to as neuroleptic medications

c. Effectively treat only the positive symptoms of schizophrenia and have no therapeutic effect on the negative symptoms

Table 9-1

Nursing Considerations for Clients Taking Antipsychotic Medications

Drug Class and Name	General Nursing Considerations and Interventions
Typical/traditional • Chlorpromazine (Thorazine) • Fluphenazine (Prolixin) • Haloperidol (Haldol) • Loxapine (Loxitane) • Molindone (Moban) • Perphenazine (Trilaton) • Thioridazine (Mellaril) • Thiothixene (Navane) • Trifluoperazine (Stelazine) **Atypical** • Clozapine (Clozaril) • Olanzapine (Zyprexa) • Quetiapine (Seroquel) • Risperidone (Risperdal) • Ziprasidone (Zeldox)	1. Assess client's response to medication and for any possible drug interactions. 2. Monitor client on antipsychotic meds for extrapyramidal side effects and other adverse reactions. 3. Administer the Abnormal and Involuntary Movement Scale (AIMS) to assess the client on antipsychotic meds for signs of tardive dyskinesia. 4. Assess for signs of NMS and access emergency care for client if NMS suspected. 5. Monitor the client's vital signs for hypotension, orthostatic hypotension, and tachycardia. 6. Monitor the client's body weight for weight gain. 7. Monitor the client for any seizure activity. 8. Instruct the client to avoid getting overheated in the sun; use sunblock; and avoid taking hot baths.
Anti-parkinsonism/anticholinergic • Benztropine (Cogentin) • Biperiden (Akineton) • Diphenhydramine (Benadryl) • Ethopropazine (Parsidol; not presently available in U.S.) • Procyclidine (Kemadrin) • Trihexyphenidyl (Artane)	1. Suggest chewing sugarless gum or hard candy to offset side effect of dry mouth. 2. Suggest rinsing mouth frequently to decrease side effect of dry mouth. 3. Encourage use of stool softners, increasing water intake, and dietary fiber to decrease side effect of constipation. 4. Suggest use of saline nasal sprays to decrease side effect of nasal congestion. 5. Instruct client to use caution due to temporary side effect of blurred vision. Vision will return to previous condition in a few weeks. 6. Instruct client to report any eye pain immediately. 7. Instruct client on need to use caution in the sun, wear sunscreen, sunglasses, and avoid becoming overheated because of side effects of photophobia and photosensitivity. 8. Instruct client to use caution with sudden changes in body positions due to possible orthostatic hypotension. 9. Monitor client for signs of urinary retention and hesitation.

How are depot injections of antipsychotic medications helpful?

d. Depot therapy injections available in a few traditional antipsychotic drugs for clients who have a poor adherence history

e. Most common side effects are the extrapyramidal side effects (EPS) (see Table 9-2)

2. Atypical antipsychotics

a. Developed and first marketed in 1990

b. Effective in treating the positive and negative symptoms of schizophrenia

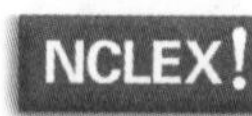

c. Minimal to no risk of developing EPS

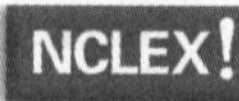

d. Decreased risk for development of tardive dyskinesia (TD)

Table 9-2

Extrapyramidal Side Effects from Antipsychotic Medications

Akathisia	Motor restlessness, inability to remain still, can also occur as subjective feeling
Akinesia	Absence of movement or difficulty with movement
Dystonias	Muscle spasms, spastic movements of the neck and back, can be painful and frightening for the client
Pseudo-parkinsonism	Shuffling and slow gait, mask-like facial expression, tremors, pill-rolling movements of the hands, stooping posture, rigidity
Tardive dyskinesia	Involuntary and abnormal movements of the mouth, tongue, face, and jaw, may progress to the limbs, irreversible condition, may occur in months after antipsychotic medication use
Neuroleptic malignant syndrome	A potentially lethal side effect of antipsychotic medication that requires emergency treatment; manifest symptoms include: hyperthermia, muscle rigidity, tremors, altered consciousness, tachycardia, hypertension, and incontinence

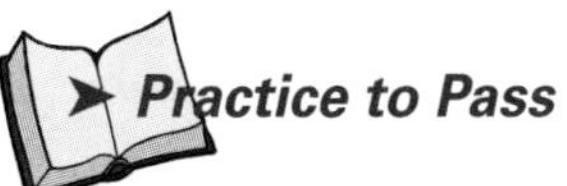

How might you assess for tardive dyskinesia?

3. Anti-parkinsonism (anticholinergics)
   - **a.** Increase dopamine levels
   - **b.** Maybe helpful in the management of negative symptoms of schizophrenia
   - **c.** Used to prevent or manage EPS of antipsychotic medications; common anticholinergeric side effects are dry mouth, blurred vision, constipation, decreased lacrimation, photophobia, urinary hesitance, tachycardia, and nausea

B. Individual and group interventions

1. Management of delusions and hallucinations
   - **a.** Establish a trusting, therapeutic relationship with the client by being honest, supportive, and consistent with the client
   - **b.** Encourage the client to express feelings and thoughts
   - **c.** Assess for signs that the client is possibly having delusions or hallucinations
   - **d.** Communicate with the client using clear, direct statements
   - **e.** Provide an environment with a low degree of stimulation
   - NCLEX! **f.** Express to the client that you understand that he or she believes the delusion or hallucination but you do not share in the delusional belief or hallucination
   - NCLEX! **g.** Avoid arguing with the client about the delusion or hallucination
   - **h.** Provide reality testing and focus on reality
   - **i.** If the client is experiencing a visual hallucination, provide a room with adequate lighting
2. General nursing considerations and interventions

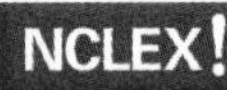

   - **a.** Provide an environment that is safe for the client and others

b. Avoid any physical contact or touching of the client

c. Encourage the client to verbalize feelings and thoughts openly

d. Utilize therapeutic communication techniques with the client

e. Identify support systems for the client

NCLEX!

f. Assess for self-destructive behaviors and provide needed precautions

g. Provide for activities of daily living (ADLs) when the client is not able to meet those needs

NCLEX!

h. Provide opportunities for the client that promote socialization and decrease isolation

i. Involve the client in setting realistic goals in the treatment plan

j. Provide daily living skills groups for the client to participate in

NCLEX!

C. ***Milieu therapy:*** a method of psychotherapy that controls the environment of the client to provide interpersonal contacts in order to develop trust, assurance, and personal autonomy

1. Provide for the client's safety and the safety of others in the milieu
2. Provide a supportive environment that is structured and predictable
3. Collaborate with the multidisciplinary team regarding the client's plan of care
4. Collaborate with the client regarding his or her plan of care
5. Encourage the client to participate in milieu groups and activities that promote socialization
6. Assist client with ADLs as needed, but encourage independence as client progresses

Practice to Pass

Schizophrenia is generally considered a chronic condition, which needs long-term management. What are some nursing interventions that may decrease relapse potential?

D. **Family therapy**

1. Involve the family to determine use of appropriate community resources
2. Educate the family about the chronic illness of schizophrenia, implications, early signs and symptoms of relapse, disease management, medication management, and community support systems available

NCLEX!

3. Provide an outlet for the family to discuss their feelings and explore alternative effective coping skills

VI. Evaluation/Outcomes

A. **Evaluation of the client's treatment and progress** is an ongoing, continual process

B. **Outcome criteria are individualized for each client** and may include the following; the client will:

NCLEX!

1. Remain free of harm, and demonstrate absence of violence toward others
2. Be able to establish a trusting, open relationship with therapist/nurse
3. Report and experience no hallucinations or diminished hallucinations
4. Report and experience no delusional thought processes

5. Demonstrate increased socialization skills and decreased isolative behavior
6. Demonstrate appropriate affect and improved thought processes
7. Report the ability to experience pleasure and improved interest in activities
8. Demonstrate an improved ability to concentrate and complete tasks
9. Demonstrate improved speech patterns and congruent communication
10. Adhere to medication schedule as prescribed
11. Demonstrate no EPS or adverse reactions to medication regime
12. Verbalize side effects and adverse reactions to report to practitioner/MD
13. Verbalize indication, dosage, route, and schedule of medication regime
14. Actively participate in plan of care
15. Demonstrate ability to meet ADLs with or without assistance
16. Demonstrate effective coping patterns
17. Utilize appropriate community resources

C. **Outcome criteria are individualized for each client's family** and may include the following; the family will:

1. Be able to verbalize and identify early signs and symptoms of disease exacerbation
2. Be able to verbalize the implications of schizophrenia as a chronic illness
3. Demonstrate effective coping patterns
4. Utilize appropriate community resources
5. Be able to verbalize client's medication regime
6. Be able to verbalize and identify signs and symptoms of EPS and neuroleptic malignant syndrome (NMS)
7. Be able to verbalize how and when to access to emergency care services

VII. Specific Disorders

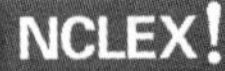

A. **Schizophrenia:** a syndrome characterized by difficulty thinking clearly, knowing what is real, managing feelings, making decisions, or relating to others

1. The positive characteristics of schizophrenia are added behaviors not normally seen, such as delusions, hallucinations, loose associations, and overactive affect
2. The negative characteristics of schizophrenia are the absence of normal behaviors, for example, flat affect, minimal self-care, social withdrawal, and concrete thinking
3. People with schizophrenia may exhibit purposeless or ritualistic behaviors or even pace for hours on end; some have bizarre facial or body movements
4. The most common type of hallucination is auditory; the next most common type is visual

5. Delusions are false beliefs that cannot be changed by logical reasoning or evidence; it is thought that they represent dysfunction in the information-processing circuits between the hemispheres
6. People with schizophrenia frequently have ineffective social skills, which increases their sense of isolation
7. Neurobiological factors of schizophrenia include genetic defects, abnormal brain development, neurodegeneration, disordered neurotransmission, and abnormal brain structures
8. Psychiatric rehabilitation emphasizes the development of skills and supports, considers the client to be in control, and promotes choices, self-determination, and individual responsibility

NCLEX!

B. Schizoaffective disorder: having clinical manifestations characteristic of both schizophrenia and a mood disorder, such as depression, mania, or a mixed episode

1. Client experiences symptoms of a mood disorder with one or more of the following:
   a. Delusions
   b. Hallucinations
   c. Disorganized speech
   d. Disorganized behavior
   e. Negative characteristics
2. Clients often have difficulty maintaining a job or functioning in school, experience problems with self-care, are socially isolated, and often suffer from suicidal ideation

C. Schizophreniform disorder: the essential features of schizophrenia are present with the exception that the duration is at least 1 month, but less than 6 months

D. Other psychotic disorders

1. Delusional disorder: the presence of non-bizarre delusions (delusions that could possibly occur in reality) that persist for at least 1 month; no other manifestations of psychosis are noted
2. Brief psychotic disorder: the presence of at least one positive symptom of schizophrenia with duration between 1 day and 1 month; the existence or absence of any stressor should be noted
3. Shared psychotic disorder (*folie a deux*): a delusional system develops in the context of a close relationship between two people who share a similar delusion
4. Substance-induced psychotic disorder: the presence of hallucinations and delusions are a direct result of the physiological effects of a substance
5. Psychotic disorder due to a general medical condition: the presence of hallucinations and delusions are a direct result of the general medical condition

Case Study

As you begin your shift as the charge nurse in an acute care psychiatric unit, you are informed in shift change report of a new client admission. The client has a medical diagnosis of schizophrenia, paranoid type and has had multiple psychiatric hospital admissions caused by poor adherence to antipsychotic medication therapy.

❶ What types of symptoms might you anticipate seeing?

❷ What are the priorities of care for the client?

❸ What are the possible nursing diagnoses?

❹ How will you approach this client to begin fostering a therapeutic relationship?

❺ What options are available to decrease incidence of poor medication adherence?

For suggested responses, see page 308.

Posttest

1 While talking with a client diagnosed with schizophrenia, you notice the client loses eye contact with you and starts staring at the wall. The client is making facial grimaces. The *most* appropriate nursing intervention would be to:

(1) End the conversation because the client is not listening to you.
(2) Administer to the client the ordered prn trihexyphenidyl (Artane).
(3) Ask the client directly, "What are you seeing on the wall?"
(4) Redirect the client's attention to continue your conversation.

2 A client taking antipsychotic medications for treatment of schizophrenia complains to the nurse of feeling nervous. The nurse notices that the client is pacing the long hallway and is unable to remain still even when other clients are talking with him. This client is *most* likely experiencing:

(1) Akathisia.
(2) Akinesia.
(3) Dystonia.
(4) Tardive dyskinesia.

3 A client is exhibiting symptoms that are characteristic of schizophrenia, but is also exhibiting manic behaviors. This client's *most* likely diagnosis is:

(1) Schizophreniform disorder.
(2) Brief psychotic disorder.
(3) Shared psychotic disorder.
(4) Schizoaffective disorder.

4 A male client on the unit has a diagnosis of paranoid-type schizophrenia. The new mental health care worker on this unit approaches the nurse and asks about the best way to work with this client. The nurse replies:

(1) "Avoid touching this client and invading personal space."
(2) "Offer back rubs at bedtime to decrease the client's anxiety."
(3) "Greet this client with a firm handshake."
(4) "Place your hand on the client very softly when you speak to him."

5 What nursing diagnosis is *most* likely to be associated with a client diagnosed as having schizophrenia, residual type?

(1) Impaired verbal communication
(2) Self-care deficit
(3) Social isolation
(4) Anxiety

6 What nursing diagnosis is *most* likely to be associated with a client diagnosed as having schizophrenia, disorganized type?

(1) Impaired verbal communication
(2) Sleep pattern disturbance
(3) Social isolation
(4) Self-care deficit

7 Which of the following statements is correct in regards to the Abnormal and Involuntary Movement Scale (AIMS)?

(1) The AIMS is used to screen for pseudoparkinsonism.
(2) The AIMS should be used yearly to screen clients taking antipsychotic agents.
(3) A rating on the AIMS of zero indicates absence of abnormal involuntary movement.
(4) The AIMS is a diagnostic tool used to identify tardive dyskinesia.

8 A female client complains to the nurse that her vision has become blurred since she started taking an anticholinergic medication. The *best* response of the nurse would be:

(1) "You need to schedule an appointment with your eye doctor to get a new prescription for your eyeglasses."
(2) "Blurred vision is a temporary side effect of your medication that usually resolves with 4 to 6 weeks."
(3) "You need to stop taking your antipsychotic medication and notify your doctor immediately."
(4) "Blurred vision is a permanent condition as a result of your medication."

9 A male client is planning to be discharged from the hospital. It is your responsibility as the nurse to educate this client regarding his medications. This client is taking an anticholinergic medication. A critical client teaching point would include:

(1) To report eye pain immediately to doctor.
(2) To take this medication on an empty stomach.
(3) To explain that the client may experience sudden changes in their bowel functioning in time.
(4) That most over-the-counter medications are compatible with this medication.

10 Which of the following is considered to be a positive symptom associated with schizophrenia?

(1) Alogia
(2) Avolition
(3) Social withdrawal
(4) Loose associations

See pages 185–186 for Answers and Rationales.

Answers and Rationales

Pretest

1 **Answer: 4** *Rationale:* Safety is always the highest priority when caring for a client with a diagnosis of schizophrenia, paranoid type. Clients with this diagnosis are potentially violent and can quickly become aggressive as a result of their psychosis. The other options (1, 2, and 3) of diagnoses are appropriate for the client's care plan but are not given the highest priority.
Cognitive Level: Analysis
Nursing Process: Planning; *Test Plan:* PSYC

2 **Answer: 1** *Rationale:* The client believes that his or her thoughts are true. Challenging the client's thoughts only increases anxiety, mistrust, and conflict for the client (option 3). Promises should never be made to a client because, if not kept, trust cannot be established (option 1). Seclusion is not an appropriate intervention for delusional thought processes (option 4).
Cognitive Level: Application
Nursing Process: Implementation; *Test Plan:* PSYC

3 **Answer: 3** *Rationale:* A blunted affect is characteristic of a negative symptom of schizophrenia. All the other options are positive symptoms associated with schizophrenia (options 1, 2, and 4).
Cognitive Level: Comprehension
Nursing Process: Assessment; *Test Plan:* PSYC

4 **Answer: 3** *Rationale:* This client is exhibiting signs and symptoms of neuroleptic malignant syndrome (NMS). This is a potentially lethal side effect of antipsychotic medications that requires immediate medical care. All the other interventions are not

appropriate and would delay appropriate treatment (options 1, 2, and 3).
Cognitive Level: Analysis
Nursing Process: Analysis; *Test Plan:* PSYC

5 **Answer: 2** *Rationale:* The precise cause of schizophrenia is unknown. The general consensus is that schizophrenia results from the interaction between factors that have been correlated with schizophrenia. Research has correlated genetic factors with schizophrenia, but more research is needed (option 1). Poor parenting skill (option 3) or early-age trauma (option 4) have not been documented in causing schizophrenia.
Cognitive Level: Application
Nursing Process: Implementation; *Test Plan:* PSYC

6 **Answer: 1** *Rationale:* Short-term goals need to be measurable and accomplished in a brief period of time. Clients need to meet short-term goals during hospitalization to promote a sense of accomplishment, which may increase their self-esteem. Options 2, 3, and 4 are less measurable then option 1.
Cognitive Level: Analysis
Nursing Process: Evaluation; *Test Plan:* PSYC

7 **Answer: 4** *Rationale:* Clients with catatonic-type schizophrenia may exhibit mutism and wax-like flexibility of the extremities. The mutism and wax-like flexibility of the extremities are not characteristic of the other diagnoses (options 1, 2, and 3).
Cognitive Level: Application
Nursing Process: Assessment; *Test Plan:* PSYC

8 **Answer: 3** *Rationale:* Clang associations are association disturbances in which schizophrenic clients rhyme words in a sentence that make no sense. Echopraxia is meaningless imitation of motions made by others (option 1). Echolalia is involuntary parrot-like repetition of words spoken by others (option 2). Neologism is the coining of a new word that is meaningless to anyone but the client (option 4).
Cognitive Level: Comprehension
Nursing Process: Assessment; *Test Plan:* PSYC

9 **Answer: 2** *Rationale:* Atypical antipsychotic medications are helpful in treating both negative (option 4) and positive (option 3) symptoms of schizophrenia. This class of medications has minimal to no risk for extrapyramidal side effects, which includes tardive dyskinesia (option 1).
Cognitive Level: Comprehension
Nursing Process: Implementation; *Test Plan:* PSYC

10 **Answer: 3** *Rationale:* Thought insertion is a thought disorder of schizophrenia that is defined as the client believing that others are putting thoughts in his or her mind against the client's will. Thought broadcasting is the belief by a client that he or she can broadcast his or her thoughts to others (option 1). Thought blocking occurs when a client's thoughts stop in midstream (option 2). Thought control is the belief that others can control their thoughts against their will (option 4).
Cognitive Level: Analysis
Nursing Process: Assessment; *Test Plan:* PSYC

Posttest

1 **Answer: 3** *Rationale:* This client is most likely experiencing a visual hallucination. First, it is important for nurses to know the content of the hallucination so they can assist the client to process the experience and prevent any aggressive behavior. After this intervention is completed, than the client should be oriented back to reality. Ending the conversation would not promote trust with the client (option 1). Trihexyphenidyl will not prevent hallucinations (option 2). The nurse should not redirect the conversation until the nurse has evaluated for hallucinations (option 4).
Cognitive Level: Analysis
Nursing Process: Implementation; *Test Plan:* PSYC

2 **Answer: 1** *Rationale:* Akathisia is an extrapyramidal side effect of antipsychotic medications that may manifest as subjective and objective restlessness. Akinesia (option 2), dystonia (option 3), and tardive dyskinesia (option 4) are also extrapyramidal side effects of antipsychotic medications, but are not characteristic of this client's symptoms.
Cognitive Level: Application
Nursing Process: Assessment; *Test Plan:* PSYC

3 **Answer: 4** *Rationale:* Schizoaffective disorder has clinical manifestations that are characteristic of both schizophrenia and a mood disorder, such as mania, depression, or a mixed episode. Schizophreniform disorder (option 1), brief psychotic disorder (option 2), and shared psychotic disorder (option 3) have other essential characteristics not indicative of what this client is exhibiting.
Cognitive Level: Application
Nursing Process: Analysis; *Test Plan:* PSYC

4 **Answer: 1** *Rationale:* Paranoid schizophrenic clients are very suspicious and potentially dangerous. It is best to avoid any physical contact with a client

that has a diagnosis of paranoid schizophrenia because the client may feel threatened. Offering a back rub (option 2), shaking hands (option 3), and placing a hand on the client (option 4) include physical contact. Also it is safer to keep a physical distance from the client in the event he or she becomes physically aggressive.
Cognitive Level: Application
Nursing Process: Planning; *Test Plan:* PSYC

5 **Answer: 3** *Rationale:* Residual-type schizophrenia manifests with socially withdrawn behavior, an inappropriate affect, and an absence of prominent psychotic symptoms. The most likely and common nursing diagnosis would be Social isolation. Impaired verbal communication (option 1), Self-care deficit (option 2), and Anxiety (option 4) are less likely with schizophrenia, residual type.
Cognitive Level: Analysis
Nursing Process: Planning; *Test Plan:* PSYC

6 **Answer: 1** *Rationale:* Schizophrenia, disorganized type, is characterized by disorganized speech patterns. Other manifestations of this diagnosis include disorganized behavior and inappropriate affect. Sleep pattern disturbance (option 2), Social isolation (option 3), and Self-care deficit (option 4) are possible, but not classic for disorganized schizophrenia.
Cognitive Level: Analysis
Nursing Process: Planning; *Test Plan:* PSYC

7 **Answer: 3** *Rationale:* The AIMS is used to screen for signs of tardive dyskinesia, which is a possible side effect of antipsychotic medications. It is not a screening tool (option 1 and option 2) or a diagnostic tool (option 4). A score of 1 to 4 on any single item indicates the need for further evaluation. A score of 0 on all items indicates no further evaluation is needed.
Cognitive Level: Comprehension
Nursing Process: Assessment; *Test Plan:* PSYC

8 **Answer: 2** *Rationale:* Blurred vision is an anticholinergic symptom/side effect that usually resolves in a few weeks. If there is no improvement with time, then the doctor should be notified. It is too early to schedule an appointment (option 1). The blurred vision is expected and usually resolves in a few weeks (option 3). Permanent condition of blurred vision is unusual (option 4).
Cognitive Level: Analysis
Nursing Process: Implementation; *Test Plan:* PSYC

9 **Answer: 1** *Rationale:* Eye pain may indicate undiagnosed narrow angle glaucoma, which needs immediate attention. This condition is known as mydriasis. It is not necessary to take anticholinergic medication on an empty stomach (option 2). Constipation is a common side effect of anticholinergic medications (option 3). Most over-the-counter medications are not compatible with anticholinergic medications (option 4).
Cognitive Level: Analysis
Nursing Process: Planning; *Test Plan:* PSYC

10 **Answer: 4** *Rationale:* Loose associations are considered to be a positive symptom associated with schizophrenia because they indicate a distortion or excess of normal functioning. Alogia (option 1), avolition (option 2), and social withdrawal (option 3) are considered negative symptoms of schizophrenia. Negative symptoms indicate a loss or lack of normal functioning. Negative symptoms develop over time and hinder the client's ability to endure life tasks.
Cognitive Level: Comprehension
Nursing Process: Analysis; *Test Plan:* PSYC

References

American Psychiatric Association (2000). *Diagnosis and statistical manual of mental disorders* (4th ed. text revision). Washinton, DC: American Psychiatric Association, pp. 288, 297–344.

Buchanan, R. & Carpenter, W. (2000). Schizophrenia: Introduction and overview. In B. Saddock & V. Saddock (Eds.). *Comprehensive textbook of psychiatry.* Philadelphia: Williams & Wilkins.

Copel, L. (1999). *Nurse's clinical guide: Psychiatric and mental health care* (2nd ed.). Springhouse, PA: Springhouse, pp. 107–116, 407.

Fontaine, K. L. (1999). Schizophrenic disorders. In K. L. Fontaine, & J. S. Fletcher (Eds.), *Mental health nursing* (4th ed.). Menlo Park, CA: Addison-Wesley, pp. 281–314.

Keltner, N. & Folks, D. (2001). *Psychotropic drugs* (3rd ed.). St. Louis: Mosby, pp. 78, 84, 90, 103, 123, 420–447.

Keltner, N., Schwecke, L. & Bostrom, C. (1999). *Psychiatric nursing* (3rd ed.). St. Louis: Mosby, p. 239.

Krupnick, S. & Wade, A. (1999). *Psychiatric care planning* (2nd ed.). Springhouse, PA: Springhouse, p. 97.

Moller, M. & Murphy, M. (2001). Neurobiological responses and schizophrenia and psychotic disorders. In G. Stuart & M. Laraia (Eds.), *Principles and practices of psychiatric nursing* (7th ed.). St. Louis: Mosby, pp. 402–437.

North American Nursing Diagnosis Association (2001). *Nursing diagnosis: Definitions and classification 2001–2002.* Philadelphia: North American Nursing Diagnosis Association.

O'Brien, S. (1998). Health promotion and schizophrenia: The year 2000 and beyond. *Holistic Nursing Practice, 12*(2):38–43.

O'Connor, F. (1998). The role of serotonin and dopamine in schizophrenia. *Journal of the American Psychiatric Nurses Association, 4*(4):30–41.

Stahl, S. (1998). What makes an antipsychotic atypical? *Journal of Clinical Psychiatry, 59*(8):403.

Townsend, M. (2001). *Nursing diagnosis in psychiatric nursing: Care plans and psychotropic medications* (5th ed.). Philadelphia: F. A. Davis, pp. 147–167.

Videbeck, S. (2001). *Psychiatric mental health nursing.* Philadelphia: Lippincott, pp. 296–323.

Wilson, B., Shannon, M, & Stang, C. (2000). *Nurses' drug guide 2000.* Stamford, CT: Appleton & Lange.

CHAPTER 10

Delirium, Dementia, and Other Cognitive Mental Disorders

Jane E. Bostick, MSN, RN

CHAPTER OUTLINE

OBJECTIVES

- Identify eight characteristics commonly seen in clients experiencing dementia.
- Describe three treatment modalities for clients with delirium and dementia.
- Differentiate between delirium and dementia.
- State examples of at least five nursing diagnoses frequently used in the management of clients with cognitive mental disorders.

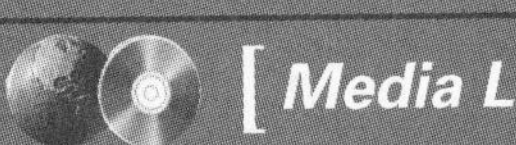

Use the CD-ROM enclosed with this text, or log onto the address given to access the free, interactive Companion Website created for this series. The CD-ROM and Companion Website accompanying this book offer additional practice opportunities and information—NCLEX Review, Case Studies, Glossary, In Depth with NCLEX, and more.

www.prenhall.com/hogan

Review at a Glance

agnosia *an inability to recognize familiar situations, people, or stimuli; not related to impairment in sensory organs*

agraphia *the inability to read or write*

alexia *the inability to identify an object or its use by sight such as a toothbrush or telephone; visual agnosia*

aphasia *a loss of the ability to understand or use language*

apraxia *an inability to carry out skilled and purposeful movement; the inability to use objects properly*

astereognosis *the inability to identify familiar objects when placed in the hand such as a comb or pencil; tactile agnosia*

auditory agnosia *the inability to recognize familiar sounds such as a ringing doorbell or telephone*

catastrophic reaction *the overreaction toward minor stresses that occurs in demented clients*

confabulation *the filling in of memory gaps with imaginary information in an attempt to distract others from observing the deficit*

delirium *an acute, usually reversible brain disorder characterized by clouding of the consciousness (decreased awareness of the environment) and a reduced ability to focus and maintain attention*

dementia *a chronic, irreversible brain disorder characterized by impairments in memory, abstract thinking, and judgment, as well as changes in personality*

hyperetamorphosis *the need to compulsively touch and examine every object in the environment*

hyperorality *the need to taste, chew, and examine any object small enough to be placed in the mouth*

perseveration phenomena *repetitive behaviors such as lip licking, finger tapping, pacing, or echolalia*

pseudodelirium *symptoms of delirium without any identifiable organic cause*

pseudodementia *a reversible disorder that frequently mimics dementia; the most common pseudodementia is depression*

sundown syndrome *disorientation that worsens at the end of the day*

Pretest

1 A client experiencing delirium will most likely have:

(1) A normal electroencephalogram (EEG).
(2) An underlying medical condition causing impairment in cerebral blood flow.
(3) Atrophy of the cerebral cortex.
(4) Plaques found on the outside of dead and damaged neurons.

2 Family members have noticed that during the bath, a client tries to chew on a bar of soap. Which term best describes this behavior?

(1) Hyperactivity
(2) Hyperetamorphosis
(3) Hyperorality
(4) Hyperemesis

3 A client who is experiencing alcohol-withdrawal delirium will typically experience which of the following behaviors?

(1) Reduced alertness or awareness of the environment
(2) Slow, dull speech pattern
(3) Lethargy and apathy
(4) Restlessness and irritability

4 A client in stage 2 of dementia of the Alzheimer's type will often wander, become lost, and confused. Which of the following nursing diagnoses would be most appropriate to address this behavior?

(1) Acute confusion related to fluid and electrolyte imbalance
(2) Anxiety related to fear of cognitive deficits
(3) Impaired verbal communication related to aphasia, agraphia, agnosia
(4) Risk for injury or trauma related to impaired judgment and cognitive deficits

5 An older adult who readily admits to memory loss may be experiencing which one of the following diseases?

(1) Dementia
(2) Depression
(3) Huntington's disease
(4) Parkinson's disease

6 Which of the following is an appropriate outcome for a client experiencing an acute episode of delirium?

(1) Client will have decreased confusion as evidenced by orientation to person, place, and time.
(2) Client will remain free from self-directed violence as evidenced by agreement to a no-suicide contract.
(3) Client will verbalize increased feelings of self-esteem as evidenced by statements acknowledging ability to perform certain tasks independently.
(4) Client will have intact tactile senses as evidenced by ability to recognize familiar objects when placed in his or her hand.

7 The nursing action most likely to be effective in improving the level of orientation of a client experiencing dementia is:

(1) Telling the client the current day of the month and time in a raised voice.
(2) Assuring the client that the deceased spouse will not be expected home soon.
(3) Turning on a radio station that plays soft rock music.
(4) Encouraging the client to discuss memories of being an elementary teacher.

8 The nurse administering which of the following medications to a client realizes that it increases the availability of acetylcholine in the synapse and leads to the recovery of some mental functioning for clients with dementia?

(1) Fluoxetine (Prozac)
(2) Trazodone (Desyrel)
(3) Haloperidol (Haldol)
(4) Donepezil (Aricept)

9 The physician orders paroxetine (Paxil) for an older client who is experiencing short-term memory loss. The rationale for this order is:

(1) To enhance circulation to the brain.
(2) To elevate acetylcholine levels in the brain.
(3) To elevate serotonin levels in the brain.
(4) To enhance oxygenation to the brain.

10 Which of the following statements communicates a caregiver's understanding of coping strategies for dealing with the care of a parent with stage 2 dementia of the Alzheimer's type?

(1) "I need to stay with my parent 24 hours a day."
(2) "I need to bathe my parent at the same time every day."
(3) "I need to postpone my vacation for a few more years."
(4) "I need to spend time with my parent doing something we both enjoy."

See page 206 for Answers and Rationales.

I. Overview/Classification

A. ***Delirium:*** an acute, usually reversible brain disorder characterized by clouding of the consciousness (decreased awareness of the environment) and a reduced ability to focus and maintain attention

NCLEX!

1. Develops over a short period of time (usually hours to days) and tends to fluctuate during the course of the day
2. Evidence from history, physical examination, or laboratory findings suggests that the disturbance is caused by the direct physiological consequences of a general medical condition
3. Types of delirium (APA, 2000)
   - **a.** Delirium due to . . . (indicate general medical condition)

b. Substance-intoxication delirium

c. Substance-withdrawal delirium

d. Delirium due to multiple etiologies

e. Delirium not otherwise specified (NOS)

B. ***Dementia:*** a chronic, irreversible brain disorder characterized by impairments in memory, abstract thinking, and judgment, as well as changes in personality

1. Chronic development of multiple cognitive deficits manifested by memory impairment and one or more of the following cognitive disturbances:

   a. **Aphasia,** a loss of the ability to understand or use language

   b. **Apraxia,** an inability to carry out skilled and purposeful movement; the inability to use objects properly

   c. **Agnosia,** an inability to recognize familiar situations, people, or stimuli; not related to impairment in sensory organs

   d. Disturbance in executive functioning (i.e., planning, organizing, sequencing, abstracting)

NCLEX!

2. Course is insidious and progressive, characterized by gradual onset and continuing cognitive decline

3. Cognitive deficits cause a significant impairment in social or occupational functioning and represent a significant decline from previous level of functioning

4. Types of dementia (APA, 2000)

   a. Dementia of the Alzheimer's type (DAT)

   b. Vascular dementia (formerly multi-infarct dementia)

   c. Dementia due to other general medical conditions

   d. Substance-induced persisting dementia

   e. Dementia due to multiple etiologies

   f. Dementia not otherwise specified (NOS)

C. Amnestic disorders

1. Development of memory impairment characterized by inability to learn new information or inability to recall previously learned information

2. Can be transient (lasting for 1 month or less) or chronic (lasting for more than 1 month)

3. Causes significant impairment in social or occupational functioning and represents a significant decline from a previous level of functioning

4. Types of amnestic disorders (APA, 2000)

   a. Amnestic disorder due to . . . (indicate the general medical condition)

   b. Substance-induced persisting amnestic disorder

   c. Amnestic disorder not otherwise specified (NOS)

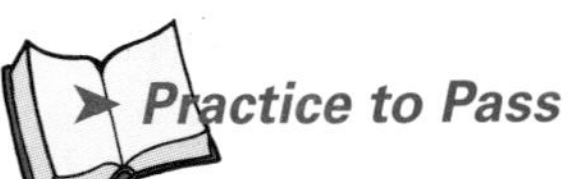

A client hospitalized with a fractured hip begins to show signs of disorientation and memory loss. What are some possible explanations for the confusion?

D. Other cognitive disorders (APA, 2000)

1. Cognitive dysfunction presumed to be caused by a direct physiological effect of a general medical condition that does not meet criteria for any of the specific delirium, dementia, or amnestic disorders previously listed

2. Cognitive disorders not otherwise specified (examples)

   a. Mild neurocognitive disorder

   b. Postconcussional disorder

II. Etiology

A. **Delirium, dementia, and other cognitive disorders** are caused by multiple etiologies that interfere with cerebral blood flow

B. **General medical conditions** causing an interference of necessary blood supply and therefore nutrients (e.g., oxygen, glucose, vitamins) to the brain can result in cognitive disorders

1. Decreased cerebral blood flow: cardiac arrhythmias or arrest, shock, hypertension, congestive heart failure, (CHF) cerebrovascular attack (CVA), transient ischemic attacks (TIA), pulmonary embolism (PE), systemic lupus erythematosus (SLE)

2. Brain hypoxia: chronic obstructive pulmonary disease (COPD), asthma, emphysema, anemia, carbon monoxide poisoning

3. Vitamin deficiency: alcoholism, pernicious anemia, Wernicke's disease, Korsakoff's syndrome

4. Infections: sepsis, subacute bacterial endocarditis, pneumonia, urinary tract infections, AIDS dementia complex (ADC)

5. Endocrine and metabolic disorders: uncontrolled diabetes mellitus, insulin shock, hypothyroidism, adrenal insufficiency, electrolyte imbalance, acidosis, alkalosis

6. Hepatic and renal failure: hepatic encephalopathy; end-stage renal disease (ESRD)

7. Trauma and tumors: traumatic brain injury (TBI), carcinomas

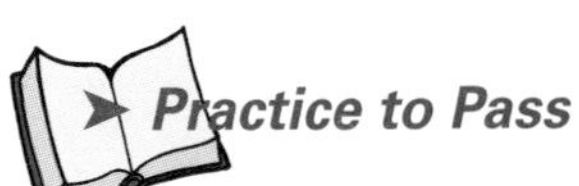

A client has just entered the Emergency Department with confusion, combativeness, and restlessness. What information should you obtain first?

C. **Substances causing toxicity to the brain** either by exposure to, high doses of, or withdrawal from the substance can lead to cognitive disorders

1. Ingestion of medications such as anticonvulsants, neuroleptics, anxiolytics, antidepressants, cardiovascular medications, antineoplastics, and hormones; or exposure to lead, aluminum or other heavy metals

2. Drugs commonly abused such as alcohol, cannabis, cocaine, hallucinogens, anxiolytics, or opioids

3. Termination or reduction in use of long-term, high-dose substances such as alcohol, sedatives, hypnotics, or anxiolytics

D. Genetic or viral diseases can cause pathological changes or biochemical imbalances in the brain that interfere with cerebral blood flow

NCLEX!

1. Dementia of the Alzheimer's type: specific cause is unknown but theories include reduction in brain acetylcholine, accumulation of aluminum in the brain, immune system alterations, head trauma, and genetic factors such as chromosome abnormalities (e.g., Down syndrome)
2. Parkinson's disease: caused by a loss of nerve cells in the substantia nigra of the basal ganglia
3. Huntington's disease: transmitted as a mendelian dominant gene, and damage occurs in the areas of the basal ganglia and the cerebral cortex
4. Pick's disease: caused by atrophy in the frontal and temporal lobes of the brain
5. Creutzfeldt-Jakob disease: caused by a transmissable virus

III. Assessment

A. Delirium has a sudden onset and an identifiable cause

1. A positive history for delirium includes:
   - **a.** A thorough medical evaluation revealing abnormal lab results

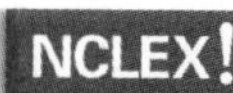

   - **b.** An electroencephalogram (EEG) confirming cerebral dysfunction
   - **c.** More than one examination at different times of the day detect fluctuations in levels of consciousness that characterize the syndrome
   - **d.** Identification of the underlying cause of delirium
   - **e.** Ruling out other reasons for delirium (depression, anxiety, dementia, or personality disorder)
2. Presenting signs and symptoms

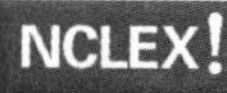

   - **a.** Fluctuating levels of consciousness (i.e., alternating periods of coherence with periods of confusion); disorientation that worsens at the end of the day, usually referred to as **sundown syndrome**
   - **b.** Alternating patterns of hyperactivity (typical of drug withdrawal) to hypoactivity (typical of metabolic imbalance)
   - **c.** Hyperactive behaviors
     1) Rambling, bizarre, incoherent, rapid, pressured, or loud speech
     2) Restlessness, picking at clothes or bed linen, irritability, euphoria
     3) Calling out for help, striking out at others, bizarre and destructive behavior, combativeness, anger, profanity
   - **d.** Hypoactive behaviors
     1) Limited, dull patterns of speech
     2) Lethargy, apathy, withdrawn behavior
     3) Reduced alertness or awareness of environment
   - **e.** Cognitive changes
     1) Disorganized thinking

2) Diminished ability to focus attention, easily distracted
3) Disorientation to time and place
4) Impairment in recent and remote memory
5) Visual or auditory hallucinations, frightening delusions

f. Sleep pattern disturbances, including vivid and terrifying dreams or nightmares

g. Predominant emotion is fear with a high level of anxiety

B. Dementia is a progressive disease and symptoms can be divided into three stages

1. Stage 1 (typically lasts 1 to 3 years)

NCLEX!

a. Difficulty performing complex tasks related to a decline in recent memory; forgetfulness, missed appointments; clients often recognize and are frightened by their confusion

b. Declining personal appearance, inappropriate dress for weather

c. Lack of spontaneity in verbal and nonverbal communication

d. Disoriented to time but can remember people and places

e. Decreased concentration, increased distractibility, impaired judgment

2. Stage 2 (lasting approximately 2 to 10 years)

a. Poor impulse control with frequent outbursts and tantrums; labile emotions; **catastrophic reactions** or overreactions to minor stresses occur frequently in demented clients

NCLEX!

b. Wandering or aggressive behavior, hallucinations, delusions

c. Aphasia, which begins with the inability to find words and eventually limits the person to as few as six words

d. Hyperorality, the need to taste, chew, and examine any object small enough to be placed in the mouth

e. Perseveration phenomena, repetitive behaviors such as lip licking, finger tapping, pacing, or echolalia

NCLEX!

f. Confabulation, the filling in of memory gaps with imaginary information in an attempt to distract others from observing the deficit

g. Agraphia, the inability to read or write

h. Agnosia (the inability to recognize familiar situations, people, or stimuli) can occur as auditory, visual, or tactile impairments

1) **Auditory agnosia** is the inability to recognize familiar sounds such as a ringing doorbell or telephone
2) **Astereognosia,** or tactile agnosia, is the inability to identify familiar objects such as a comb or pencil when placed in the hand
3) **Alexia,** or visual agnosia, is the inability to identify an object or its use by sight such as a toothbrush or telephone

3. Stage 3 (lasting 8 to 10 years before death occurs)
   a. Kluver-Bucy syndrome develops, which includes the continuation of hyperorality and the development of binge eating
   b. **Hyperetamorphosis,** the need to compulsively touch and examine every object in the environment
   c. Progressive deterioration in motor ability including inability to walk, sit up, or even to smile
   d. Progressive decrease in response to environmental stimuli leading to total nonresponsiveness or vegetative state
   e. Severe decline in cognitive function, losing ability to recognize others or even self
   f. May scream spontaneously or be able to say only one word; frequently becomes mute

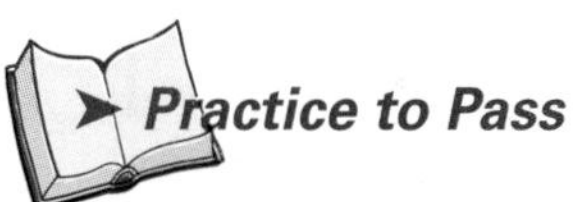

A client becomes increasingly confused as the day goes on. What can you do to provide a safe and secure environment?

C. **Screening tools**

1. Folstein Mini-Mental State Examination: an organic screening tool useful for differentiating dementia from functional states (see Box 10-1 for sample items)
   a. Total score of 30 points
   b. Score of 9–12 indicates a high likelihood of organic illness
2. Cognitive Performance Scale: a subscale from the nursing home Minimum Data Set (MDS)
   a. Ranges from: 0 (cognitively intact) to 6 (very severe cognitive impairment)
   b. Items assessed on the MDS include comatose, short-term memory, decision making ability, making self understood, eating self-performance

Box 10-1

Sample Items from the Mini-Mental State Examination (MMSE)

Orientation to Time

"What is the date?"

Registration

"Listen carefully, I am going to say three words. You say them back after I stop. Ready? Here they are . . .

HOUSE (pause), CAR (pause), LAKE (pause). Now repeat those words back to me." [Repeat up to 5 times, but score only the first trial.]

Naming

"What is this?" [Point to a pencil or pen.]

Reading

"Please read this and do what it says." [Show examinee the words on the stimulus form.]
CLOSE YOUR EYES

3. Geriatric Depression Screening Scale (GDS)

   a. Useful screening tool specifically developed for older adults to screen for possible depression (which can mimic dementia)

   b. A 15- or 30-item questionnaire with dichotomous "yes" or "no" answers; easy to administer in approximately 15 to 20 minutes; certain items are reverse-scored for more accurate assessment

   c. Results indicate absence of or mild depression (0 to 10), moderate depression (11 to 20) or severe depression (21 to 30) (when using the longer 30-item questionnaire)

D. Differentiating between delirium and dementia

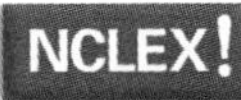

1. Delirium may coexist with dementia, making accurate assessment and appropriate treatment difficult; see Table 10-1 for comparisons between delirium and dementia

2. The most prevalent primary dementia is dementia of the Alzheimer's type (DAT) which occurs in 50 percent of older adults; vascular dementia resulting

Table 10-1 Comparisons between Delirium and Dementia

Delirium	Dementia
Onset is usually sudden; acute development	Onset is insidious and progressive; chronic development
Caused by temporary, reversible disturbance in brain function	Caused by irreversible alteration of brain function
Duration: hours to days	Duration: months to years
EEG: diffuse slowing of fast cycles related to state of excitement	EEG: normal or mildly slow
Disturbed attention, learning, and thinking, poor perception Impaired memory, both recent and remote	Disorientation, impairments in judgment, abstract thinking, and learning Impaired memory (recent memory affected before remote memory)
Orientation: fluctuates throughout day; periods of lucidity; sundown syndrome (worsens at night)	Progressively loses orientation to person, place, and time—loses time orientation first, then place, then person; sundown syndrome
Hallucinations, delusions, illusions	Change in personality; normal peculiarities are exaggerated: suspicious—paranoid, compulsive—rigid, orderliness
Labile affect	Labile affect; prone to apathy, depression, withdrawal, stubbornness in attempt to cope with surroundings and decreased abilities
Act on impulse, loss of usual social behavior	Decreased inhibitions; restlessness, agitation, especially if coerced; inflexible—routine important, anxiety, rage, despair
Coping mechanisms—none, no psychological impairment	Uses denial and repression—confabulation to make up for memory loss
Normal or mild misnaming of objects	Aphasia, agnosia, agraphia in later stages
Nursing Interventions	
Maintain nutrition and fluid balance, could be life-threatening	Not usually life-threatening
Restrain only when necessary since it increases agitation and fear; safety is a priority, one-on-one observation	Individualized attention, consistent social interaction, group activities, exercise, stimulation of senses, active during the day
Repetitive orientation, don't reinforce hallucinations; lighted room, family members present	Lighted room, personal belongings, clear simple instructions; find out source of anxiety, try to alleviate—coping mechanisms to defend self become emphasized during anxiety

from narrowing of the arteries is prevalent in 20 to 50 percent of older adults; less common forms of dementia stem from degenerative nervous system disorders (e.g., Parkinson's disease) and other pathological processes (e.g., AIDS dementia complex)

E. ***Pseudodementia:*** a reversible disorder that frequently mimics dementia

NCLEX!

1. Depression, the most common pseudodementia, is frequently misdiagnosed or overlooked in the older adult; see Table 10-2 for comparisons between dementia and depression
2. Drug toxicity
3. Metabolic disorders
4. Infections
5. Nutritional deficiencies
6. Chronic lung disease and heart disease

F. ***Pseudodelirium:*** symptoms of delirium without any identifiable organic cause

1. Symptoms may occur from psychosocial stress, sensory deprivation or sensory overload (e.g., ICU psychosis)
2. A preexisting biochemical imbalance such as mood disorder, anxiety, schizophrenia, or dementia can make persons vulnerable to pseudodelirium

IV. Nursing Diagnoses/Analysis

A. Priority nursing diagnoses for persons with delirium

1. Acute confusion related to alcohol or drug abuse, medication ingestion, fluid and electrolyte imbalances, infection

Table 10-2

Comparisons between Dementia and Depression

Dementia	Depression
Onset slow and progressive, difficult to pinpoint onset	Onset relatively rapid, can be traced to distressing event or situation
Recent memory is impaired, attempts to hide cognitive losses with confabulation	Readily admits to memory loss; other cognitive impairments may or may not be present; can recall recent events
Affect is shallow and labile	Depressed mood is pervasive
Attention and concentration may be impaired	Attention and concentration usually intact
Unable to recognize familiar people and places, may get lost easily, disoriented to time	Oriented to person, place, and time
Approximate "near miss" answers are common, tries to answer	"Don't know" answers are common, refuses to participate in activities, prefers to be left alone
Changes in personality (from cheerful and easy-going to angry to suspicious)	Personality remains stable
Struggles to perform ADLs, is frustrated as a result	Apathetic to performing ADLs, loses interest in appearance
Appetite and sleep patterns may not be affected	Changes in appetite, weight, and sleep pattern

2. Anxiety related to fear of cognitive and behavioral deficits

3. Altered thought processes related to distractibility, decreasing judgment, memory loss, confabulation, delusions, hallucinations, illusions

4. Bathing/hygiene/dressing/grooming/feeding self-care deficit related to inability to sequence skills necessary to perform these skills

5. Impaired verbal communication related to aphasia, agraphia, agnosia

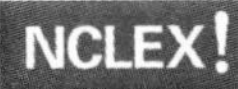

6. Risk for injury or risk for trauma related to aggressive behavior, labile emotions, impaired judgment, illusions, delusions, or hallucinations

7. Sleep pattern disturbance related to fear, anxiety, sundowning, agitation

B. Priority nursing diagnoses for persons with dementia

1. All of the previous nursing diagnoses for persons with delirium are also appropriate for persons with dementia, plus the following:

2. Compromised/disabling ineffective family coping related to changing roles, physical exhaustion, financial problems

3. Risk for and/or caregiver role strain related to lack of respite resources or support from significant others, unpredictable illness course, insufficient finances, aggressive behavior or emotional outbursts of care receiver

4. Visual/auditory/tactile sensory/perceptual alterations related to biochemical imbalances for sensory distortion, agnosia, astereognosia, alexia

5. Self-esteem disturbance related to loss of independent functioning, loss of capacity for remembering, loss of capability for effective verbal communication

NCLEX!

6. Risk for violence: self-directed or directed at others related to confusion, agitated state, suicidal ideation, delusions, hallucinations, illusions

V. Planning and Implementation

A. Specific treatment modalities

1. Psychopharmacology

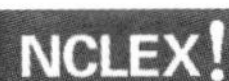

a. Cholinesterase inhibitors can slow down progression of mild to moderate dementia

1) Tacrine (Cognex) effects can be seen in 6 weeks; can cause elevation in liver enzymes, discontinue therapy if occurs

2) Donepezil (Aricept), slows deterioration of mild to moderate dementia without serious liver toxicity attributed to tacrine

b. Management of anxiety, aggression, and agitation

1) Lorazepam (Ativan) 0.5 mg p.o.; less drug accumulation and less confusion than longer-acting anxiolytics; watch for sedation and falls

2) Trazodone (Desyrel) 25 to 500 mg/day; can decrease agitation and aggression without decreasing cognitive performance

3) Buspirone (Buspar) 10 to 60 mg/day; not sedating and has fewer side effects, preferable to benzodiazepines

A client who has been medicated for agitation begins to develop a stiff neck and has difficulty swallowing. You also notice tremors of the hands and strange facial movements. What do you suspect is happening? How would you respond?

c. Management of depression

NCLEX!

1) Selective serotonin reuptake inhibitors (SSRIs) are better tolerated in older adults than tricyclic antidepressants (TCAs), which have high anticholinergic and cardiac side effects

2) Common SSRIs include: fluoxetine (Prozac), paroxetine (Paxil), sertraline (Zoloft), and nefazodone (Serzone)

d. Management of psychotic features (hallucinations and delusions)

1) Atypical antipsychotic agents are more effective in managing positive and negative symptoms without extra-pyramidal side effects

2) Common atypical antipsychotics include: olanzapine (Zyprexa), quetiapine (Seroquel), and risperidone (Risperdal)

NCLEX!

3) Use of haloperidol (Haldol), a potent neuroleptic, is controversial and has been known to cause tardive dyskinesia in older adults; small doses (0.5 mg) may help to regulate sleep

2. Behavior modification

NCLEX!

a. Use of physical restraints should be carefully evaluated and used as a last resort; sensor devices that alert staff when a client is out of bed or going outside should be installed to manage risks to safety from wandering behavior

NCLEX!

b. Reality orientation in the form of labels on objects in the environment, and large-print calendars and clocks can be gentle reminders of information; discuss meaningful topics such as significant life events, family, work, or hobbies to promote the person's identity; avoid arguing with or convincing persons with dementia about actual reality; communicate in a calm, quiet voice with simple, clear instructions

3. Group and individual therapies

NCLEX!

a. Reminiscence or life review therapy: facilitate discussion of topics dealing with specific life transitions such as childhood, adolescence, marriage, childbearing, grandparenthood, and retirement; pets, music, and special foods can be used to evoke memories from client's past; share positive and negative feelings

NCLEX!

b. Validation therapy: interacting with clients on a topic they initiate, in a place and time where they feel most secure; reflecting the underlying feelings of concern (e.g., "You miss your husband. You must be feeling lonely here."); reality orientation is geared toward the person and place rather than to the time

4. Milieu therapy (see Box 10-2)

a. Special care units (SCU): environmentally designed and specifically programmed to serve needs of residents with Alzheimer's disease and related dementias

b. Design components of SCU

NCLEX!

1) Safe, secure, specially adapted physical environment to accommodate wandering behavior inside and outside (circular design, secure walkway and patio)

Box 10-2

Nursing Interventions for Clients with Cognitive Impairment

The following interventions should be incorporated into the care of confused clients:

- Provide simple, clear instructions focusing on one task at a time.
- Break tasks into very small steps.
- Speak slowly and in a face-to-face position when communicating with clients known to have a hearing loss. Shouting causes distortion of high-pitched sounds and can frighten the client.
- Allow the client to have familiar objects around him or her to maintain reality orientation and enhance self-worth and dignity.
- Discuss topics that are meaningful to the client such as significant life events, family, work, hobbies, and pets.
- Refrain from arguing or convincing client that delusions are not real.
- Provide a simple, structured environment with consistent personnel to minimize confusion and provide a sense of security and stability in the client's environment.
- Encourage reminiscence and discussion of life review by sharing picture albums.
- Discuss family traditions and holidays, memories of school, courtship, dating rituals, favorite pets, and other past events.
- Encourage family/caregivers to express feelings, particularly frustration and anger.
- Provide a list of community resources and support groups available to assist in decreasing stress and role strain for the family/caregiver.

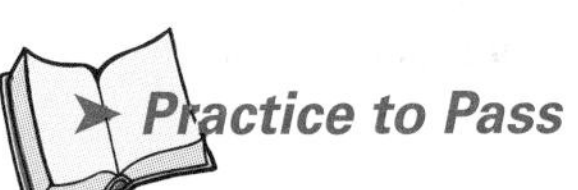

You are the nurse manager of a special care unit for clients with dementia. The wife of a newly admitted client approaches you and says, "I can't take care of him all by myself any longer, but I feel that I am betraying him by placing him in a nursing home." How would you respond?

2) Personalized rooms with own furniture and familiar belongings
3) Clean, well-maintained, well-lit environment with windows
4) Stimuli from birdcage, fish aquarium, or other pets
5) Location adjacent to child daycare programs so that multigenerational interaction occurs

c. Structured programs and activities that provide quality interaction between staff, residents, and families

d. Caring staff: special training programs leading to certification for all levels of education (RN, LPN, CNA); consistent staffing pattern with stable personnel assignments

VI. Evaluation/Outcomes

NCLEX!

A. Client will remain free of injury as evidenced by absence of falls, fractures, bruises, contusions, or burns

B. Client will participate in self-care at optimal level with appropriate degree of supervision and guidance to maintain independence

C. Client will communicate basic needs with the use of visual and verbal clues when needed

D. Caregivers will demonstrate adaptive coping strategies for dealing with the stress of the caregiver role

E. Client will interact with others in group activities, maintaining anxiety at minimal level in response to frustrating situations

F. Client will sleep 5 to 7 hours per night and nap 1 to 2 hours per day

G. Client will maintain stable vital signs and weight

VII. Specific Disorders

A. Labels for specific disorders are those identified in the *Diagnostic and Statistical Manual of Mental Disorders Text Revision* (APA, 2000); descriptions are adapted and summarized

B. Delirium (APA, 2000)

1. Due to (general medical condition): there is evidence from history, physical assessment, or laboratory test results that the disturbance is directly caused by a general medical condition (e.g., delirium due to hepatic encephalopathy)
2. Substance-intoxication delirium: symptoms developed during substance intoxication or medication use (e.g., alcohol intoxication delirium)
3. Substance-withdrawal delirium: symptoms developed during, or shortly after, a withdrawal syndrome (e.g., alcohol withdrawal delirium)
4. Delirium due to multiple etiologies: symptoms developed because of a general medical condition plus substance intoxication or medication side effect
5. Delirium not otherwise specified (NOS): symptoms are suspected to be caused by a general medical condition or substance use, but there is insufficient evidence to establish a specific etiology

C. Dementia (APA, 2000)

1. Dementia of the Alzheimer's type (DAT): cognitive deficits are not caused by other central nervous system conditions known to cause progressive deficits in memory or cognition (e.g., cerebrovascular disease, Parkinson's disease, Huntington's disease, subdural hematoma, normal-pressure hydrocephalus, brain tumor) or systemic conditions known to cause dementia (e.g., hypothyroidism, vitamin deficiencies, hypercalcemia, neurosyphilis, HIV infection) or substance-induced conditions (e.g., dementia of the Alzheimer's type with early onset; with depressed mood)

   NCLEX!

   a. Senile dementia of the Alzheimer's type (SDAT): occurs in people over age 65; characteristic findings are loss of nerve cells and the presence of plaques on neurons and tangles on neuron fibers (see Figure 10-1)

   b. Presenile dementia: occurs in people under age 65

   NCLEX!

   c. Diagnosis is usually made by ruling out causes for clients' symptoms; the only definitive method is a postmortem examination of brain tissue

2. Vascular dementia (formerly multi-infarct dementia): focal neurological signs and symptoms or laboratory test results indicative of cerebrovascular disease are judged to be etiologically related to the disturbance (e.g., vascular dementia, uncomplicated)
3. Dementia due to other general medical conditions: physiological evidence that the disturbance is directly the result of HIV disease, head trauma, Parkinson's disease, Huntington's disease, Pick's disease, Creutzfeldt-Jakob disease, hypothyroidism, brain tumor, or vitamin deficiency (e.g., dementia due to HIV disease)
4. Substance-induced persisting dementia: physiological evidence that the deficits are caused by the persisting effects of substance use (e.g., a drug of abuse, a medication) (e.g., alcohol-induced persisting dementia)

Figure 10-1

Neuron with neurofibrillary tangles seen in Alzheimer's disease.

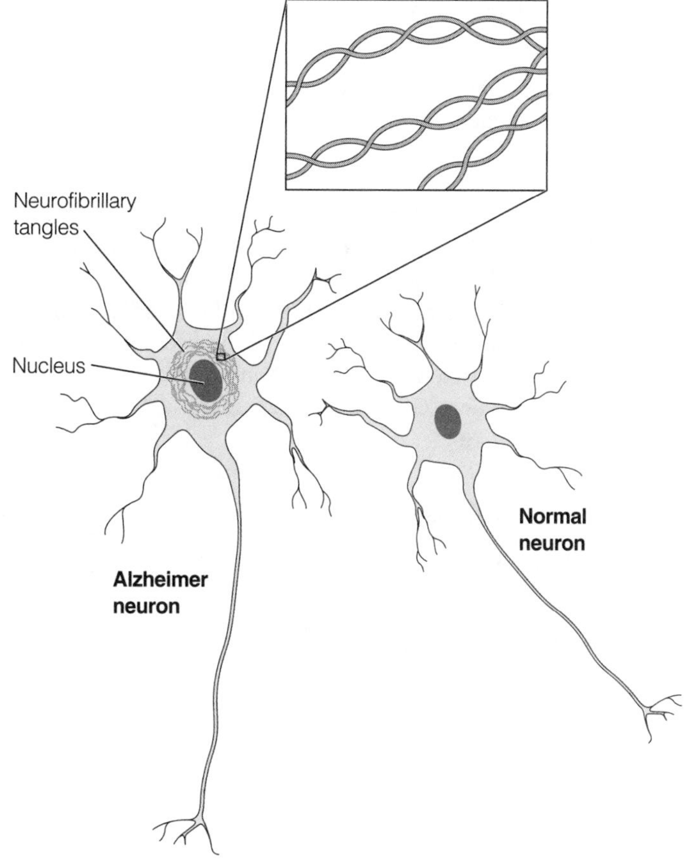

5. Dementia due to multiple etiologies: physiological evidence that the disturbance has more than one etiology (e.g., head trauma plus chronic alcohol use, dementia of the Alzheimer's type with subsequent development of vascular dementia)

6. Dementia not otherwise specified (NOS): clinical presentation of dementia for which there is insufficient evidence to establish a specific etiology

C. Amnestic disorders (APA, 2000)

1. Amnestic disorder due to (general medical condition): there is evidence from history, physical assessment, or laboratory findings that the disturbance is directly caused by a general medical condition (e.g., amnestic disorder due to head trauma)

2. Substance-induced persisting amnestic disorder: physiological evidence that the memory disturbance is related to the persisting effects of drug abuse or medication use (e.g., alcohol-induced persisting amnestic disorder)

3. Amnestic disorder not otherwise specified: clinical presentation of amnesia for which there is insufficient evidence to establish a specific etiology

D. Cognitive disorder not otherwise specified (APA, 2000)

1. Mild neurocognitive disorder: impairment in cognitive functioning as evidenced by neuropsychological testing or clinical assessment accompanied by

objective evidence of a general medical condition or central nervous system dysfunction

2. Postconcussional disorder: following a head trauma, impairment in memory or attention with associated symptoms

Case Study

G. B., an 85-year-old female client, was admitted to the hospital 2 weeks ago with a possible diagnosis of viral pneumonia and acute delirium caused by brain tissue inflammation. Although her medical condition improved markedly, she still had intervals of disorientation, confusion, and memory impairment, particularly at night. You are the nurse working in the skilled nursing facility where G. B. has been transferred.

❶ What initial assessments will you make when G. B. is admitted to your unit?

❷ Identify three nursing diagnoses appropriate in the care of G. B.

❸ What outcome/evaluation criteria might be appropriate for G. B.?

❹ List and describe at least four nursing interventions aimed at promoting safety and security for G. B. and her family.

❺ When G. B.'s daughter asks you about what to do when G. B. insists her deceased husband is away at work and will be coming home soon, how would you respond?

For suggested responses, see pages 308–309.

Posttest

1 **The client with dementia of the Alzheimer's type says to the nurse, "I have a date tonight for the Valentine's dance." The most appropriate response is:**

(1) "You're confused. This isn't Valentine's Day."
(2) "I didn't think your spouse was still living. Who is your date with?"
(3) "I think you need some more medication. I'll be right back with your shot."
(4) "Today is January 11th. Tell me about some of the other dances you've been to."

2 **Which of the following interventions is most appropriate in helping a client with early dementia complete activities of daily living (ADLs)?**

(1) Perform ADLs for the client.
(2) Provide a written list of activities to be completed.
(3) Give the client ample time to perform the ADLs as independently as possible.
(4) Tell the client to finish the ADLs by 9:00 A.M. or else a nurse aide will do them.

3 **The *primary* nursing intervention in working with a client who has a diagnosis of dementia is ensuring that the client:**

(1) Receives favorite foods and drinks to increase nutrition and hydration.
(2) Meets other clients with dementia to prevent social isolation.
(3) Discusses feelings of fear and loss to prevent low self-esteem and anxiety.
(4) Remains in a safe and secure environment to prevent injury.

4 **A client who is fighting against his restraints and shouting incoherently is brought by ambulance to the Emergency Department, accompanied by his girlfriend. She reports that he seemed fine until he took some pills that he had purchased that afternoon, but an hour later "he went crazy." Which of the following actions should the nurse take *first*?**

(1) Take his vital signs.
(2) Check his orientation.
(3) Start intravenous (IV) fluids.
(4) Administer sedative medication.

5 **A client was recently released from wrist and ankle restraints. Suddenly the client begins to beat the sheets and yell, "Get those bugs away from me. They're all over. Get them!" The best initial response by the nurse is:**

(1) "What kind of bugs are on you?"
(2) "Don't worry, those are just little bugs, they won't hurt you."
(3) "You're seeing bugs because you are sick, but I don't see any bugs on you."
(4) "Just hold very still and the bugs will crawl away."

6 **An appropriate nursing diagnosis for a client with a medical diagnosis of delirium caused by a systemic infection is:**

(1) Self-esteem disturbance related to loss of independent functioning.
(2) Risk for caregiver role strain related to lack of respite and financial resources.
(3) Disabling ineffective family coping related to changing roles and financial strain.
(4) Altered thought processes related to elevated temperature.

7 **When working with a client suspected of having Alzheimer's disease, the nurse needs to be alert for increasing agitation that worsens at night, known as:**

(1) Pseudodementia.
(2) Pseudodelirium.
(3) Catastrophic reaction.
(4) Sundown syndrome.

8 **A client with dementia has been admitted to a nursing home. Which of the following nursing actions will help the client maintain optimal cognitive function?**

(1) Discuss pictures of children and grandchildren with the client.
(2) Play word games and do crossword puzzles with the client.
(3) Watch the evening news on the television with the client.
(4) Provide the client with a list of tasks to perform each day.

9 **Which of the following nursing actions would be *most* effective for improving a confused client's level of hydration?**

(1) Place a pitcher of water at the bedside.
(2) Offer a choice of fruit juice, soft drinks, and water every 2 hours while awake.
(3) Instruct all staff members to stop by and offer fluids prn.
(4) Instruct a family member to sit with the client and offer fluids frequently.

10 **A client who scores 11 out of 30 on the Mini-Mental State Examination has a high likelihood of:**

(1) Poor education.
(2) Bipolar disease.
(3) Organic disease.
(4) Low self-esteem.

See pages 206–207 for Answers and Rationales.

Answers and Rationales

Pretest

1 **Answer: 2** ***Rationale:*** Delirium is caused by an underlying physiological condition that can usually be identified and treated. An abnormal EEG is seen during states of arousal in delirium. Atrophy of the cerebral cortex and neuronal plaques are common sequelae associated with Alzheimer's disease.
Cognitive Level: Knowledge
Nursing Process: Assessment; ***Test Plan:*** PSYC

2 **Answer: 3** ***Rationale:*** During stage 2 of Alzheimer's disease, clients have a need to place objects in the mouth so they can taste or chew them, causing a health hazard. This behavior is called hyperorality. Hyperactivity is behavior characterized by decreased attention span, increased impulsivity, and emotional lability. Hyperetamorphosis is the need to compulsively touch and examine every object in the environment. Hyperemesis is characterized by excessive vomiting.
Cognitive Level: Application
Nursing Process: Assessment; ***Test Plan:*** PSYC

3 **Answer: 4** ***Rationale:*** Presenting signs and symptoms of delirium, particularly caused by withdrawal from a substance, include hyperactive behaviors such as restlessness and irritability. Hypoactive behaviors are typical of delirium caused by a metabolic disorder.
Cognitive Level: Application
Nursing Process: Assessment; ***Test Plan:*** PSYC

4 **Answer: 4** ***Rationale:*** Wandering behavior poses a potential risk for injury or trauma because clients experiencing dementia get lost easily and are unable to retrace their steps back home. Although the other nursing diagnoses apply, maintaining the safety of these clients is of utmost importance.
Cognitive Level: Analysis
Nursing Process: Analysis; ***Test Plan:*** PSYC

5 **Answer: 2** ***Rationale:*** Clients with dementia caused by neurological impairment (e.g., secondary to Huntington's disease or Parkinson's disease) may not readily admit to memory loss and use confabulation to fill the deficit. Depression, a form of pseudodementia, can mimic dementia and can cause temporary memory deficits, which are usually acknowledged by the client.
Cognitive Level: Application
Nursing Process: Analysis; ***Test Plan:*** PSYC

6 **Answer: 1** ***Rationale:*** Clients experiencing acute episodes of delirium will have periods of lucidity and will regain full orientation when the underlying cause of the delirium is identified and treated. Suicidal ideation, low self-esteem, and tactile agnosia are problems commonly seen with dementia but not usually associated with delirium.
Cognitive Level: Application
Nursing Process: Planning; ***Test Plan:*** PSYC

7 **Answer: 4** ***Rationale:*** Remembering accomplishments and shared joys helps distract client from deficit and gives meaning to existence. Speaking loudly, arguing, and listening to meaningless music are not effective ways to communicate with or improve the orientation of a client with dementia.
Cognitive Level: Application
Nursing Process: Implementation; ***Test Plan:*** PSYC

8 **Answer: 4** ***Rationale:*** Donepezil (Aricept) is a cholinesterase inhibitor that appears to slow down cognitive deterioration in individuals with mild to moderate dementia. All other options may be prescribed for clients with dementia but have no proven effect for regaining cognitive function.
Cognitive Level: Comprehension
Nursing Process: Implementation; ***Test Plan:*** PHYS

9 **Answer: 3** ***Rationale:*** Short-term memory loss is a sign of depression in the older adult that can be caused by a deficit of serotonin in the brain. Paroxetine (Paxil) blocks the reuptake of serotonin resulting in elevated levels of serotonin in the brain.
Cognitive Level: Comprehension
Nursing Process: Analysis; ***Test Plan:*** PHYS

10 **Answer: 4** ***Rationale:*** Spending nonstressful time with the client helps diminish feelings of resentment, isolation, and alienation. Regular periods of respite are necessary to help caregivers prevent burnout and allow them to continue participating in their life.
Cognitive Level: Analysis
Nursing Process: Evaluation; ***Test Plan:*** PSYC

Posttest

1 **Answer: 4** ***Rationale:*** Option 4 uses a method of reality orientation that increases self-worth and personal dignity. Rumination of delusional thinking, as suggested in option 2, promotes disorientation. Option 1 is demeaning and belittling to the client. No in-

jection, as suggested in option 3, will improve the client's dementia symptoms.
Cognitive Level: Analysis
Nursing Process: Implementation; ***Test Plan:*** PSYC

2 **Answer: 3** ***Rationale:*** Clients with dementia need extra time to perform tasks; therefore, option 3 is the most appropriate response. A written list or an ultimatum to perform ADLs within a strict time frame may be overwhelming to the client and increase confusion. Performing ADLs for the client does not promote an ability for independent action.
Cognitive Level: Analysis
Nursing Process: Implementation; ***Test Plan:*** PSYC

3 **Answer: 4** ***Rationale:*** Client safety and security are nursing priorities for clients with disorientation, confusion, and memory deficits seen in dementia; therefore, option 4 should take precedence over all other interventions.
Cognitive Level: Analysis
Nursing Process: Implementation; ***Test Plan:*** PSYC

4 **Answer: 1** ***Rationale:*** The highest priority is given to nursing interventions that will maintain life; therefore, basic physiological needs must be addressed initially with baseline vital signs. Nutrition and fluid balance may be maintained by IV therapy once vital signs are evaluated and a physician's order is obtained. Checking the level of orientation is important but does not provide any new information to the nurse. Sedative medications may complicate an attempt to identify the original cause of the confusion.
Cognitive Level: Analysis
Nursing Process: Implementation; ***Test Plan:*** PSYC

5 **Answer: 3** ***Rationale:*** The most appropriate response is option 3, which orients the client to the reality of being sick and reassures the client of safety. By agreeing with the client that the bugs exist, as in options 1, 2, and 4, the nurse is communicating that the hallucinated objects are real and can make the client feel even more frightened.
Cognitive Level: Application
Nursing Process: Implementation; ***Test Plan:*** PSYC

6 **Answer: 4** ***Rationale:*** Most cognitive impairments seen in delirium are physiological in origin; therefore, the identified problem and all its effects should be reflected in a complete nursing diagnosis found in option 4. Options 1, 2, and 3 are more reflective of the psychosocial processes associated with dementia.
Cognitive Level: Application
Nursing Process: Analysis; ***Test Plan:*** PSYC

7 **Answer: 4** ***Rationale:*** Clients with dementia often experience extreme agitation at the end of the day, probably as a result of tiredness and fewer orienting stimuli such as planned activities and contact with people. This restless and agitated behavior worsens at night and is commonly referred to as sundown syndrome. Pseudodementia is a reversible disorder that mimics dementia. Pseudodelirium is characterized by symptoms of delirium without any identifiable organic cause. Catastrophic reaction is the overreaction toward minor stresses that occurs in demented clients.
Cognitive Level: Comprehension
Nursing Process: Analysis; ***Test Plan:*** PSYC

8 **Answer: 1** ***Rationale:*** Recent memory loss is a common problem found in dementia; therefore, the client may be frustrated when constantly confronted with evidence of failing memory. The activities suggested by options 2, 3, and 4 rely on recall of recent memories rather than remote memories and can cause increased anxiety and confusion. Pictures of family members can encourage a discussion of remote memories that will help the client feel less anxious while promoting a sense of pleasure from discussing past experiences.
Cognitive Level: Application
Nursing Process: Implementation; ***Test Plan:*** PSYC

9 **Answer: 2** ***Rationale:*** When working with a confused client, the most effective nursing action is simple, direct, and unambiguous. Option 2 is the most effective nursing action designed to increase the client's fluid intake.
Cognitive Level: Application
Nursing Process: Implementation; ***Test Plan:*** PSYC

10 **Answer: 3** ***Rationale:*** A Mini-Mental State Examination score of less than 20 usually indicates the presence of dementia or delirium and requires further investigation. The Mini-Mental State Examination does not measure education, bipolar disorder, or self-esteem.
Cognitive Level: Application
Nursing Process: Assessment; ***Test Plan:*** PSYC

References

American Psychiatric Association (2000). *Diagnostic and statistical manual of mental disorders* (4th ed. text revision). Washington, DC: American Psychiatric Association, pp. 35–80.

Cleary, B. & Fontaine, K. (1999). Cognitive impairment disorders. In K. Fontaine & J. Fletcher (Eds.), *Mental health nursing* (4th ed.). Menlo Park, CA: Addison-Wesley, pp. 373–398.

Ebersole, P. & Hess P. (2001). *Geriatric nursing and healthy aging.* St. Louis: Mosby, pp. 436–459.

Garand, L., Gerdner, L., Wakefield, B., & Buckwalter, K. (1998). Neuropsychiatric disorders. In M. Boyd & M. Nihart (Eds.), *Psychiatric nursing: Contemporary practice.* Philadelphia: Lippincott-Raven, pp. 612–666.

Glendon, K. & Ulrich, D. (2001). *Unfolding case studies: Experiencing the realities of clinical nursing practice.* Upper Saddle River, NJ: Prentice-Hall, Inc., pp. 85–87, 101–105.

Keltner, N. & Folks, D. (2001). Dementia and delirium. In N. Keltner & D. Folks (Eds.), *Psychotropic drugs* (3rd ed.). St. Louis: Mosby, pp. 213–245.

Laraia, M. & Sundeen, S. (2001). Cognitive responses and organic mental disorders. In G. Stuart & M. Laraia (Eds.), *Principles and practice of psychiatric nursing* (7th ed.). St. Louis: Mosby, pp. 460–484.

LeMone, P. & Burke, K. (2000). *Medical-surgical nursing: Critical thinking in client care* (2nd ed.). Upper Saddle River, NJ: Prentice Hall-Health, Inc., pp. 1818–1827.

North American Nursing Diagnosis Association (1999). *NANDA nursing diagnoses: Definitions and classification, 1999–2000.* Philadelphia: North American Nursing Diagnosis Association, pp. 34–136.

Pace-Murphy, K., Dyer, C., & Gleason, M. (2000). Delirium, dementia, and amnestic and other cognitive disorders. In K. Fortinash & P. Holoday-Worret (Eds.), *Psychiatric mental health nursing* (2nd ed.). St. Louis: Mosby, pp. 386–414.

Townsend, M. (2000). *Psychiatric mental health nursing: Concepts of care* (3rd ed.). Philadelphia: F. A. Davis, pp. 339–356.

Townsend, M. (2001). *Nursing diagnoses in psychiatric nursing: Care plans and psychotropic medications* (5th ed.). Philadelphia: F. A. Davis, pp. 95–112.

Varcarolis, E. (1998). Cognitive disorders. In E. Varcarolis (Ed.), *Foundations of psychiatric mental health nursing* (3rd ed.). Philadelphia: W. B. Saunders, pp. 681–718.

Varcarolis, E. (2000). *Psychiatric nursing clinical guide: Assessment tools and diagnoses.* Philadelphia: W. B. Saunders, pp. 323–352.

CHAPTER 11

Substance Use Disorders

Ann Koranda, RN, CNS, LADC, CGP

CHAPTER OUTLINE

OBJECTIVES

- Discuss at least six causative factors associated with substance abuse or dependence.
- Identify five behavior patterns of substance use of clients with substance abuse.
- Differentiate between psychological and physical dependency.
- State examples of at least five nursing diagnoses frequently used for clients exhibiting clinical symptoms of psychoactive substance abuse or dependency.
- Describe four treatment modalities for acute intoxication and detoxification.

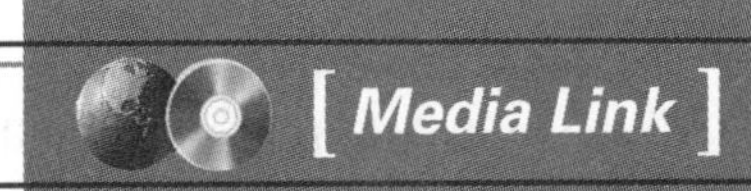

Use the CD-ROM enclosed with this text, or log onto the address given to access the free, interactive Companion Website created for this series. The CD-ROM and Companion Website accompanying this book offer additional practice opportunities and information—NCLEX Review, Case Studies, Glossary, In Depth with NCLEX, and more.

www.prenhall.com/hogan

Review at a Glance

abstinence *a term that indicates someone has quit or stopped their addictive behavior; is not synonymous with recovery or healing from addiction*

chemical dependence *a chronic, progressive disease that can be fatal if left untreated*

craving *a psychological "hungry" feeling to engage in addictive behavior even if an individual was not originally planning to use, or thinking about using the substance or engaging in the addictive behavior*

dependence *a diagnostic term that means an individual's chemical use patterns or addictive behavior meets three of the seven criteria needed to make the diagnosis of dependence*

physical dependence *a physiological adaptation to the drug; withdrawal can occur only when an individual acquires physical dependence*

process addiction *a behavioral syndrome characterized by preoccupation with the activity and compulsion to engage in the activity despite negative consequences*

recovery *a term that means someone is abstinent and working a program of personal growth and self discovery*

relapse *a term used to describe someone who has returned to active addictive behavior*

substance abuse *the purposeful use, for at least 1 month, of a drug that results in adverse effects to oneself or others*

substance dependence *occurs when drug use is no longer under control and continues despite adverse effects*

tolerance *reduced response to a drug's action; it can be biologically inherited or developed gradually over time*

withdrawal *a condition that occurs after a person who has used a substance regularly and heavily has recently decreased or stopped use, and now demonstrates a pattern of signs and symptoms that in general are the opposite of the acute effects of the drug*

Pretest

1 **A nurse is teaching a new group of inpatients about addiction. The clients say they can stop drinking whenever they want. These clients still lack the understanding that addiction is a disease in which individuals lose permanent ability to:**

(1) Regulate their addictive and impulsive behaviors.
(2) Recognize that their addictive behavior is harmful to themselves and others.
(3) Act sober even if they are not.
(4) Identify with a higher power.

2 **The clients in a psycho-education class on addiction express the feeling that they cannot relate with other clients who do not have the same kind of addictions as they do. The nurse teaches about the similarities and the differences between process and chemical addictions. The nurse would evaluate that the clients understand the difference between process addictions and chemical addictions when they say,**

(1) "Withdrawal is not associated with process addictions."
(2) "Intoxication is not associated with process addictions."
(3) "Tolerance is not associated with process addictions."
(4) "There is a difference between process and chemical addictions."

3 **Upon orientation to the addiction treatment unit the nurse informs the client of the family program and suggests that the client invite his son to the sessions. The client questions why his 13-year-old son needs to participate, as he has not seen his father drunk. The nurse's *best* response would be:**

(1) "There generally are no consequences from the addictive behavior because the parent is usually sober when they are with the children."
(2) "There generally are no consequences from the addictive behavior because the parents are using responsibly when they are with the children."
(3) "There are generally consequences from the addictive behavior because the child knows they are using even if they do not see it."
(4) "There are generally consequences from the addictive behavior because parents are impaired whether they are actively using or recovering from use."

4 The nurse provides an inservice on impaired nursing practice. The nurse evaluates teaching as effective, when the staff is able to identify that the *most* influential risk for impaired nursing practice is that:

(1) "Most nurses are adult children of alcoholics or dysfunctional families and are at risk for developing addiction."
(2) "Most nurses have exposure to various substances and believe they are not at risk to develop the disease."
(3) "Most nurses have preconceived ideas about 'what kind of people' get addictions."
(4) "Most nurses are codependent in their personal and professional relationships."

5 A client comes to day treatment intoxicated but says he is not. The nurse's evaluation of his symptomatology reveals:

(1) Denial.
(2) Reaction formation.
(3) Transference.
(4) Countertransference.

6 A client expresses to the nurse that he feels his family and friends are against him. They have expressed concern that his continued drinking could be fatal given that he has developed alcoholic cardiomyopathy. The *best* response by the nurse would be:

(1) "The person expressing concern has a problem with his or her own drinking."
(2) "The person expressing concern has no right to judge another person's drinking."
(3) "The person expressing concern may be jealous that the client can drink more than they can."
(4) "The person expressing concern has noticed the client's drinking creates consequences for them."

7 A client who presents in the psychiatric unit tells the admitting nurse she is having a hard time staying sober and is very depressed. The rationale for treating the depression in a client with substance abuse is:

(1) Depression can often keep an individual from working on a recovery program.
(2) Depression should be treated only after the client has been sober for 1 month.
(3) Depression is a symptom of substance abuse.
(4) Depression is an expected outcome of substance abuse recovery.

8 The student nurse has to go to an Alcoholics Anonymous (AA) meeting as part of the clinical rotation and report back what he or she finds out about the meeting. The student finds that the Twelve Steps of AA teaches that:

(1) Once an individual has learned to be sober, they can graduate from the program.
(2) Once an individual has learned to be sober, they can remain at risk to use.
(3) Acceptance of being an alcoholic will prevent urges to drink.
(4) A Higher Power will protect individuals if they feel like using.

9 The nurse working in obstetrics is reinforcing the physician health teaching about the risks of using substances during pregnancy. The client states that she only drinks a little beer and wine and would never use any dangerous drugs. The nurse then assesses for use of which drug that causes the most physical, cognitive, and growth and developmental problems to the fetus?

(1) Benzodiazepines
(2) Hallucinogens
(3) Alcohol
(4) Cocaine

10 A client who was discharged from addiction treatment on disulfiram (Antabuse) medication 3 months ago, returns to the liver service for his follow-up appointment. During the nursing assessment, the nurse prepares the chart for review and notices the lab work from last week indicates that the GGT is as high as the GGT from his inpatient addiction treatment. The nurse would could infer that the client is:

(1) Drinking or experiencing liver problems from the Antabuse.
(2) Using marijuana or experiencing liver problems from the Antabuse.
(3) Eating fatty foods, not exercising, or experiencing problems from the Antabuse.
(4) Recently exposed to measles or experiencing problems from the Antabuse.

See pages 230–231 for Answers and Rationales.

I. Overview

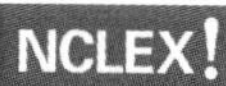

A. ***Substance abuse*** is defined as the purposeful use, for at least 1 month, of a drug that results in adverse effects to oneself or others

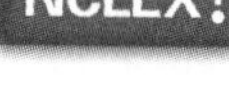

B. ***Substance dependence*** occurs when the use of the drug is no longer under control and continues despite adverse effects

C. ***Chemical dependence*** is a chronic, progressive disease that can be fatal if left untreated

1. A medical and spiritual illness with well-defined signs and symptoms including denial and relapse

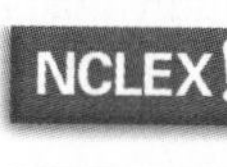

2. Disease progression and course of illness is predictable and treatable

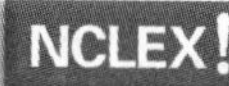

3. Treatment focus is **abstinence** (voluntarily going without drugs), medications as appropriate, education, lifestyle change, and increasing self-awareness and personal growth

D. Statistics

1. Substance use disorders in the United States cost over $300 billion a year

2. Alcoholism is a major health problem, one that is responsible for 100,000 deaths annually in the United States

3. 7.5 percent of the population is chemically dependent

4. 1 out of every 10 persons is said to be alcoholic

E. Types and various diagnoses of addiction

1. Addictive substances and **process addictions** syndrome are characterized by preoccupation with and compulsion to engage in an activity (see Box 11-1 for a list of addictive substances and process addictions)

a. Substances

1) Depressants (opiate/opioids/sedatives/hypnotics)

2) Stimulants

3) Cannabinoids/hallucinogens

4) Inhalants

Box 11-1

A List of Addictive Substances and Process Addictions

Top Three Most Abused Substances

1. Alcohol
2. Nicotine
3. Caffeine

Top Twenty Most Abused Controlled and Illicit Substances

1. Cocaine
2. Heroin
3. Marijuana
4. Alprazolam (Xanax)
5. Diazepam (Valium)
6. Lorazepam (Ativan)
7. Clonazepam (Klonopin)
8. Methamphetamine
9. Codeine combinations
10. Unspecified benzodiazepines
11. D-Propoxyphene (Darvon, Darvocet)
12. PCP and PCP combinations
13. Hydrocodone (Vicodin, Lorcet, Lortab)
14. Amphetamine
15. Hashish
16. Temazepam (Restoril)
17. Oxycodone (Percodan, Percocet, Tylox, Roxicodone, OxyContin)
18. LSD
19. Chlordiazepoxide (Librium, Libritabs)
20. Methadone

Top Five Process Addictions

1. Eating disorders
2. Pathological gambling
3. Compulsive sexual behaviors
4. Compulsive shopping/spending
5. Compulsive internet use

b. Processes

1) Eating disorder

2) Compulsive gambling

3) Compulsive sexual disorders

4) Compulsive shopping/spending

5) Compulsive internet use

2. Definitions of substance use disorders

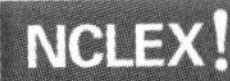

a. DSM-IV clinical syndromes

1) Intoxication

2) Withdrawal

3) Abuse

4) Dependence

b. The American Society of Addiction Medicine (ASAM) defines chemical dependence as a *primary,* chronic relapsing *disease* with genetic, psychosocial, and environmental factors influencing it; the disease is often *progressive and fatal;* it is characterized by continuous periodic *impaired control* over the substance; *preoccupation* with the substance; use of the substance despite *adverse consequences;* and distortions in thinking, most notably denial; inherent in the definition are the concepts of **tolerance, withdrawal, physical dependence,** and psychological dependence

NCLEX!

c. American Nurses Association and National Nurses Society on Addictions (ANA and NNSA) define addiction as an illness characterized by compulsion, loss of control, and continued pattern of abuse despite perceived negative consequences; obsession with a dysfunctional habit; the dysfunctional patterns include patterns of alcoholism, drug abuse, misuse of tobacco, eating disorders, excessive gambling or spending, and certain compulsive sexual disorders

F. **Medical theory of addiction:** Jellinek four phases of alcoholism

1. Prealcoholic symptomatic phase
   a. Distinct symptoms that the social drinker does not experience
   b. Drinking to cope with emotions
   c. Lack of recognition that tension is caused by drinking
   d. Phase lasts several months to 2 years
2. Prodromal phase
   a. Begins drinking in secret
   b. Gulps first few sips
   c. Attachment to alcohol present
   d. Access to alcohol involved in planning all social activities
   e. Tolerance develops (needing more alcohol to get the same effect)
   f. Continue engaging in drinking despite negative consequences
   g. Feels guilty about drinking
   h. Isolated and withdrawn
   i. Mood swings, diminished self-esteem
   j. Phase lasts 6 months to 5 years
3. Crucial phase

NCLEX!

   a. Beginning of disease process and psychological dependence
   b. Intermittent loss of control ensues when drinking (uses more than intended)
   c. Preoccupation with use develops
   d. Use of defense mechanisms
   e. Experiences craving triggers to use
   f. Concern over drinking expressed by others
   g. Anger, alienation of family and friends
   h. Drops all non-drinking socialization including friends who don't drink
   i. Activities of daily living (ADLs) suffer: sleep, appetite, and energy problems present
   j. Family issues surface: alienation, anger, role and relationship problems
4. Chronic phase
   a. Drinks to blackout/pass-out/incapacitation

b. Cognitive, physical, emotional, health deterioration

c. Reverse tolerance may develop (less quantity than previously required to bring intoxication)

d. Life begins to fall apart

5. Jellinek's theory can be applied to chemical dependency and process addiction

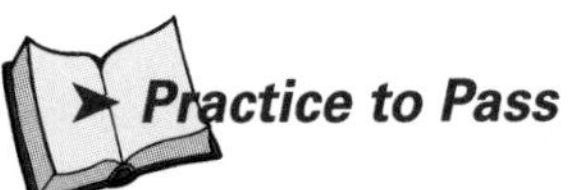

Your client's son arrives intoxicated to visit his medically ill father on the unit. The client is concerned, starts crying, and asks you for your assistance. How would you respond?

G. Jellinek model applied to process addictions

1. Contact phase

   a. Discover that engaging in addictive behavior is fun

   b. Finds that it gives pleasure or reduces pain

2. Serendipitous phase: discovers that engaging in addictive behaviors helps person cope with distress

3. Instrumental phase

   a. Consciously uses addictive behavior to cope with distress

   b. Behavior becomes routine

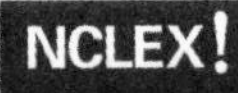

4. Dependent phase

   a. Unable to cope with life without engaging in the addictive behavior

   b. Experiences intermittent loss of control

   c. Unable to stop despite negative consequences

II. Etiology

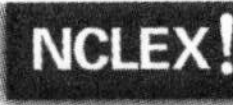

A. **Addiction is a chronic brain disease** evidenced by abnormalities in the neuronal activities of the Brain Reward System (BRS)

B. Brain structures involved in the addiction process

1. Ventral tegmental area
2. Nucleus accumbens
3. Mesolimbic dopaminergic pathways
4. Endogenous opioid and serotonin system
5. Neurotransmitters and receptor sites

C. Process of BRS activation

1. All drugs affect the cells in some way, either increasing or decreasing some cellular activities

2. Use of mood-altering substances or engaging in addictive behaviors causes increased availability of dopamine/serotonin/opioid peptides and facilitates other neurotransmitter (gamma-aminobutyric acid, glutamate, acetylcholine) dysregulation

3. Short-term euphoric response is generated by this activity, which eventually leads to the symptoms of addictive thinking, denial, and impaired control

4. Euphoric response engenders the immediate and profound desire for readministration (**cravings** that are like a psychological "hunger," triggers, and urges)

5. The positive immediate short-term euphoria overshadows any long-term consequences associated with engaging in addictive behaviors
6. Continued use leads to development of tolerance
7. Experience of tolerance leads to increased dose and frequency of use
8. Physical dependence and withdrawal syndrome may develop
9. Psychological dependence develops

D. Genetic/biologic risk

1. No one specific marker is responsible for addictions—the more risk factors the greater the risk for developing the disease

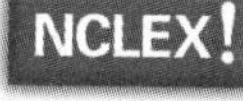

2. Genetics: twins studies demonstrate a 30 to 50 percent vulnerability for addictions; sons and daughters of alcoholics have a four and three times higher tolerance and occurrence of addiction over sons and daughters of nonalcoholic parents
3. Biology: intrapersonal genetic vulernabilities leading to BRS abnormalities

E. Psychosocial risk

1. Personality traits: individuals with certain personality traits are thought to be susceptible to the reinforcing effects of engaging in addictive behaviors
   - **a.** Antisocial: lack of responsiveness to people, places, and things in their environment; persons with antisocial personality traits experience a positive response to the psychoactive properties of engaging in addictive behavior
   - **b.** Introversion: feelings of inadequacy or low self-esteem are mediated by the euphoric effect of engaging in addictive behavior
   - **c.** Impulsiveness: impulsivity is reinforced because of the inability to anticipate impending negative consequences of use
2. Developmental failures: individuals who have lived with painful experiences are at risk to self-medicate or misuse their medication
   - **a.** Abuse survivors—may experience disturbances in their sense of self
   - **b.** Lack of nurturance in childhood—may lead to an inability to self-soothe
   - **c.** Coping skills deficit
   - **d.** Positive coping skills may not have been learned in the person's family of origin
   - **e.** The learning of positive coping skills may have been inhibited because of the positive reinforcing effect of euphoria when using an addictive drug or behavior to cope with feelings

F. Dual disorders risk

1. At least 33 percent of individuals with a psychiatric disorder develop addiction
   - **a.** Individuals with psychiatric disorders are at risk for developing addictive disorders
   - **b.** Initially drugs and alcohol may have been used to help individuals deal with being depressed, being anxious, or having painful memories
   - **c.** With continued use addiction develops for individuals at risk

NCLEX!

2. Individuals with addiction are at risk for developing psychiatric disorders

a. At least 33 percent of individuals with addiction develop a psychiatric disorder

b. Substance use can induce the development of psychiatric illness as the nucleus accumbens and the ventral tegmental area (plays a role in cognition, motivation and learning) and the neurotransmitter system (plays a role in mood regulation) are affected

c. Any one of a number of psychiatric disorders can develop

3. Individual with addictive disorders may be misdiagnosed as some disorders mask addiction (see Table 11-1 for disorders that can mask addiction or coexist with addiction)

a. Mood disorders

b. Anxiety disorders

c. Adjustment disorders

d. Sleep disorders

e. Personality disorders

f. Antisocial disorders

g. Psychotic disorders

h. Chronic pain

i. Disorders of delirium, dementia, amnesia and other cognitive disorders

NCLEX!

4. Individuals with dual diagnosis and who are intoxicated are at increased risk of suicide

NCLEX!

5. Treatment for dual diagnosis is more successful if both illnesses are treated concurrently

G. Environmental risk

1. Social learning theory: use of addictive substances is a learned behavior

a. Normalized behavior: engaging in addictive behavior is influenced by exposure to peer pressure, role models, societal norms

b. Culture: engaging in addictive behaviors is influenced by culture; certain cultural groups have use patterns that put them at risk for developing addiction (e.g., Finnish, British, Native American)

NCLEX!

2. Profession: healthcare professionals (HCPs) are at risk to develop addictive disorders because the high stress and pressure of their jobs and exposure to substances; HCPs also believe their knowledge about the disease and health protects them from the euphoric reinforcing effects of self-medicating and addictive behaviors

NCLEX!

a. The impaired nurse: nurses are at risk for developing addictive disorders

1) 10 percent of nurses working in most specialties and 15 percent of nurse anesthetists develop addiction

Table 11-1 **The Process of Dual Diagnosis: Differences among Chemical Dependency, Anxiety, Depression, and Chronic Pain**

Dynamics	Chemical Dependency	Anxiety	Depression	Chronic Pain
Contributing factors to the development of disease	Alcohol and other drug use Changes in brain chemistry and function Biology Environment Psychosocial Factors	Alcohol and other drug use Changes in brain chemistry and function Biology Environment Psychosocial factors	Alcohol and other drug use Changes in brain chemistry and function Biology Environment Psychosocial factors	Multiple non-malignant medical problems Changes in brain chemistry and function
Symptoms	Sleep/appetite disturbance Tolerance/withdrawal/progression Loss of control of substance use and behavior; preoccupation with use Continued use despite negative consequences Denial: distortions in thinking, feeling, and behavior Physical, interpersonal, social occupational, legal, and spiritual problems Hospitalization, incarceration, thoughts of suicide Feelings of helplessness/hopelessness	Muscle tension and overactive bodily responses: pounding heart, panic, trembling Hypervigilance Distortions in thinking, feeling, and behavior Avoidance of feared situations Physical, interpersonal, social, occupational, legal, and spiritual problems Hospitalization, immobilization, thoughts of suicide Feelings of helplessness/hopelessness	Appetite disturbance and sleep, decreased energy level Sad or irritable mood Loss of pleasure or interest in most enjoyable activities Distortions in thinking, feeling, and behavior Physical, interpersonal, social, occupational, legal, and spiritual problems Hospitalization, immobilization, thoughts of suicide Feelings of helplessness/hopelessness	Tolerance/withdrawal Medication misuse Anxiety, worry, frustration Sad or irritable mood Distortions in thinking, feeling, and behavior Loss of pleasure or interest in most enjoyable activities Physical, interpersonal, social, occupation, legal, and spiritual problems Hospitalization, immobilization, thoughts of suicide Feelings of helplessness/hopelessness
Recovery components	Abstinence: medications to help stop using mood-altering substances Social support: 12-step group Cognitive restructuring Relaxation training Education: disease/recovery process Practice recovery skills Coping skills training Psychotherapy: group therapy/group counseling Exercise/nutrition/sleep Changes in negative lifestyle habits	Nonaddictive anti-anxiety medications Social support Cognitive restructuring Relaxation training Education: disease/recovery process Practice recovery skills Coping skills training Psychotherapy: group therapy/group counseling Exercise/nutrition/sleep Changes in negative lifestyle habits	Antidepressant medication Social support Cognitive restructuring Relaxation training Education: disease/recovery process Practice recovery skills Coping skills training Psychotherapy: group therapy/group counseling Exercise/nutrition/sleep Changes in negative lifestyle habits	Nonaddictive pain medications Social activity Cognitive restructuring Relaxation training Education: disease/recovery process Practice recovery skills Coping skills training Group support/group counseling Exercise/nutrition/sleep Changes in negative lifestyle habits

2) Nursing practice is impaired when an individual is unable to meet the requirements of the professional code of ethics and standards of practice because of cognitive, interpersonal, or psychomotor skills affected by conditions of the individual (psychiatric illness, excessive alcohol or drug use or addiction) in interaction with the environment

b. Risk factors for vulnerability

1) Access to drugs
2) Long hours
3) Tremendous responsibility
4) Job-related stress
5) Family history of chemical dependence

c. Signs and symptoms of the nurse who abuses drugs and alcohol

1) Increased irritability with clients and colleagues
2) Mood swings, may be shifting rapidly; might be calm after taking drugs
3) Withdrawn, isolated: wants to work night shift; avoids informal staff get-togethers
4) Purposely waits until alone to open the narcotic cabinet
5) Late for work; misses work; elaborate excuses for missing work
6) Work quality decreases
7) Charting is illegible
8) Signs out more narcotics than other nurses on the unit

d. System response

1) Intervention and immunity from prosecution
2) In most states, there is opportunity for supportive intervention rather than loss of licensure if the impaired nurse seeks treatment and follows the monitoring recommendation from the Board of Nursing in the state in which he or she practices

III. Assessment

A. Commonly abused substances and addictive behaviors: addictive use patterns are gathered from a standardized screening and assessment tool and nursing baseline assessment

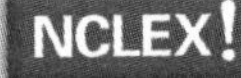

1. Screening/assessment tools

a. CAGE

1) Have you ever:
   a) Attempted to *Cut back* on your alcohol?
   b) Been *Annoyed* by comments made about your drinking?
   c) Felt *Guilty* about your drinking?
   d) Had an *Eye-opener* in the morning to calm your nerves?
2) A positive answer for two of the screening questions indicates a need for further assessment

An elderly client is confused about the reason why he was transferred to the inpatient addictions unit. She says she only has two drinks a night. What additional assessment data do you need before you can respond to her concern?

b. Michigan Alcoholism Screening Test (MAST)

c. Addiction Severity Index (ASI)

B. **Nursing admission assessment data** that focuses on use of mood-altering chemicals

1. Physical assessment/systems review

a. Blackout or lost consciousness: blacking out or passing out can be related to a person's use of alcohol or other substances

b. Changes in bowel movement: persons using alcohol and/or drugs frequently can experience changes in bowel movement; changes range from diarrhea because of drinking to constipation from using pain medications frequently; withdrawal from narcotics can cause diarrhea

c. Weight loss or weight gain: persons using alcohol or drugs regularly may experience weight loss/gain and/or poor nutritional balance

d. Experiencing stressful situation: stress can precipitate an increase in drinking; stress can also result from drinking or using drugs regularly

e. Sleep problems: persons using alcohol and/or other drugs experience all sorts of sleep problems; one may start using alcohol to promote sleep, but once someone develops tolerance, sleep is more difficult

f. Chronic pain: persons experiencing chronic pain may use drugs and/or alcohol to self-medicate

g. Concern over substance use: if friends and relatives worry about substance use, it is generally because there is something to be concerned about

h. Cutting down on alcohol consumption (or drug use, prescription medication use, gambling, or addictive behavior): if one feels that he or she must cut down, it is usually because there are problems

2. Personal family assessment: persons with positive family history are at risk for developing an addictive disorder

NCLEX!

3. Chemical use assessment: key elements

a. Identify type of substance used

b. Identify type of compulsive behavior

c. Pattern and frequency of substance use

d. Amount

e. Age at onset

f. Age of regular use

g. Changes in use patterns

h. Periods of abstinence in history

i. Previous withdrawal symptoms

j. Date of last substance use/compulsive behavior

k. Ask about each substance or behavior separately

l. Ranges of illicit drugs can be ingested into the body in numerous ways; remember that about 33 percent of alcohol users also use another substance

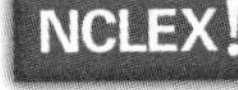

4. Medication assessment

   a. Ask about pain-relief medications, laxatives, cold medications, sleep and/or stay awake medications, and/or anxiety/nerve control medications

   b. Prescribed dose is now not enough to control pain/anxiety even though it might have helped at the beginning

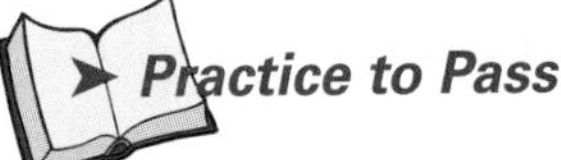

A client is not experiencing pain relief from the Darvocet that you administered 90 minutes ago. What are you concerned about?

   c. Runs out of medication early and needs a refill early

   d. Pain medication that is used for physical pain is now used for emotional pain

   e. Medication is used for dealing with "stress" or stressful events

   f. More medication was taken than intended

   g. Laxatives are used regularly because the pain medications cause constipation or because the individual has difficulty having bowel movements without the use of laxatives

   h. Cold tablets or cough syrup are taken more frequently than expected

5. Over-the-counter (OTC) or nutritional supplement assessment: use of any herbal, vitamin or OTC products to help with sleep, weight loss, staying awake, giving more energy, stabilizing mood and/or improving mood, or making client feel a certain way?

6. Social history assessment: persons experiencing physical, sexual, or emotional abuse may medicate internal distress by using mood-altering substances

7. Laboratory value assessment: laboratory values that may be abnormal in substance abusers:

   a. Gamma glutamyl transferase (GGT)

   b. Aspartate aminotransferase (SGOT/SGPT)

   c. Alkaline phosphatase (AK)

   d. Lactate dehydrogenase (LD)

   e. Mean corpuscular volume (MCV)

   f. Urine toxicology and blood screen for drugs of abuse is also an essential component of the substance use evaluation

IV. Nursing Diagnoses/Analysis

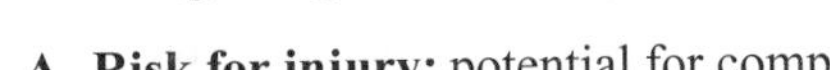

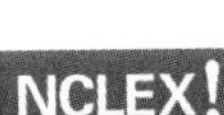

A. **Risk for injury:** potential for complications of substance withdrawal

B. **Risk for injury:** potential for relapse

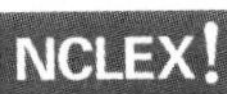

C. **Altered family process:** addictive disorder

D. **Knowledge deficit:** addictive disorder

E. **Anxiety:** a vague, uneasy feeling, feeling of discomfort or dread accompanied by an autonomic response, the source of which is often non-specific or unknown to the individual; a feeling of apprehension caused by anticipation of danger; it is an alerting signal that warns of impending danger and enables the individual to take measures to deal with threat (NANDA, 20001, p. 19)

F. **Ineffective coping:** inability to form a valid appraisal of the stressors, inadequate choices of practical responses, and/or inability to use available resources (NANDA, p. 54)

G. **Impaired social interactions:** an individual participates in an insufficient or excessive quantity or ineffective quality of social exchange (NANDA, p. 171)

H. **Ineffective denial:** an attempt to disavow the knowledge or meaning of an event to reduce anxiety/fear to the detriment of health (NANDA, p. 63)

I. **Self-esteem disturbance:** negative self-evaluation and feelings about self or self-capacities, which may be directly or indirectly expressed

J. **Dysfunctional grieving:** extended unsuccessful use of intellectual and emotional responses by which individuals attempt to work through the process of modifying self-concept based upon the perception of loss (NANDA, p. 88)

K. **Impaired adjustment:** inability to modify his or her lifestyle or behavior in a manner consistent with a change in health status (NANDA, p. 15)

L. **Disturbed sleep pattern:** time-limited disruption of sleep (natural, periodic suspension of consciousness) amount and quality (NANDA, p. 169)

M. **Chronic pain:** an unpleasant sensory and emotional experience arising from actual or potential tissue damage or described in terms of such damage (International Association for the Study of Pain); sudden or slow onset of any intensity from mild to severe, constant or recurring, without being anticipated or having a predictable end; has a duration of greater than 6 months (NANDA, p. 130)

N. **Altered health maintenance:** inability to identify, manage, or seek out help in order to achieve or maintain recovery

O. **Hopelessness:** state in which an individual sees limited/no alternatives/personal choices available and is unable to mobilize energy on own behalf (NANDA, p. 94)

P. **Powerlessness:** a perception that one's own action will not significantly effect an outcome; a perceived lack of control over or influence on a current situation or immediate happening (NANDA, p. 141)

Q. **Spiritual distress:** disruption in the life principle that pervades a person's entire being and that integrates and transcends a person's biological and psychosocial nature (NANDA, p. 175)

V. Planning and Implementation

A. Nursing care in acute stage of abuse

1. Care of the client during intoxication

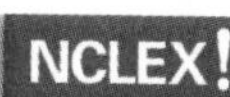

a. Focus is on safety

b. Interventions

1) Maintain safe environment

2) Orient to time, place, and person

3) Maintain adequate nutrition and fluid balance

4) Monitor for beginning of withdrawal signs and symptoms

c. Outcome: client remains safe during periods of intoxication

2. Care of the client experiencing withdrawal from mood altering substances: focus is safe withdrawal process

NCLEX!

a. Interventions

1) Maintain safe environment

2) Create a low-stimulation environment

3) Monitor vital signs and withdrawal symptoms

a) Nausea/vomiting

b) Tremor

c) Paroxysmal sweats

d) Anxiety

e) Agitation

f) Tactile disturbances

h) Auditory disturbances

i) Visual disturbances

i) Headache or fullness in head

j) Disorientation and sensorium

4) Some clients who might be opiate-dependent may be managed long-term with the use of methadone; the methadone may be initially prescribed for withdrawal but then the client will be maintained on a certain daily dose; contrary to popular belief many people who are maintained on methadone do a very fine job with recovery

NCLEX!

5) The nurse must be careful in assessing the chronic pain client for withdrawal as some of the pain that the client is experiencing is related to his or her chronic pain and is not an acute withdrawal symptom

6) While female clients may have been initially screened for pregnancy, they should be screened later in the episode of care to be sure that any medication use potentially harmful to the fetus is minimized; alcohol is the most harmful drug of all and the most harmful to the fetus of any drug

7) Monitor for delirium tremens, psychotic symptoms, and suicide/seizure risk

8) Administer the withdrawal medication: anticonvulsants; benzodiazepines; sedative vitamins; or other medications as ordered; thiamine help to prevent confusion and other mental status changes

NCLEX!

a) Benzodiazepines are the drug of choice for alcohol or benzodiazepine withdrawal

b) It is preferable to give the longer-acting agent so the tapering process is smoother for the client with a longer-acting medication

9) Maintain adequate nutrition and fluid intake

10) Maintain normal comfort measures

11) Monitor for covert substance use during detoxification period
12) Provide emotional support and reassurance to client and family
13) Provide reality orientations and address hallucinations in a therapeutic manner
14) Advise client of the depressive uneasy feelings and the fatigue that is usually experienced during withdrawal
15) Begin to educate the client about the disease of addiction and the initial treatment goal of abstinence

c. Outcome

1) Safe withdrawal from drugs and alcohol
2) Oriented to reality
3) Begin to develop motivation and commitment for abstinence and **recovery** (abstinence plus working a program of personal growth and self-discovery)

B. Nursing care in the rehabilitative stages of abuse

NCLEX!

1. Focus is on teaching about the disease/recovery process and building on the client's motivation for abstinence, lifestyle change, and recovery

2. Interventions

a. Assist client to complete detoxification from all mood-altering substances; monitor for suicide and/or seizure risk

b. Promote abstinence from all mood-altering substances

c. Administer medications for enhancing abstinence/treatment of mood/anxiety and/or thought disorders as applicable

d. Assist clients to put structure and discipline back into their life

e. Facilitate hope

f. Teach disease/recovery dynamics

g. Teach about how the disease has impacted the roles and functions for the individual and the family

h. Provide therapeutic interaction/group counseling to:

1) Process losses (i.e., loss of independence)
2) Discuss memories and flashback
3) Address shame and guilt
4) Educate about disease/recovery
5) Facilitate acceptance of illness

i. Teach and encourage practice of recovery skills

1) Encourage daily commitment to sobriety and recovery
2) Build/utilize sober support networks (i.e., AA or other 12-step groups)
3) Teach the importance of honesty and making amends

4) Encourage daily prayer/mediation
5) Teach drink refusal skills and managing cravings
6) Enhance coping/communication/problem-solving skills
7) Practice asking for help
8) Recognition of signs of impending **relapse** (return to addictive behavior)
    a) Hungry
    b) Angry
    c) Lonely
    d) Tired
    e) Having thoughts about using but not telling anyone
    f) Slipping back into using old defensive mechanisms as opposed to honesty and openness

NCLEX!

j. Help the client to develop an emergency plan, which is a list of things the client would do and people he or she would call if they felt like using or actually used

k. Demonstrate how to utilize affirmations, slogans, and the serenity prayer

l. Initiate random breathalyzers and urine drug screens to objectively assess for sobriety/substance use

1) Breathalyzers are an inexpensive way to do random checks to see if individuals are coming to program sober; because many clients have high tolerance it is difficult to determine if they have been drinking
2) Random urine drug screen test provides the client with objective evidence of sobriety or use (urine collection procedure: instruct the client not to turn on the water or flush the toilet until the specimen is given to the nurse)

m. The client with eating disorders will need to work with the dietician and family physician about increasing/decreasing caloric intake and discontinuing laxative use; they will need to increase their daily water and fiber intake

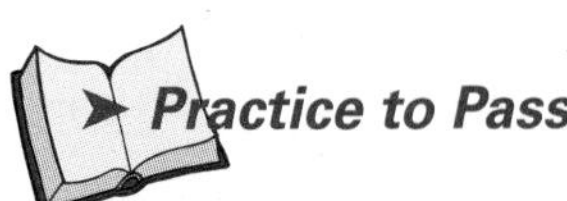

A client who was just discharged from outpatient services on 250 mg of disulfiram a day calls to say she is breaking out in a red rash all over her face. The client stated she was cleaning light fixtures. What is your concern and what will you advise the client to do?

n. Clients who have experienced multiple relapses and seem to have severe addiction may not have a goal of immediate total abstinence; their goals may be to increase the number of sober days within a specific period of time or reduce the number of drinks/money gambled at one sitting; this goal is developed from the Harm Reduction Model, which basically says "there certainly is a beneficial effect to the general public if someone reduces the number of drinks each time they drink"; while this is not an ideal goal for CD clients it certainly makes sense to decrease risk of more serious consequences if someone is using less cocaine

C. Treatment modalities and nursing interventions

1. Medical model: teach the disease and recovery dynamics

2. Assist the client to comply with treatment recommendations

3. Assist with dual diagnosis treatment
4. Detoxification/abstinence/medications
   a. Disulfiram (Antabuse): usual dose is 250 mg/day
      1) Prevents breakdown of alcohol
      2) Person who drinks alcohol becomes very sick (flushing, weakness, nausea/vomiting)
      3) Teach about monitoring for use of alcohol in products/food containing alcohol
      4) Can elevate liver enzymes
   b. Naltrexone (ReVia) usual dose is 50 mg/day orally
      1) Prevents or diminishes cravings/euphoric effect of engaging in addictive behavior (i.e., alcohol/drugs/gambling)
      2) Can elevate liver enzymes
   c. Antidepressant/antianxiety medications
      1) Enhances and stabilizes mood and diminishes anxiety
      2) Teach about the decreased effectiveness of the medication if there is use of mood-altering substances
      3) To discontinue medication it should be tapered slowly
5. The 12-step model
   a. Teach that there is no effective cure for addiction
   b. Encourage 12-step involvement
   c. Regular meeting attendance diminishes ambivalence and promotes acceptance about never engaging in addictive behaviors again
   d. Key elements of 12-step framework are acceptance, surrender, processing grief, higher power, and power of the group
6. Cognitive behavioral model
   a. Develop and use positive coping skills
   b. Implement specific skill training
      1) Assertiveness
      2) Drink refusal
      3) Problem-solving
      4) Cognitive restructuring
      5) Mood management
      6) Anger problems
      7) Social skills
      8) Listening-communication skills
   c. Identify and change behaviors associated with addictive behaviors (i.e., going into the liquor store to buy soft drinks)

NCLEX!

NCLEX!

NCLEX!

7. Relapse prevention model
   a. Identify situations and factors that contribute to relapse
   b. Increased positive self-efficacy expectations about the ability to achieve abstinence
   c. Identify the euphoric recall about engaging in addictive behavior, which can serve to keep someone actively engaging in addiction
8. Motivational enhancement/stages of change
   a. Utilize various types of reflective listening and other specialized communication strategies to help build a client's commitment to change
   b. Express empathy; ambivalence is a normal part of the change process
   c. Help to develop discrepancy between the way the clients see themselves and the way they really are
   d. Avoid getting in to arguments over things, especially labels
   e. Roll with resistance; resistance is a sign to change strategies
   f. Support the client's self efficacy
9. Assess the client's stage of change and apply nursing interventions according to the stage of change the client is in
   a. Pre-contemplation: "We are blind to our problems"
   b. Contemplation: "We are not ready to change"
   c. Determination/preparation: "We are getting ready to change"
   d. Action: "We are learning how to change; we are doing it"
   e. Maintenance: "We make changes stick"

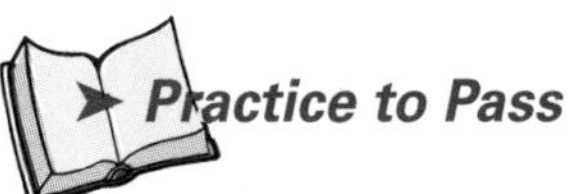

A young teen was just admitted to your addiction program; she is not happy to be here and feels she is too young to be an alcoholic. She "drinks the same amount as everyone else" she knows and believes she was just unlucky to be involved in a traffic accident. What education will you provide to the client? What approach will you use?

VI. Evaluation/Outcomes

A. **Completes the withdrawal process safely**

B. **Makes a commitment to sobriety** and participates in the treatment process

C. **Learns about the dynamics of addiction** and the recovery skills necessary to recover from this disease

D. **Begins to identify the consequences of the substance use** or addictive behaviors

E. **Begins to practice** some recovery behaviors while in treatment

F. **Begins to accept** having an addictive disorder and never being able to use safely or engage in addictive behavior again

G. **Identifies coping behaviors** to address cravings, thoughts, and triggers to use or engage in addictive behaviors

VII. Dual Disorder Issues

A. **Focus is on teaching** that each disorder is an illness that requires co-occurring treatment and building on the client's motivation for abstinence, remissions of mental illness, lifestyle change, and the recovery process

B. Additional interventions

1. Discuss the physiological aspects of mental illness and substance abuse and of the interaction effects
2. Teach that psychiatric medications are nonaddictive and can enhance recovery
3. Medication teaching includes focus on the fact that drinking or drug use will interfere with the efficacy of the psychiatric medication and that medication use and drinking should not mix

VIII. Family Issues

A. Anger/alienation of the chemically dependent person

B. Teach disease dynamics

1. Family rules/communication
2. Family members' dysfunctional behaviors and denial about the addiction of their family member

C. Problematic coping skills

D. Mood adjustment problems

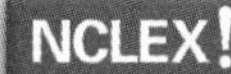

E. Codependency and low self-esteem

F. Learning and practicing recovery dynamics and skills

1. Self-love and self-care
2. Utilizing support groups (i.e., Al-Anon)
3. Establishing healthy relationships/boundaries
4. Daily prayer/meditation
5. Improved coping/problem-solving
6. Asking for help
7. Confronting dysfunctional beliefs and learning how to change them
8. Affirmations, slogans, serenity prayer

G. Processing anger and losses/memories

1. Confronts substance abuser about the consequences of his or her use and how it affected the family
2. Processing emotional distance between family members
3. Processing loss of "helper/competent" role now that the recovering family member is taking back some of his or her lost family roles

Case Study

A client in her early 20s comes to the Emergency Department complaining of rapid heart rate and states she has passed out a couple of times recently. You suspect her symptoms are related to substance use.

❶ What additional information will you gather from this client?

❷ What body system will you focus your nursing assessment on?

❸ What laboratory values would help you determine if substance use played a role in the development of your client's symptoms?

❹ The client's symptoms are related to substance use. What information will you use to differentiate which substance the client may be abusing?

❺ What nursing interventions will you need to deliver to this client?

For suggested responses, see pages 309–310.

Posttest

1 The nurse instructs the client about addiction. The nurse determines that the client understands the instructions given when the client says:

(1) "Addiction is a moral disease."
(2) "Addiction is a medical illness."
(3) "Addiction is a behavioral habit."
(4) "Addiction is an emotional attachment."

2 A client says he takes a drink every morning to calm his nerves and stop his tremors. The nurse realizes that the client is at risk for:

(1) An anxiety disorder.
(2) A neurological disorder.
(3) Physical dependence.
(4) Psychological dependence.

3 A young female presents for her school checkup. She denies any medical problems or taking any medications, but she does acknowledge daily laxative use. As the school nurse, what other symptoms or problems would you expect to find?

(1) Headaches
(2) Altered sleep patterns
(3) Abnormal eating patterns
(4) Intermittent chest pain

4 A client with a long history of relapsing from cocaine dependence states he wants to be sober and doesn't understand why he keeps thinking about using. Education about the role the Brain Reward System (BRS) plays in maintaining addiction could help the client understand the disease better. The nurse will evaluate the client's understanding of this education if the client states that the role BRS plays is to:

(1) "Reinforce the use patterns of role models."
(2) "Mediate job stress and pressure."
(3) "Facilitate the intoxication process."
(4) "Facilitate cravings and triggers for readministration."

5 A client is asking about the detoxification process and withdrawal from a benzodiazapine. The *best* response by the nurse is that the client will:

(1) Be placed on a rapid detoxification schedule.
(2) Experience the start of withdrawal immediately upon discontinuation.
(3) Be placed on a similar medication for detoxification.
(4) Sleep almost continuously for the first 24 hours.

6 A nurse is assigned to five clients in various stages of inpatient treatment today. In caring for a chemically dependent client requiring acute care, the nurse's primary role is to:

(1) Deliver psycho-education on the dangers of drug and alcohol use.
(2) Review the problems in the client's relapse prevention plan.
(3) Facilitate administration of anti-craving medications.
(4) Monitor and provide withdrawal care based on unit protocol.

7 A client with chronic headaches is detoxifying from alcohol and will require medications to treat the withdrawal. When assessing the client's withdrawal symptoms the priority of nurse would be to assess:

(1) The level of pain the client is experiencing according to the pain scale.
(2) The difference between the client's current level of pain and the usual level of pain.
(3) Whether the client is experiencing more pain than usual because of tolerance.
(4) The defense mechanisms the client uses and how that influences the level of pain.

8 A nursing educator is teaching a group of community health nurses on moderating alcohol use. The nurse educator evaluates the group's understanding of "harm reduction" if the group is able to identify which group is not appropriate for "harm reduction"?

(1) Individuals with tolerance
(2) Individuals with alcohol abuse
(3) Individuals unable to control use
(4) Individuals with high-dose use

9 Some adolescent clients relapse because they feel pressured by their peers. Which skill training could the nurse plan for adolescents in order to assist them in relapse prevention?

(1) Vocational skills
(2) Drinking refusal skills
(3) Problem-solving skills
(4) Communication skills

10 A family member identified a drinking problem in your client. This client was admitted to the medical unit for chest pain and is undecided regarding the desire for chemical dependence treatment suggested by the addiction consultation team. An additional nursing diagnosis for the client would be:

(1) Impaired family process: alcoholism.
(2) Ineffective management of therapeutic regimen: individual.
(3) Risk for injury: potential for relapse.
(4) Decisional conflict.

See pages 231–233 for Answers and Rationales.

Answers and Rationales

Pretest

1 **Answer: 1** *Rationale:* The key symptom of addiction is impaired control, or the inability to regulate one's addictive behavior. While persons with addiction don't always recognize consequences of their behavior (option 2), it is not because they lose this ability. Acting sober is an addictive behavior (option 3). Identifying with a higher power is the next step after developing understanding of lack of control (option 4).
Cognitive Level: Comprehension
Nursing Process: Evaluation; *Test Plan:* PSYC

2 **Answer: 2** *Rationale:* The DSM-IV describes intoxication as a reversible substance-specific syndrome because of recent ingestion or exposure to a substance. Withdrawal (option 1) and tolerance (option 3) can occur for process addictions even though one may not always think of them as being true for behavioral addiction. Primarily there is no difference between process and chemical addictions (option 4).
Cognitive Level: Analysis
Nursing Process: Evaluation; *Test Plan:* PSYC

3 **Answer: 4** *Rationale:* The quality of the parental relationship will be impaired while there is regular dependent drinking taking place. Alcohol impairs and affects the brain's capacity to function and cope with activities of daily living. Children are able to sense the differences in their relationship with their parents

when they are drinking or recovering from its effects; however, the change in relationship is the primary cause of the consequences (option 3). In regard to consequences of use, anyone who has dependent drinking will experience the negative consequences (options 1 and 2).
Cognitive Level: Analysis
Nursing Process: Implementation; ***Test Plan:*** PSYC

4 **Answer: 2** ***Rationale:*** Nurses' exposure to substances, knowledge about specific effects of certain drugs, and belief that they can handle drug and alcohol use safely to deal with their problems has the greatest impact on the risk for becoming dependent. Some nurses are adult children of alcoholics (option 1) and some may have problems with codependence (option 4), but this does not put them at more risk than those in the general public who have similar problems. Preconceived ideas about what kind of people become addicted does have a role in risk but not as great as access (option 3).
Cognitive Level: Analysis
Nursing Process: Evaluation; ***Test Plan:*** PSYC

5 **Answer: 1** ***Rationale:*** It would not be unusual for a client who has severe addiction to come to day treatment intoxicated and deny it. Denial would cause a client to insist he or she is not intoxicated or doesn't have a problem with alcoholism despite concrete evidence of the problem. Reaction formation is a defense mechanism that causes people to act exactly opposite to the way they feel (option 2). Transference is the unconscious process of displacing feelings for significant people in the past onto the nurse in the present relationship (option 3). Countertransference is the nurse's emotional reaction to clients based on feelings for significant people in the nurse's past (option 4).
Cognitive Level: Application
Nursing Process: Assessment; ***Test Plan:*** PSYC

6 **Answer: 4** ***Rationale:*** Concern expressed about drinking is one of the four screening items on the CAGE questionnaire. The other options (1, 2, and 3) support the client's belief that others are against him or have no business being concerned.
Cognitive Level: Application
Nursing Process: Implementation; ***Test Plan:*** PSYC

7 **Answer: 1** ***Rationale:*** Antidepressant medication and the treatment of depression can enhance sobriety for individuals suffering from depression. Treating one without the other may result in poor outcomes (option 2). Depression may be a symptom of substance abuse or substance abuse may be a symptom of depression, but this can only be assessed after a time of sobriety (option 3). Depression is common in substance abuse recovery but is not necessarily an expected outcome (option 4).
Cognitive Level: Comprehension
Nursing Process: Analysis; ***Test Plan:*** PSYC

8 **Answer: 2** ***Rationale:*** AA teaches that the alcoholic can never safely return to social drinking and that total abstinence is the only course for the addiction. When sobriety has been achieved people don't "graduate" (option 1); they stay and help others achieve sobriety. Acceptance and Higher Power are active concepts in AA, but practicing these principles does not remove urges to drink (option 3) or guarantee sobriety (option 4).
Cognitive Level: Knowledge
Nursing Process: Analysis; ***Test Plan:*** PSYC

9 **Answer: 3** ***Rationale:*** Alcohol use during pregnancy causes dysmorphic prenatal and postnatal difficulties and CNS dysfunction. Other substances cause significant health concerns as well, but not quite as many different kinds of problems (options 1, 2 and 4).
Cognitive Level: Analysis
Nursing Process: Assessment; ***Test Plan:*** PSYC

10 **Answer: 1** ***Rationale:*** Antabuse and alcohol use cause elevated liver enzymes. Marijuana use (option 2), eating fatty foods (option 3) or being exposed to measles (option 4) does not cause elevated GGT.
Cognitive Level: Analysis
Nursing Process: Assessment; ***Test Plan:*** PHYS

Posttest

1 **Answer: 2** ***Rationale:*** Alcoholism was officially listed as a disease in 1956 and Jellinek's identification of the four phases of disease progression in 1960 reinforced the disease concept. The general public continues to view addiction as a moral weakness (option 1). Addiction does include behavioral habits (option 3) and emotional attachment (option 4) but is seen first as a medical disease.
Cognitive Level: Application
Nursing Process: Evaluation; ***Test Plan:*** PSYC

2 **Answer: 3** ***Rationale:*** Taking a drink in the morning to steady one's nerves is a sign of physical dependence. With physical dependence the person begins to drink to avoid withdrawal symptoms. Tremors are one of the ten symptoms of alcohol withdrawal listed in the Clinical Institute Withdrawal Assessment of

alcohol symptoms. People with anxiety may have tremors, but they wouldn't be specific to only mornings (option 1). Tremors can be caused by movement disorders for which alcohol may suppress the tremors; however, if one had a movement disorder, the tremors would not just occur in the morning (option 2). Psychological dependency (option 4) is the belief that the client has to have the substance in order to survive; this client is drinking in the morning to calm his nerves.
Cognitive Level: Application
Nursing Process: Assessment; ***Test Plan:*** PHYS

3 **Answer: 3** ***Rationale:*** Laxative abuse is a method used to control weight by anorexics and bulimics. Eating disorder clients may have cardiac rhythm disturbances but not necessarily chest pain (option 4), headaches (option 1), or altered sleep (option 2) as a result of their disordered eating.
Cognitive Level: Application
Nursing Process: Assessment; ***Test Plan:*** PHYS

4 **Answer: 4** ***Rationale:*** Cravings appear to be the result of pleasurable memories engendered from the psycho-activating effect of engaging in addictive behaviors. It's true that environment and role models influence use patterns, and that we use addictive behaviors to self-medicate stress and pressure we experience (options 1 and 2). The act of being intoxicated does not necessarily lead to thought, triggers, or urges to use (option 3).
Cognitive Level: Application
Nursing Process: Evaluation; ***Test Plan:*** PSYC

5 **Answer: 3** ***Rationale:*** Withdrawal from depressants is generally treated by substitution with a longer-acting drug in the same class. Clients are usually medicated on a fixed schedule dosing pattern or a symptom-triggered approach with the client receiving a specific dose of medication depending on the severity of the withdrawal symptoms. Onset of withdrawal symptoms and the time it takes to complete withdrawal would depend on the half-life of the benzodiazepines on which the client depends. The symptoms from depressants are activating kinds of symptoms such as nausea, vomiting, and tremor. Withdrawal symptoms are generally the opposite symptoms of the drug someone is addicted to.
Cognitive Level: Application
Nursing Process: Implementation; ***Test Plan:*** PHYS

6 **Answer: 4** ***Rationale:*** Acute care is defined as care of the client experiencing intoxication and withdrawal. Beginning education about the disease (option 1) and interventions (options 2 and 3) to help someone stay sober are introduced at the end of the active phase and become the focus of treatment during the rehabilitative phase of treatment.
Cognitive Level: Application
Nursing Process: Planning; ***Test Plan:*** PHYS

7 **Answer: 2** ***Rationale:*** Headaches are a symptom of detoxification from alcohol. A client with chronic headaches would be expected to have headaches so the nurse would need to assess the difference between the pain level of usual headaches and the withdrawal headaches. Initially, assessment of pain using the pain scale will not provide the difference between the types of pain (option 1). Clients experiencing pain who are addicted may need more pain medication than the non-addicted client because of tolerance regardless of level of pain (option 3). How an individual appraises the symptoms of stress could influence defense and coping mechanisms they might use, but it wouldn't be specific to the one symptom of pain (option 4).
Cognitive Level: Application
Nursing Process: Assessment; ***Test Plan:*** PHYS

8 **Answer: 3** ***Rationale:*** Clients who are unable to control their use or are unable to learn strategies to reduce intake and/or harm caused by their use, are not good candidates for this approach. People with tolerance (option 1), alcohol abuse (option 2), and high dose use (option 4) may be successful in decreasing the frequency and quantity of alcohol they drink.
Cognitive Level: Application
Nursing Process: Evaluation; ***Test Plan:*** PSYC

9 **Answer: 2** ***Rationale:*** The quality of an adolescent's recovery environment can be helpful or hurtful to someone attempting to maintain sobriety. Friends or acquaintances may encourage a recovering person to use. The recovering adolescent may want to refuse but may not know how. Behavioral rehearsal, saying "no thanks" to an offer to engage in addictive behavior, can increase a recovering person's confidence. Vocational skills will not help the adolescent refuse a drink (option 1). Problem-solving skills (option 3) and communication skills (option 4) may be useful but not as helpful as skills directly related to refusing to drink.
Cognitive Level: Application
Nursing Process: Planning; ***Test Plan:*** PSYC

10 **Answer: 4** ***Rationale:*** The definition for decisional conflict is uncertainty about a course of action to be taken when choice among competing actions involve risk, loss, or challenge to personal life values. Im-

paired family process: alcoholism, may apply, but it is more appropriate for the family than the individual (option 1). Ineffective management of therapeutic regimen (option 2) and risk for injury (option 3) imply that the client has already made a commitment to recovery.
Cognitive Level: Analysis
Nursing Process: Analysis; ***Test Plan:*** PSYC

References

Boyd, M. A. & Nihart, M. A. (1998). *Psychiatric nursing contemporary practice.* Philadelphia: Lippincott.

Carson, V. B. (2000). *Mental health nursing: The nurse-patient journey* (2nd ed.). Philadelphia: W. B. Saunders Company, pp. 721–772.

Fontaine, K. L. (1999). Substance-related disorders. In K. L. Fontaine & J. S. Fletcher (Eds.), *Mental health nursing* (4th ed.). Menlo Park, CA: Addison-Wesley, pp. 315–352.

Fontaine, K. L. & Fletcher, J. S. (1999). *Mental health nursing* (4th ed.). New York: Addison-Wesley.

Fortinash, K. M. & Holoday-Worret, P. A. (2000). *Psychiatric mental health nursing.* St. Louis: Mosby, pp. 354–385.

Jack, L. (1990). *The core curriculum of addictions nursing.* Skokie, IL: Midwest Education Association, pp. 49–82.

Keltner, N. L., Schwecke, L. H., & Bostrom, C. E. (1999). *Psychiatric nursing* (3rd ed.). Chicago: Mosby.

NANDA. (2001). *Nursing diagnoses: Definitions and classification 2001–2002.* Philadelphia: North American Nursing Diagnosis Association.

O'Brien, P. G., Kennedy, W., & Ballard, K. (1999). *Psychiatric nursing—An integration of theory and practice.* St. Louis: Mosby, pp. 263–276.

Stuart, G. W. & Laraia, M. T. (2001). *Principles and practice of psychiatric nursing* (7th ed.). St. Louis: Mosby, pp. 485–569.

Sullivan, E. J. (1995). *Nursing care of clients with substance abuse.* St. Louis: Mosby, pp. 47–70, 191–233.

Townsend, M. C. (2000). *Psychiatric mental health nursing* (3rd ed.). Philadelphia: F. A. Davis, pp. 357–399.

CHAPTER 12

Victims of Abuse

Marybeth O'Neil, RN, MSN, CS

CHAPTER OUTLINE

OBJECTIVES

- Differentiate the different types of abuse.
- Identify characteristics of the victim and perpetrator.
- Analyze clinical signs and symptoms of abuse.
- Determine appropriate nursing diagnoses applicable to victims of abuse.
- Formulate a plan of care for a victim of abuse.
- Identify expected outcomes for victims of abuse.

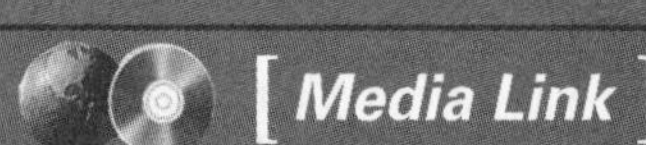

Use the CD-ROM enclosed with this text, or log onto the address given to access the free, interactive Companion Website created for this series. The CD-ROM and Companion Website accompanying this book offer additional practice opportunities and information—NCLEX Review, Case Studies, Glossary, In Depth with NCLEX, and more.

www.prenhall.com/hogan

Review at a Glance

abuse *a pattern of behavior that dominates, controls, lowers self-esteem, or takes away choice*

assault *threat of violence*

battering *repeated violence against a person*

child abuse *inflicting injury to a child or adolescent that can range from minor bruise to severe neurological trauma or death*

domestic violence *abuse that happens within the confines of a family system*

elder abuse *physical, emotional, psychological, or sexual injury to a person over the age of 65, most often inflicted by family members*

incest *sexual relations between a child or adolescent and a relative or surrogate relative before the child is 18 years of age*

mandatory reporting laws *laws that require the reporting of certain types of abuse, such as child, elder, or vulnerable adult abuse*

Munchausen's syndrome by proxy *a form of child abuse where the primary caregiver reports or induces symptoms in a child which necessitate medical intervention; the caregiver does this for his or her own emotional gratification*

neglect *a condition in which a caregiver does not provide for the needs of an individual in his or her care, can be physical, emotional, economic, social, educational*

partner abuse *physical or psychological violence toward an intimate partner intended to intimidate or degrade the partner*

perpetrator *the person who commits an act of abuse*

post-traumatic stress disorder *psychiatric condition that occurs after a traumatic event characterized by hyperarousal, irritability, hypervigilance, poor sleep, intrusive thoughts, nightmares, flashbacks, difficulty concentrating, avoidance and numbing*

rape *forced sexual intercourse*

shaken baby syndrome *syndrome resulting from violent shaking of young infants that results in whiplash-like closed head and neck injuries, can result in death caused by hemorrhage or cerebral edema*

sexual assault *forceful genital, anal, or oral penetration of the victim by any object, including a penis*

victim *person who experiences abuse*

Pretest

1 **A mother tells the nurse during an admission interview that her 2-year-old, who has numerous bruises, has fallen down stairs frequently. The mother is able to provide few details. The nurse evaluates this as:**

(1) Possible child abuse.
(2) Knowledge deficit pertaining to home safety.
(3) Normal behavior for a 2-year-old.
(4) Possible attention deficit disorder.

2 **An 85-year-old female is brought to the Emergency Department after a fall at home. The client appears confused, malnourished, dehydrated, and is reluctant to explain how the fall happened. The client's 62-year-old daughter frequently interrupts the client and does not allow the client to answer questions. Which of the following nursing interventions is a *priority*?**

(1) Take the history from the daughter because the client is confused.
(2) Provide the daughter with nutritional teaching.
(3) Request a psychiatric evaluation for the client.
(4) Interview the client alone first and assess for abuse.

3 **A 5-year-old girl is brought to the clinic for symptoms of a urinary tract infection (UTI). The nurse's assessment reveals bruises in the child's genital and rectal areas. The mother reports that she had left the little girl with her boyfriend the night before. The nurse's *first* priority with this client is:**

(1) Obtain a urine sample to confirm a UTI.
(2) Teach the mother about symptoms of UTI.
(3) Report suspected sexual abuse to protective services.
(4) Assess the child for other health problems.

4 **A female comes to the Emergency Department with a broken wrist and severe bruises from a beating by her husband. She states that she does not want to leave the relationship at this time. The *most* appropriate response by the nurse is:**

(1) "You need to leave the relationship."
(2) "I will call a lawyer for you."
(3) "Let's develop a safety plan for repeated violence."
(4) "Here is a list of services that can help you."

5 A nurse is teaching a class on domestic violence to high school students. Which of the following statements by a student would indicate to the nurse that further teaching is needed?

(1) "Violence often begins in a dating relationship."
(2) "The abuser will often apologize and promise to stop."
(3) "If you are educated and have money, abuse does not happen."
(4) "Abusers are often excessively jealous and possessive."

6 The nurse is interviewing a female client who has experienced both physical and psychological abuse. Which of the following statements by the client indicates the greatest need for more teaching about abuse?

(1) "Now that I have left him, I don't need to worry."
(2) "This is the third time I've left; I hope it works."
(3) "I feel like the abuse was my fault."
(4) "He will try to take the children away from me if I don't go back."

7 The nurse is teaching the mother of a young child, who has just been removed from the home because of sexual abuse by the stepfather, about the consequences of abuse. Which of the following should the nurse include in the teaching?

(1) Since the child was removed there will be no long-term consequences.
(2) Because it was someone the child trusted, it will not be as traumatic.
(3) The child will be at risk for depression in the future.
(4) The child will become an abuser in the future.

8 A 15-year-old female student comes into the school nurse's office asking to be tested for pregnancy. She confides to the nurse that her boyfriend forced her to have sex against her will. The *most* appropriate intervention by the nurse would be:

(1) Administer a pregnancy test.
(2) Do teaching on safe sex.
(3) Do teaching on birth control methods.
(4) Identify the student's immediate concerns.

9 A pregnant female comes to the Emergency Department with bruises on her arms and abdomen after a fight with her boyfriend. The nurse would determine which of the following to be the *priority* for teaching with this client?

(1) Risks of pregnancy complications caused by abuse
(2) Assertiveness training to deal with the boyfriend
(3) Childbirth classes to prepare for the birth
(4) Instructions on the use of resources available to her

10 The nurse is assessing the family of a child brought in for severe injuries. What behavior by the parents would indicate probable abuse?

(1) A delay in seeking treatment for the child's injuries
(2) A detailed description of the events prior to the injuries
(3) An anxious, concerned attitude
(4) Encouraging the child to explain the injuries

See page 256 for Answers and Rationales.

I. Overview of Abuse

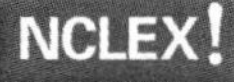

A. ***Abuse:*** the willful infliction of physical injury, emotional anguish, or both on another person

B. Violence: the physical force exerted for the purpose of dominating, controlling, lowering self-esteem or taking away choice

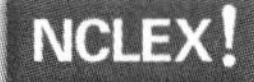

C. ***Domestic violence:*** violence that occurs within a family system; is often used interchangeably with abuse; it includes physical abuse, neglect, psychological abuse, economic abuse, and sexual abuse

D. ***Perpetrator*** **(or abuser):** the person who inflicts violence or abuse on another

E. ***Victim:*** the person who is scapegoat, target, or recipient of the abuse or violence

F. Abuse is one of the fastest-growing public health problems today:

1. It cuts across all socioeconomic lines

2. It includes all age groups and relationship types
3. Drug and alcohol use is often involved
4. Societal factors that contribute to abuse
    a. Divorce and blended families
    b. Lack of nuclear family for support
    c. Social isolation
    d. Economic strain
5. Elders are living longer and becoming more dependent on children for care
6. Emergency Department is often place of interface with the health system
7. Victims may present with injuries or health problems
8. Abuser's behavior is often cyclic and escalates in frequency and intensity over time
9. Victim may blame self in an attempt to control the situation
10. Victim may try to protect the perpetrator or be reluctant to identify the abuser
11. Nurses must be aware of possible abuse, particularly if injuries are unexplained or explanation does not match physical picture

NCLEX!

12. **Mandatory reporting laws** require nurses report suspected abuse in all states; there are civil and criminal penalties for not reporting

G. Types of abuse

1. Physical abuse: physical harm or injury caused by beating, hitting, cutting, shooting, burning, or raping; **assault** is a threat of violence; **battering** is repeated physical abuse
2. **Sexual assault:** pressured or forced sexual contact, including sexually stimulated talk or actions, inappropriate touching or intercourse, incest, and **rape** (forced sexual intercourse)
3. Emotional or psychological abuse
    a. Intimidation or the attempt to instill fear
    b. Social isolation of victim
    c. Violation of personal rights, such as refusing to allow victim contact with family, friends, and others
4. Economic abuse: financial exploitation of a victim by restricting access to money, food, clothing, or transportation

NCLEX!

5. **Neglect:** withholding or failing to provide proper personal care in any of the following areas:
    a. Physical: not providing needed food, clothing, or shelter
    b. Emotional: not providing needed love and nurturance
    c. Medical: not providing needed medical care or prescriptions

   d. Education: failure to enroll child in school

   e. Abandonment: leaving without proper supervision

H. Victims

1. Children and adolescents
2. Siblings
3. Partners (heterosexual and homosexual)
4. Elders

I. Physiological responses to abuse

1. Multiple injuries: especially to head, face, throat, trunk, or sexual organs
2. Unexplained bruises, lacerations, abrasions, head injuries, fractures
3. Malnutrition, dehydration
4. Stress-related responses such as headaches, GI symptoms, anxiety, depression, chronic pain, insomnia, menstrual problems
5. Eating disorders: anorexia and bulimia
6. Death

J. Psychological responses to abuse

1. Fear
2. Lowered self-esteem
3. Behavioral problems in children
4. Helplessness
5. Hopelessness
6. Depression
7. Isolation
8. Difficulties with problem-solving and decision-making

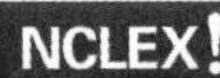

9. **Post-traumatic stress disorder:** psychiatric condition that occurs after a traumatic event, characterized by hyperarousal, irritability, hypervigilance, poor sleep, intrusive thoughts, nightmares, flashbacks, difficulty concentrating, avoidance, and numbing

K. Etiology/psychopathology

1. Characteristics of victims

   a. Low self-esteem and feelings of helplessness and hopelessness

   b. Feelings of powerlessness, guilt, and shame

   c. May protect perpetuator and accept responsibility for abuse

   d. May blame self in an attempt to control situation

   e. May deny severity of situation and feelings of anger and terror

2. Characteristics of perpetrators
   a. Use threats and intimidation to control the victim
   b. Often suffered from abuse, neglect, or severe discipline as a child
   c. May be hostile and blame others or circumstances for own problems
   d. Impulsive and immature with low self-esteem
   e. Have unmet dependency needs

NCLEX!

   f. Are extreme disciplinarians who believe in physical punishment
   g. Poor parenting skills and high expectations of child
   h. Concerned about child's gender or performance before birth
   i. May have had difficult pregnancy and/or labor and delivery
   j. May have substance abuse problems
   k. Have high expectations of others' behavior
   l. Are generally law abiding and only a danger to family
3. Characteristics of family systems where abuse occurs
   a. Socially isolated

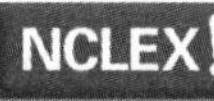

   b. Multigenerational transmission: family history of abuse
   c. Rigid family rules and external boundaries
   d. Use and abuse of power by family authority figure
   e. Drug and alcohol use prevalent

II. Theories of Abuse

A. **There is no single theory about the causes of abuse;** it is most probable that numerous factors are involved

B. **Some current theories include the following:**

1. Neurobiological
   a. Biologists believe aggression is inherent in humans and regulated by hormones such as testosterone; increased levels affect aggression
   b. Neurophysiologists believe it is related to imbalances of neurotransmitters, such as serotonin
2. Social learning theory
   a. Violence is a learned behavior, learned by observation, modeling, and direct experience
   b. Intergenerational transmission; poor parenting skills contribute to it
   c. A culture that accepts and promotes violence and media that desensitizes through repeated exposure to violence both play a role
   d. Violence is part of our socialization process
3. Psychological or interpersonal theories
   a. Etiology lies in the personality of the abuser

- **b.** Abusers may have psychiatric illness such as personality disorder
- **c.** Abusers have poor impulse and anger control
- **d.** Abusers have poor coping skills
- **e.** Abusers have low esteem and fears of abandonment
- **f.** Abusers suffered early emotional deprivation

4. Feminist theories

- **a.** The sexist structure of society contributes to abuse
- **b.** Women are controlled and subordinated by power and privilege of males
- **c.** Abuse is about gender and power
- **d.** Power inequities between victim and perpetrator contribute
- **e.** Devaluation of women by society contributes

5. Sociologic: societal issues promote abuse

- **a.** Unemployment
- **b.** Poverty
- **c.** Crime
- **d.** Teen pregnancy
- **e.** Isolation

III. Abuse in Special Populations

NCLEX!

A. ***Child abuse:*** physical, emotional, sexual, or psychological damage done to a child

1. Abuse can range from mild to severe physical injuries including death, and mild to severe psychological damage

2. Children exposed to domestic violence demonstrate more behavioral and emotional problems than other children; abused children are more likely to have cognitive deficits and are at higher risk for becoming batterers

NCLEX!

3. Witnessing violence can have negative psychological effects on children

4. Adolescents who kill parents have often been severely abused

5. Types of abuse

- **a.** Physical abuse: inflicting injury to a child that can range from minor to severe including death; see Table 12-1 for signs of physical child abuse
- **b.** Emotional or psychological abuse: causing psychological harm by demeaning or intimidating treatment that undermines a child's sense of safety or competence; see Box 12-1 for behavioral signs of emotional abuse
- **c.** Physical neglect: harm or threatened harm to a child's health or welfare by a parent or guardian through failure to provide adequate food, clothing, shelter, proper supervision, or medical treatment; see Box 12-2 for signs of physical neglect
- **d.** Emotional neglect: chronic failure to provide a nurturing supportive environment needed for necessary growth and development; parental signs of

Table 12-1

Physical and Behavioral Signs of Physical Abuse in Children

Physical Signs	Behavioral Signs
Bruise in various stages of healing, often on head and neck	Behavioral extremes aggressive to passive
Bite marks	Fear of parents or caregiver
Burns in shape of objects or glove-like from immersion in hot liquids	Extreme rage or passivity
Fractures, scars or serious internal injuries	Apprehension when other children cry
Lacerations or welts	Verbal reports of abuse
Bald spots from hair being pulled	Hyperactivity, distractibility or hypervigilance
	Disorganized thinking, self-injurious or suicidal behavior
	Running away from home or illegal behaviors
	Cheating, lying, low academic performance
	Poor relationships with peers
	Inappropriately dressed for weather
	Regressive behaviors (such as enuresis, encopresis)

emotional neglect include: parent ignoring the child's presence or rebuffing child's attempts to interact; ignoring social, educational, or recreational needs, or denying the child opportunity to receive positive reinforcement

6. Sibling abuse: harm inflicted on a child by a sibling
   a. Most unrecognized type of child abuse
   b. May be physical, emotional, or sexual
   c. Parents may think of sibling violence as part of normal development

   NCLEX!

   d. Children hit by parents more likely to abuse siblings
7. Child sexual abuse: involvement of a child or adolescent in sexual activity that they do not fully comprehend and to which they do not fully consent
   a. Two types: sexual abuse by a non-relative and **incest,** sexual contact between relatives or surrogate relatives with a child or adolescent before the age of 18

Box 12-1

Behavioral Signs of Emotional Abuse in Children

Behavior inappropriate for age, either precocious or regressed
Anxiety
Behavioral extremes
Self-destructive behaviors
Inappropriate affect
Vandalism, cheating, lying, stealing
Excessive self-soothing behaviors such as thumb-sucking and rocking
Anorexia or bulimia

Box 12-2

Signs of Physical Neglect in Children

Inappropriately dressed for season, or ill-fitting or dirty clothing
Malnourished, always hungry, hoarding, or stealing food
Medical problems such as infected sores or poor dental health
Delinquent behavior—stealing or drug use
Poor school performance, truancy
Poor peer relations
Listless and tired
Poor hygiene
Failure to thrive in infants

b. See Table 12-2 for physical and behavioral indicators of child sexual abuse

c. Child sexual abuse can have long-term behavioral effects such as: post-traumatic stress disorder (see Chapter 5), sexual problems in adulthood, difficulties trusting others, anxiety and panic attacks, depression, substance abuse, eating disorders (particularly bulimia), and self-destructive behaviors such as cutting or burning self

d. Abuse usually develops over time; perpetrator wins child's confidence and trust and may bribe child with gifts and money

e. Perpetrator imposes secrecy with threats of harm to child or family

f. The earlier the abuse the more profound the damage

g. If the abuser is a trusted friend or relative, the violation of trust is most traumatic

Table 12-2

Physical and Behavioral Signs of Child Sexual Abuse

Physical Signs	Behavioral Signs
Frequent urination or dysuria	Overly sexualized behavior, seductive or advanced sexual knowledge
Venereal disease or gonorrhea of throat	Promiscuity or prostitution
Pain or difficulty walking or sitting	Fear of particular person or place
Foreign matter in bladder, rectum, urethra, or vagina	Compulsive masturbation or precocious sexual play
Sleep problems: insomnia or nightmares	Sexually abusing another child
Rashes or itching in genital area	Unexplained gifts or money from questionable sources
Bruises, edema or pain in genital area, rectum, or vagina	Drop in school performance
Scarred labia or rectal fissures	Sudden onset of enuresis
Pregnancy	Excess anxiety
	Compulsive bathing
	Running away from home
	Suicide attempts and self-destructive behaviors, such as head banging

8. Etiology and psychopathology

a. Characteristics of individuals who sexually abuse children

1) 90 percent of abusers were severely sexually abused as children

2) Are experiencing stressful life situations

3) Have few support systems; socially isolated

4) Are lacking in adaptive coping mechanisms and have low self-esteem

5) Have unusually high expectations of child

6) Have poor impulse control and low self-esteem

7) May abuse substances

b. Characteristics of incestuous family systems (family systems theory)

1) Father domineering, impulsive, and physically abusive

2) Mother passive and submissive, may be battered

3) System closed with rigid rules; external boundaries are rigid

4) Enmeshed family system: within system, individual boundaries are poorly defined and characterized by excessive dependence on family members for physical and psychological needs

5) Role reversal may take place, child caring for parent

c. See Box 12-3 for risk factors that may predispose individuals to abuse

9. Assessment of the physically or emotionally abused child

a. Observe for physical and behavioral signs as previously outlined in Table 12-1

b. Be concerned if there has been a delay in seeking treatment

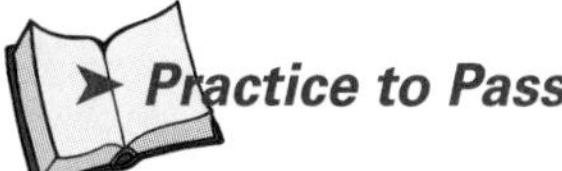

You are caring for a young child who is a suspected victim of sexual abuse by a parent. What would you assess for in the child and the parents?

NCLEX!

NCLEX!

Box 12-3

Risk Factors That May Predispose Individuals to Abuse Children

- Suffered abuse or neglect themselves
- Hostile, blaming others
- Low self-esteem
- Impulsive, immature
- Prenatal issues such as depression, unwanted pregnancy, fear of labor and delivery or difficult delivery
- Burdened by caring for parents
- High expectations of others' behaviors
- Overwhelmed by care needs of others
- Unmet emotional needs of their own
- Substance abuse problems
- Extreme disciplinarian with poor parenting skills
- Experiencing increased socioeconomic stress
- Family pattern of violence
- Need to maintain control

NCLEX!

c. Vague accounts of events around injuries

NCLEX!

d. Injuries that do not match report of cause

NCLEX!

e. Resistance to leaving child alone with healthcare provider

f. Assess relationship of child to caregiver

g. Assess for **shaken baby syndrome**

1) Whiplash-like closed head and neck injuries that can result in death caused by hemorrhage or cerebral edema

2) Caused by violent shaking of young infants

NCLEX!

3) Respiratory distress and retinal bleeding are key indicators; it is a medical emergency

h. Be alert to **Munchausen's syndrome by proxy:** injuries or illness induced in child by caregiver in order to meet caregiver's needs to be important and receive positive reinforcement from healthcare providers

10. Priority nursing diagnoses

a. Pain related to the infliction by parent or guardian of physical or emotional pain or injury with the intent to cause harm

b. Anxiety related to underdeveloped ego or punitive superego, inadequate parenting skills, or high expectation of children's behavior

NCLEX!

c. Ineffective family coping related to inadequate support systems or poor parenting skills

d. Post-trauma response related to having been the victim of physical and/or emotional abuse

e. Social isolation related to inadequate support systems or being prevented from interacting with peers or others

NCLEX!

f. Self-esteem disturbance related to unmet dependency needs, repeated abuse, dysfunctional family system, or not being valued by parents or guardian

11. Planning and implementation

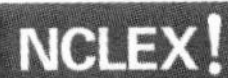

a. Report to child protective services according to facility policy and current laws

b. Provide treatment and medication for injuries

c. Encourage child to discuss fears

d. Reassure child that he/she is not to blame

e. Assess parents/caregivers' ability to cope with situation

f. Use a nonpunitive approach with parents/caregivers

g. Provide parent education, including information on normal growth and development, anger management, appropriate discipline methods, and parenting skills

h. Provide referral for community resources such as support groups, Parents Anonymous, parenting classes, and employment counseling

You are caring for the family of a young child who has been physically abused by the parents. What would your plan of care for the family include?

12. Evaluation: ongoing evaluation of child's safety and parent's ability to cope with situation; follow through with plans and protect child; verbalization of normal growth and development; utilization of appropriate community resources; stress reduction; improved parenting skills; and increased ability to manage anger

B. *Partner abuse*

1. Description: partner abuse is the physical or psychological violence toward an intimate partner intended to intimidate or degrade the partner
2. Victims
   - **a.** Can be from all socioeconomic and educational levels and any ethnic, religious, or racial background
   - **b.** Abuse may occur within a heterosexual or homosexual relationship
   - **c.** Victims may be male or female
   - **d.** Most frequent abuse is male on female
     1) 95 percent of victims of reported domestic or partner abuse are female
     2) 50 percent of female homicide victims are killed by partners
     3) 53 percent of males who abuse partners abuse their children
   - NCLEX! **e.** Victims are 15 times more likely to abuse alcohol or drugs and 5 times more likely to commit suicide than the average population
3. Abuse
   - **a.** Can be physical, economic, emotional, social, or sexual
   - **b.** First incidence of violence often occurs in dating relationship
   - **c.** Frequency varies from several times a year to weekly
   - **d.** Attacks escalate in severity and frequency over time
   - **e.** Violence often follows a pattern of escalating tension, abuse, and remorse, whereby abuser promises to change and treats victim well for brief periods
   - NCLEX! **f.** Psychological abuse may be the most devastating with constant threats of violence or even death
   - **g.** Abuser may make threats of removing children, killing or injuring family pets, or having victim committed for mental health treatment to intimidate and control victim
4. Psychological responses
   - **a.** Victim may leave abuser and return several times in an attempt to get the abuser to change his or her behavior, testing own abilities to cope and testing children's response
   - **b.** See Box 12-4 for reasons victims may have difficulty leaving abusive relationships
   - **c.** Leaving an abusive relationship is a process that happens over time
   - NCLEX! **d.** The most dangerous period is when victim leaves the relationship

Box 12-4

Reasons Victims May Have Difficulty Leaving Abusive Relationships

Financial dependency

Religious beliefs about marriage

Emotional attachment to spouse or partner

Not wanting to view the relationship as pathological

The cycle of violence contains a period of time where abuser promises to change or reform and begs forgiveness and treats victim well

Victim may blame self and feel if he or she only does better the abuse will stop

Fears for safety—abusers often threaten to kill partners if they leave; abuser may harm or kill family pets to illustrate this

Not wanting to disrupt children's lives; abuser often threatens to take children away

Abuser may threaten to have victim committed as mentally ill

Shame involved in admitting abuse

5. Etiology and psychopathology same as presented in abuse overview

6. Assessment

  a. Identification is of ultimate importance

  b. Observe for physical and emotional signs of abuse as previously noted in Table 12-1

  c. Assess history of intimate attachment relationship

  d. Observe for extreme jealousy or passiveness

  e. Determine whether conflict resolution styles are authoritative or equal

  f. Do not ask client about whether he or she is being abused, since client may not identify the behavior as abuse; ask instead more general questions

    1) "Have you ever been pushed or shoved during an argument?"

    2) "Has anyone ever hit, punched, kicked, or slapped you?"

    3) "How are disagreements dealt with in the home?"

  g. Assess beliefs about abuse and responsibility for violent acts

7. Priority nursing diagnoses

  a. Pain related to the infliction by partner of physical or emotional pain or injury with the intent to cause harm

  b. Anxiety related to underdeveloped ego or punitive superego or fear of revealing the abuser and the consequences

NCLEX!

  c. Ineffective family coping related to inadequate support system, poor relationship skills, or unrealistic expectations of either the relationship or the partner

  d. Self-esteem disturbance related to unmet dependency needs, repeated abuse, or dysfunctional family system

  e. Hopelessness related to belief in lack of options or inadequate support system

NCLEX!

f. Powerlessness related to lifestyle of helplessness, low self-esteem, or lack of support network of caring others

g. Altered family processes related to inadequate caretaking or dysfunctional family relationships

h. Social isolation related to inadequate social support or being prevented from interacting with family, friends, or others

8. Planning and implementation

a. Treat existing injuries

NCLEX!

b. Assess imminent danger

1) Is victim planning to leave abuser?

2) How frequent and severe are attacks; are they escalating?

3) Are there weapons in the home?

4) Is the abuser using drugs or alcohol and is use increasing?

5) Has the abuser threatened to kill the victim or self?

c. Client education

1) Assure the client that he or she is not to blame for the abuse

2) Provide information to client about laws, ordinances, and their rights

3) Provide referral and phone number of community resources such as women's shelters or safe houses even if the victim does not want to use them presently

4) Use mutual goal setting—allow the client to decide on goals; this empowers the victim and validates his or her strengths

5) Assist client to mobilize available support systems

6) Assist with development of a safety plan if returning to previous environment (see Box 12-5)

9. Evaluation: client verbalizes feelings of fears and anxiety; acknowledges danger of situation; develops a safety plan; begins using community resources provided; engages natural support systems such as family and friends

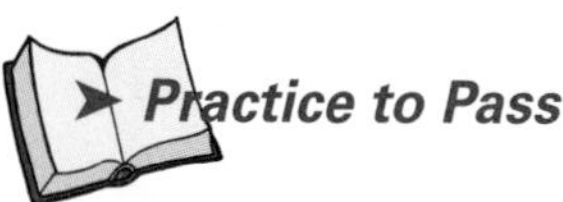

You are discharging a client after treatment of injuries from domestic abuse. The client is returning to the same environment. What would your priorities be for discharge planning?

Box 12-5

Safety Plan for Continued Violence

Ask neighbors to phone police if violence begins.

Establish code with family and friends to signify violence.

Plan an escape route to use if the abuser blocks main exit.

Identify a place to go and how to get there.

Have an escape bag that has extra clothing for self and children.

Have children's favorite toys available in a safe place.

Have extra copies hidden and available of important papers, such as driver's licenses, birth certificates, marriage license, insurance papers, social security numbers, bank account numbers, and important phone numbers and extra cash.

C. Elder abuse

1. **Elder abuse:** physical, emotional, psychological, or sexual injury to an elderly person (over age 65); recent findings indicate that 60 percent of elder abuse is done by spouse so it may overlap with partner abuse; is one of the most under-reported crimes

NCLEX!

2. Elder abuse takes many forms and may be difficult to identify due to elders' reluctance to reveal information out of fear of abandonment or retaliation
   - **a.** Physical abuse: violence that results in bodily harm or injury
   - **b.** Emotional or psychological abuse includes the following
     1) Verbal assaults, threats, or intimidation
     2) Social: restriction of social contacts
     3) Violation of personal rights: forced to act against their will
     4) Unreasonable confinement, forced isolation or denying privacy
     5) Abandonment or threats of abandonment
   - **c.** Neglect: not providing needed care
     1) Deprivation of proper medical care
     2) Providing unsafe environment
     3) Economic: strict control of money, food, clothing, or transportation
3. There are no federal laws specifically to protect elders but most states have laws for the protection of vulnerable adults; nurses need to be familiar with their state statutes governing reporting of this type of abuse
4. Etiology and psychopathology
   - **a.** Perpetrators are usually family members
   - **b.** Abuser may have personal problems and a lack of support
   - **c.** Abuser may be stressed by caring for elder
   - **d.** There may be a history of family violence
   - **e.** There may be unresolved previous conflicts and power struggles
   - **f.** Abuse may be in retaliation for past behavior of elder
   - **g.** Cultural devaluation of elders
5. Assessment
   - **a.** Physical signs as noted in overview of abuse
   - **b.** Assess for symptoms of mental illness in both victim and abuser
   - **c.** Determine if victim is financially dependent on suspected abuser

NCLEX!

   - **d.** Assess interactions within family system for signs of aggression
   - **e.** Establish a trusting relationship, as victim may be hesitant to disclose abuse for fear of abandonment or placement in a long-term care facility

f. Assess for symptoms of neglect

1) Malnutrition and/or dehydration

2) Untreated medical conditions and poor dental hygiene

3) Reports of being locked in a room

g. Assess for substance abuse in both caregiver and victim

6. Priority nursing diagnoses

a. Fear related to the infliction by caretaker of physical, emotional, or financial abuse with the intent to cause harm or abandonment

b. Anxiety related to fear of revealing the abuser and the consequences

c. Chronic pain related to poor health and illness or repeated infliction of physical or emotional pain over an extended period of time

d. Post-traumatic stress response related to having been the victim of physical, emotional, and/or financial abuse

e. Ineffective coping: individual or family related to inadequate support systems, poor follow-up care, or dysfunctional family relationships

f. Risk for violence related to being vulnerable, socially isolated, or having inadequate support systems

g. Low self-esteem related to unmet dependency needs, or being physically, emotionally, or financially abused

h. Hopelessness or powerlessness related to lifestyle of helplessness, low self-esteem, or lack of support network of caring others

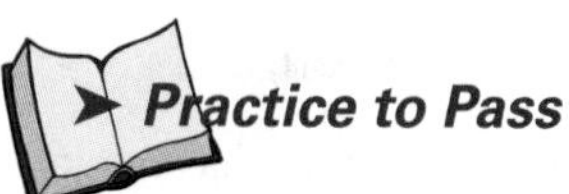

An elderly client, with numerous unexplained bruises, is brought to the Emergency Department by a caregiver. What factors would you assess to determine if the client had been abused or neglected?

7. Planning and implementation

a. Treat existing injuries

b. Assess for untreated medical conditions

c. Assess imminent danger

1) How frequent and severe are attacks?

2) Are there weapons in the home?

3) Does the victim fear for own life?

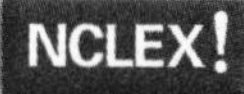

d. Is the victim considered a vulnerable adult: most states have mandatory reporting procedures for vulnerable adults

e. Provide referral to social services

8. Evaluation: the client verbalizes fears and feelings; medical condition improves; client's ability to care for self improves; client regains dignity and autonomy; family improves coping style or elder is placed in alternative living situation

D. Abuse of pregnant women

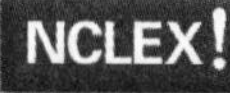

1. Pregnancy is a time of increased risk of abuse

2. A pregnant woman is most often beaten in the stomach, which can lead to complications of pregnancy, such as placenta abruptio, premature labor, miscarriage and fetal loss, or maternal injury such as fractures of the pelvis, rupture of the uterus, and hemorrhage

3. Etiology: abuse can be related to feelings of ambivalance about the pregnancy or partner feeling threatened by attention the woman is receiving due to the pregnancy

4. Assessment, diagnosis, and interventions are the same as in partner abuse with the additional need to assess partner's attitude regarding pregnancy, assessing the fetus' health and well-being, and interventions that include prenatal care

IV. Sexual Abuse

A. Description: sexual abuse includes sexual harassment, rape, sexual assault, and child sexual abuse; it is an act of violence, not of sexuality, intended to injure and intimidate the victim

B. Types

1. Sexual harassment: unwelcome sexual advances or conduct of a sexual nature on the job that creates an intimidating or offensive work environment; is considered a form of discrimination by the Equal Employment Opportunities Commission

   a. Two types of sexual harassment

   1) Quid pro quo: Latin for "this for that" when a person in authority suggests that a job, promotion, or salary will be given or withheld in exchange for sexual favors

   2) Hostile environment: sexually offensive conduct that permeates the workplace, making it difficult or unpleasant for an employee to do his or her job

2. Rape: a forced act of sexual intercourse

   a. Rape is a crime of violence: 93 percent of victims are women and 90 percent of perpetrators are men but either can be a victim or a perpetrator

   b. There is no typical rapist; victims can be children through elderly

   c. Types

   1) Date or acquaintance rape: the rapist is known to the victim; this form of rape is underreported

   2) Marital rape: occurs within marriage, this is the most prevalent and underreported form of rape, often with concurrent physical abuse

   3) Statutory rape: victim under the age of consent; this includes consensual sex between an underage victim and an adult

   4) Gang rape: a group of perpetrators often in a ritual manner

   5) Sexual assault: forceful genital, anal, or oral penetration of the victim by any object including a penis

   d. Between one-third and one-half of battered women are raped by their partners

   e. Male victims are more likely to be beaten and more reluctant to report

3. Immediate consequences of rape: in addition to physical injury, pregnancy and sexually transmitted disease can result; victims of rape can experience rape-trauma syndrome

NCLEX!

   a. Initial response may be deceptively calm, but this usually masks distress, denial, or emotional shock
   b. 25 percent of victims can have impairment that continues up to 1 year
   c. There is high level of anxiety and fear related to future attacks
   d. Victim may develop phobic reactions

NCLEX!

   e. Have difficulty with decision-making
   f. Flashbacks, violent dreams, and preoccupation with future danger are common
   g. Experience guilt, doubts, fear, anger, and hatred of the perpetrator
   h. Have problems with intimate relationship

NCLEX!

4. Long term consequences
   a. Depression (see Chapter 4)
   b. Feelings of helplessness and vulnerability
   c. Post-traumatic stress disorder (see Chapter 5)
   d. Problems with sexuality
5. Cultural specific issues with rape
   a. United States has a higher reported rate of rapes than other developed countries
   b. In countries where a young woman's worth is related to her virginity, rape is particularly devastating; to save the family reputation male members of a family may kill the woman or force the woman to marry the rapist
6. Etiology and psychopathology
   a. Intrapersonal theory
      1) Rapist is emotionally immature, powerless, and unsure of self
      2) Uses rape as a method to exert power, intimidate, or inflict pain
   b. Interpersonal theory
      1) Rapists do not have normal interpersonal involvement
      2) Rapist is preoccupied with own fantasies
   c. Social learning theory
      1) Society accepts and glamorizes violence
      2) Aggression is learned through family, peers, and culture
   d. Feminist
      1) Rape is the result of deep-rooted socioeconomic tradition of male dominance
      2) Women are devalued by society

7. Assessment

NCLEX!

a. Clients that are brought to Emergency Department by police after rape or sexual assault are easily identifiable; other victims may not be; *all* clients should be assessed for current or past sexual abuse

b. Questions need to be broadly stated: "Has anyone ever forced you to have sex when you did not want to?"

c. This can be followed with more broad open-ended questions to elicit further history

d. Explain that this line of questioning is routine and done with every client

e. Assess for physical injuries and behavioral signs of abuse as noted previously

f. In situations of criminal rape, evidence needs to be gathered; this may be done by specialized teams of nurses and doctors

NCLEX!

g. Permission *must* be obtained prior to the gathering of evidence and taking of photos for evidence

h. Give the client as much control as possible during the assessment process

8. Priority nursing diagnoses

a. Pain related to the infliction of sexual, physical, and/or emotional abuse by a predator

b. Anxiety related to fear of loss of control, fear of repeated abuse, or fear of revealing the abuser and the consequences

c. Rape trauma syndrome related to having been the victim of sexual violence executed with the use of force and against one's personal will and consent

d. Self-esteem disturbance related to unmet dependency needs, questioning of self-efficacy, or unrealistically blaming self

9. Planning and implementation

a. Initial response must include nonjudgmental listening and psychological support

NCLEX!

b. Identify immediate concerns and priorities

c. Allow client to discuss feelings about assault

NCLEX!

d. Support decision-making and active problem-solving using mutual goal setting; client's goals may differ from nurse's

e. If the attack was recent, evidence may need to be gathered; follow facility policies regarding gathering of evidence; obtain permission from client

f. Test for pregnancy and sexually transmitted diseases

g. Client education

NCLEX!

1) Reassure client that rape is not her or his fault and survival was the most important outcome

2) Advise about potential for pregnancy and sexually transmitted disease

3) Provide information about community services, such as survivors groups, shelters for battered women (men) and legal service, and encourage their use

4) If sexual assault is by a partner, identify and provide education about options, including staying with client when the abuser is present, removing abuser through arrest, obtaining protective orders to keep abuser away, or leaving abuser

h. Assist with development of a safety plan if the victim is returning to the environment with the abuser as noted in previous section on partner abuse

10. Evaluation: client expresses feelings about the incident, which may include anger, fear, guilt and vulnerability; seeks appropriate medical care for problems related to the assault; develops a safety or escape plan; identifies support systems and people that are available to assist in dealing with crisis; and actively is involved in mobilizing support systems

You are discharging a client who had been raped. What teaching would you do with this client?

Case Study

You are doing an admission assessment on a child who has multiple bruises on his body. You suspect the child may have been abused.

1. What information will you gather from the mother?
2. What physical signs will you look for in the child?
3. What behavioral signs will you look for in the child?
4. What are your priority interventions in caring for this child?
5. What things will you teach the mother?

For suggested responses, see page 310.

Posttest

1 An elderly man has been admitted to the hospital for dehydration. The client is poorly dressed, has body odor, appears unkempt, and has unexplained bruises. The nurse's *priority* action would be to:

(1) Determine if the client is experiencing abuse or neglect.
(2) Take a social history.
(3) Assess history of present illness.
(4) Inquire about medications the client is taking.

2 The nurse is caring for a client who is being treated for migraine headaches. Upon physical exam the nurse assesses old scars on the client's arms and legs. The client confides memories of sexual abuse as a child perpetrated by her father. The nurse's *immediate* response should be:

(1) "Tell me more about your migraines."
(2) "How did you get the scars?"
(3) "How old were you when the abuse stopped?"
(4) "Are you comfortable discussing the abuse?"

3 A mother brings her 2-year-old son in for his immunizations along with his 7-year-old brother. The nurse observes the mother ignoring the 7-year-old, who is pushing and slapping the 2-year-old. What would be the *most* appropriate intervention?

(1) Teach the mother this is normal sibling rivalry.
(2) Encourage the younger son to stand up for himself.
(3) Tell the mother it is best if they work this out themselves.
(4) Teach the mother this behavior may indicate sibling abuse.

4 A mother brings in an 8-month-old infant who is having difficulty breathing. The nurse assesses bleeding in the baby's retinas. The child was being cared for by the father while the mother was out. Which of the following would be the *most* appropriate action by the nurse?

(1) Question the mother about the events prior to the respiratory distress.
(2) Identify this as a potential medical emergency.
(3) Do a neurological exam on the baby.
(4) Administer oxygen to the baby.

5 The nurse evaluates a 5-year-old child who is still wearing diapers, sucking his thumb, rocking, and banging his head. The child has normal language skills. The nurse reports this behavior as:

(1) Mental retardation.
(2) Possible emotional abuse or neglect.
(3) An indication of autism.
(4) Pervasive developmental delay.

6 An adult survivor of child abuse states "Why couldn't I make him stop the abuse? If I were a stronger person, I would have been able to make him stop. Maybe it was my fault he abused me." Based on this data, which would be the *most* appropriate nursing diagnosis?

(1) Ineffective family coping
(2) Social isolation
(3) Chronic low self-esteem
(4) Anxiety

7 The nurse is assessing a normal appearing 6-year-old brought to the Emergency Department by the mother, who reports that the child vomits every time she eats. The child's history reveals no positive findings as well as several previous similar visits. The mother is very concerned and insists that the child be admitted for a full GI workup. The nurse reports this as possible:

(1) Anxiety disorder.
(2) Bulimia nervosa.
(3) Munchausen's syndrome by proxy.
(4) Severe food allergies.

8 The nurse is counseling an extremely distressed female victim immediately after a rape. What would the nurse's *most* important intervention be?

(1) Reassure the victim that the rape was not her fault.
(2) Begin gathering evidence.
(3) Test for pregnancy.
(4) Teach about sexually transmitted diseases.

9 The nurse is evaluating a family in which child abuse has occurred. What outcome would indicate progress for the parents?

(1) Parents report continued use of spanking for discipline.
(2) Both parents are attending parenting classes.
(3) Parents report high expectations for their children.
(4) Parents report an understanding of normal growth and development.

10 A teenage female is brought to the Emergency Department following a suicide attempt. During the interview the client reports to the nurse that she is doing poorly in school, is engaging in high-risk sexual activity, and has a history of running away from home. The nurse should assess for:

(1) Pregnancy.
(2) Physical abuse.
(3) Sexual abuse.
(4) Sexually transmitted disease.

See pages 256–257 for Answers and Rationales.

Answers and Rationales

Pretest

1 **Answer: 1** ***Rationale:*** The numerous bruises and the mother's vague explanations of the injuries indicate possible child abuse. Home safety is important but not as important as the child's safety (option 2). Falling down stairs frequently is not normal behavior for a 2-year-old (option 3), nor is it a symptom of attention deficit disorder (option 4).
Cognitive Level: Application
Nursing Process: Analysis; ***Test Plan:*** PHYS

2 **Answer: 4** ***Rationale:*** The symptoms, client's behavior, and daughter's behavior would indicate possible abuse or neglect. The daughter may be the abuser, and it is necessary to first interview the client apart from the daughter to assess for abuse. Nutritional assessment and teaching may follow (option 2), but the client's safety is more important at this time. Confusion alone is not a symptom of mental illness (option 4).
Cognitive Level: Application
Nursing Process: Assessment; ***Test Plan:*** PHYS

3 **Answer: 3** ***Rationale:*** The child's examination shows signs of sexual abuse, which must be reported. Further data gathering (options 1 and 4) and teaching (option 2) would be a second priority.
Cognitive Level: Application
Nursing Process: Analysis; ***Test Plan:*** SECE

4 **Answer: 3** ***Rationale:*** The client's safety is of utmost importance; if she decides to return to the violent environment, she must have a safety plan. Instructing her to leave the relationship (option 1) will not help if she is not ready. Providing legal assistance (option 2) and a list of services that are available (option 4) are appropriate but secondary.
Cognitive Level: Analysis
Nursing Process: Planning; ***Test Plan:*** PHYS

5 **Answer: 3** ***Rationale:*** Education and money do *not* make persons immune from violence. It crosses all socioeconomic lines. Violence does often begin in dating relationships (option 1); abusers do apologize and promise to stop (option 2); abusers are often excessively jealous and possessive (option 4).
Cognitive Level: Analysis
Nursing Process: Evaluation; ***Test Plan:*** HPM

6 **Answer: 1** ***Rationale:*** The most dangerous time in an abusive relationship is when the victim leaves; having left, the victim is in greater danger. It often takes several times (option 2) before victims are able to leave. Victims often feel that the abuse is their fault (option 3). Abusers will make threats of removing children from the victim to intimidate and control the victim (option 4). Options 3 and 4 can be addressed once safety has been addressed.
Cognitive Level: Analysis
Nursing Process: Analysis; ***Test Plan:*** PHYS

7 **Answer: 3** ***Rationale:*** The child will be at risk for depression. There are many long-term consequences of child abuse (option 1). Abuse is more devastating if the abuser is a person the child trusted (option 2). Not all abused children go on to become abusers (option 4).
Cognitive Level: Application
Nursing Process: Implementation; ***Test Plan:*** HPM

8 **Answer: 4** ***Rationale:*** The client has been raped and nurse needs to respond to the client's immediate concerns. Testing (option 1) and teaching (options 2 and 3) are secondary interventions.
Cognitive Level: Application
Nursing Process: Assessment; ***Test Plan:*** PSYC

9 **Answer: 1** ***Rationale:*** It is vital that the client understand that the pregnancy may be in danger from the abuse. The client will need resources (option 4), childbirth classes (option 3) and assertiveness training (option 2) in the future, but she must first understand the risk to the baby in order to motivate her.
Cognitive Level: Analysis
Nursing Process: Implementation; ***Test Plan:*** HPM

10 **Answer: 1** ***Rationale:*** A delay in seeking treatment for serious injuries is an indication of abuse. Anxiety and concern upon the parents' part would be expected (option 3). Vague descriptions of the injuries with little detail are more likely to indicate abuse than a detailed description (option 2). Preventing the child from explaining the injuries, not encouraging explanation, would be an indication of abuse (option 4).
Cognitive Level: Analysis
Nursing Process: Assessment; ***Test Plan:*** PHYS

Posttest

1 **Answer: 1** ***Rationale:*** Initial observations of dehydration, unexplained bruises and poor hygiene indicate possible abuse or neglect, which would need to be immediately assessed and reported. The nurse would then proceed with a history of present illness (option 3), determination of which medications the

client is taking (option 4) and social history (option 2).
Cognitive Level: Analysis
Nursing Process: Assessment; ***Test Plan:*** PSYC

2 **Answer: 4** ***Rationale:*** The migraines may be the presenting problem but the client is indicating a need to discuss the abuse (option 1). A nonjudgmental approach considering the client's comfort level would be best to prevent the client from feeling guilt and shame. The age the abuse stopped (option 3) and how the scars occurred (option 2) are secondary at this point.
Cognitive Level: Application
Nursing Process: Implementation; ***Test Plan:*** PSYC

3 **Answer: 4** ***Rationale:*** The physical abuse goes beyond sibling rivalry (option 1). The younger boy would not be able to stand up to someone older and larger than he (option 2), nor would he be mature enough or have the language skills needed to work things out with his sibling (option 3). Sibling abuse is often unrecognized and can lead to serious injury if not addressed.
Cognitive Level: Application
Nursing Process: Implementation; ***Test Plan:*** PHYS

4 **Answer: 2** ***Rationale:*** The events leading up to the distress are relevant (option 1) but secondary at this time; the respiratory distress and retinal bleeding are symptoms of shaken baby syndrome and represent a medical emergency. The neuro exam (option 3) and oxygen (option 4) would be the next steps.
Cognitive Level: Analysis
Nursing Process: Analysis; ***Test Plan:*** PHYS

5 **Answer: 2** ***Rationale:*** The regressive behaviors would indicate probably abuse or neglect. With mental retardation (option 1), autism (option 3), or pervasive developmental delay (option 4), the child's language skills would be affected.
Cognitive Level: Analysis
Nursing Process: Analysis; ***Test Plan:*** PSYC

6 **Answer: 3** ***Rationale:*** Inappropriate self-blame and feelings that a child could have stopped an adult's abuse indicate a low self-esteem. Options 1, 2, and 3 are possible diagnoses for adult survivors of abuse; there is not enough evidence supporting these diagnoses. More data would be needed.
Cognitive Level: Application
Nursing Process: Analysis; ***Test Plan:*** PSYC

7 **Answer: 3** ***Rationale:*** Munchausen's Syndrome by proxy is characterized by the caregiver reporting or producing symptoms in a child that require hospitalization and invasive procedures. The reports by the mother and indication of several other attempts by the mother to have the child hospitalized point to Munchausen's. The physical appearance of the child and the previous negative physical findings would rule out anxiety disorder (option 1), bulimia (option 2), and food allergies (option 4).
Cognitive Level: Analysis
Nursing Process: Analysis; ***Test Plan:*** PSYC

8 **Answer: 1** ***Rationale:*** The client needs to be reassured that the rape was not her fault. Teaching and testing (options 3 and 4) are secondary interventions after the client is calmer. Gathering evidence would proceed only after reassuring the client and obtaining permission to gather evidence (option 2).
Cognitive Level: Application
Nursing Process: Implementation; ***Test Plan:*** PSYC

9 **Answer: 4** ***Rationale:*** The spanking indicates the parents have not learned alternative discipline methods (option 1) and attending classes does not illustrate understanding of the concepts (option 2). Having unreasonably high expectations for children is a continued risk factor for abuse (option 3). Understanding normal growth and development will help the parents have more reasonable expectations of the children.
Cognitive Level: Application
Nursing Process: Evaluation; ***Test Plan:*** PSYC

10 **Answer: 3** ***Rationale:*** The sexual behavior, suicide attempt, and running away indicate possible sexual abuse. Assessment for physical abuse (option 2), pregnancy (option 1), and sexually transmitted diseases (option 4) would be secondary.
Cognitive Level: Analysis
Nursing Process: Assessment; ***Test Plan:*** PHYS

References

Boyd, M. (1998). Biopsychosocial aspects of caring for abused persons. In M. Boyd & M. Nihart (Eds.), *Psychiatric nursing: Contemporary practice.* Philadelphia: Lippincott, pp. 1052–1077.

Fishwick, N., Parker, B., & Campbell, J. (2001). Care of survivors of abuse and violence. In G. Stuart & M. Laraia (Eds.), *Principles and practice of psychiatric nursing* (7th ed.). St. Louis: Mosby, pp. 824–840.

Fontaine, K. (1999). Domestic violence. In K. Fontaine & J. Fletcher (Eds.), *Mental health nursing* (4th ed.). Menlo Park, CA: Addison-Wesley, pp. 428–447.

Fontaine, K. (1999). Sexual violence. In K. Fontaine & J. Fletcher (Eds.), *Mental health nursing* (4th ed.). Menlo Park, CA: Addison-Wesley, pp. 450–479.

Thobaben, M. (1998). Survivors of violence or abuse. In N. Frisch & L. Frisch (Eds.), *Psychiatric mental health nursing.* Boston: Delmar, pp. 561–600.

Townsend, M. (2000). Problems related to abuse or neglect. In M. Townsend (Ed.), *Psychiatric mental health nursing: Concepts of care* (3rd ed.). Philadelphia: F. A. Davis, pp. 739–757.

Urbancic, J. (2000). Survivors of family violence. In K. Fortinash & P. Holoday-Worret (Eds.), *Psychiatric mental health nursing* (2nd ed.). St. Louis: Mosby, pp. 618–647.

CHAPTER 13

Loss, Grief, and Death

George Byron Smith, ARNP, PhD(c), Cm

CHAPTER OUTLINE

OBJECTIVES

- List at least five physiologic and at least four psychological responses to loss and grief.
- Discuss the differences between normal and pathologic or dysfunctional grief.
- Differentiate between the grief experienced by males and the grief experienced by females.
- Identify at least three behaviors associated with uncomplicated, delayed, distorted, and disenfranchised grief.
- Explain the purpose of an advance directive.
- Discuss nursing management of a client experiencing grief, loss, or death.
- Identify expected outcomes for the client experiencing grief, loss, or death.

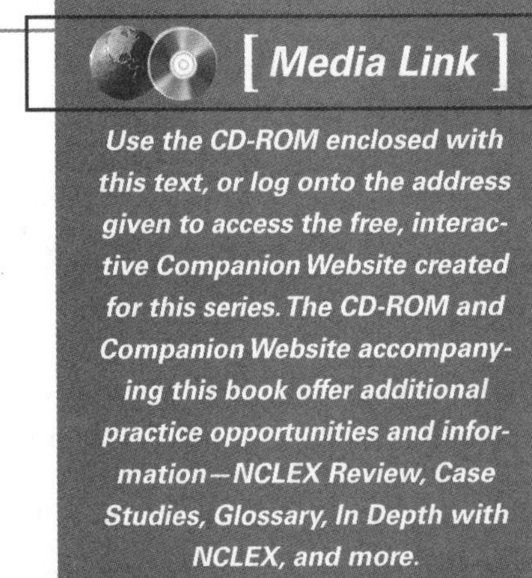

Review at a Glance

abbreviated grief *mild anxiety and sorrow experienced for a brief period but genuinely felt*

advance directive *a general term that refers to a client's written instructions about future medical care, in the event that the client becomes unable to speak or is incapacitated; each state regulates the use of advance directives differently*

anticipatory grief *anxiety and sorrow experienced prior to an expected loss or death*

bereavement *the status of having lost a family member, friend, colleague, or other significant person through death*

closed awareness *the client and family are unaware of impending loss or death*

death *cessation of physiologic processes that sustain life; a passing or parting; letting go of this life, or loss of life*

delayed grief *postponed response in which the bereaved person may have a reaction at the time of the loss, but it is not sufficient to the loss; a later loss may trigger a reaction that is out of proportion to the meaning of the current loss*

disenfranchised grief *a response to a loss or death in which the individual is not regarded as having the right to grieve or is unable to acknowledge the loss to other persons*

do-not-resuscitate order (DNR) *a physician's order of "no code" or "do not resuscitate" for clients who are in a stage of terminal, irreversible illness, or expected death*

dying *the dynamic and individualized process of death*

dysfunctional grief *unresolved or inhibited grief that does not lead to a successful conclusion*

euthanasia *the act of painlessly putting to death persons or animals suffering from incurable or distressing disease*

grief *a pervasive, individualized, and dynamic process that may result in physical, emotional, or spiritual distress because of loss or death of a loved one or cherished object*

healthcare proxy *a document appointing someone else (e.g., a relative or trusted friend) to manage health care treatment decisions when the client is unable to do so*

inhibited grief *suppressed response that may be expressed in other ways, such as somatic complaints (e.g., physically symptomatic on the anniversary of a loss or during holidays)*

living will *provides specific instructions about what medical treatment the client chooses to omit or refuse (e.g., ventilator support) in the event that the client is unable to make those decisions*

loss *the actual or potential situation in which something that is valued is changed, no longer available, or gone*

mourning *the expression of the sorrow of loss and grief in a manner understood and approved by the culture*

mutual pretense *a state in which the client, family, and healthcare provider know that the prognosis is terminal but do not talk about it and make an effort not to raise the subject*

open awareness *a state in which the client and individuals involved know about the impending loss or death and feel comfortable discussing it, even though it may be difficult*

unresolved grief *grief that is prolonged or extended in length and severity of response*

Pretest

1 An average-sized client who describes a loss in body image related to viewing him- or herself as "too fat" may be experiencing what type of loss?

(1) Actual
(2) Perceived
(3) Anticipatory
(4) Permanent

2 In counseling parents who have recently lost a child to death, it is important for the nurse to have already dealt with personal feelings about death, grief, and loss in children. This self-awareness would:

(1) Assist the nurse in helping the parents to express their grief fully.
(2) Prevent the nurse from being personally affected by the loss.
(3) Prevent the nurse from sharing any personal feelings with the parents.
(4) Assist the nurse in avoiding discussion of unpleasant feelings with the parents.

3 A young woman who comes to a routine medical visit appears depressed and tells the nurse she is having difficulty dealing with the death of her infant son. The nurse learns the infant died 30 months ago in a automobile accident. The initial nursing diagnosis is Dysfunctional grieving. The statement by the client that supports this diagnosis would be:

(1) "I do not let my children play in playgrounds because it makes me angry that my son will never be able to play like other children."
(2) "I haven't been able to remove any items from my baby's room."
(3) "I watch other toddlers in the neighborhood play, and I can't help but cry and wish my son was still alive."
(4) "I think of my son and am sad that my new baby will never be able to know his brother."

4 A middle-aged client has not eaten for 3 days, appears disheveled, continuously experiences uncontrolled crying spells, and refuses to leave her bedroom. She has been unable to return to work since her husband's funeral 4 months ago. Which of the following nursing diagnoses is most appropriate at this time?

(1) Grieving related to recent loss of spouse and inability to leave bedroom
(2) Anticipatory grieving related to failure to return to work
(3) Anxiety related to refusal to eat and uncontrollable crying spells
(4) Dsyfunctional grieving related to developmental regression, isolation, and failure to return to work

5 An Africian-American family gathered around their dying grandmother's bed refuses to allow a feeding tube to be removed and to stop feeding her, even after the healthcare team has stated that there was nothing else to be done. The nurse understands the family's resistance to removal of the feeding tube is most likely caused by:

(1) Their refusal to accept the finality of death.
(2) Their need to try every possible solution.
(3) Their spiritual and cultural beliefs.
(4) Their distrust of the healthcare system.

6 A father who recently lost his eldest son to cancer refuses to share his feelings in a support group and has not shown any tears related to the loss. The nurse recognizes this behavior as:

(1) A common expression of how men grieve loss and death.
(2) Dysfunctional expression of grief and the client should be referred to counseling.
(3) A common expression of denial and refusal to accept death or loss.
(4) The father's attempt to be strong for the rest of the family.

7 A child, age 5, expresses the belief that if he wishes hard enough he will be able to bring his father back from the dead. The nurse understands that the child is:

(1) Expressing magical thinking common to much older children.
(2) Voicing thoughts that are normal for children his age.
(3) Delusional and should be evaluated by a psychiatrist.
(4) Making up the story in order to avoid feeling sad and scared.

8 While visiting their dying mother in the hospital, the adult children tell the nurse that they do not want the mother to be told she is dying and that they will not talk about dying or death in front of their mother. The nurse understands this as:

(1) Closed awareness.
(2) Mutual pretense.
(3) Mutual awareness.
(4) Open awareness.

9 A frail older female calls the home health nurse and tells the nurse, "I am a failure, and I can no longer care adequately for my husband who has Alzheimer's disease." She has been his primary caregiver for over 5 years; now he has become despondent, is unable to ambulate, and is difficult to manage. The most applicable nursing diagnosis would be:

(1) Ineffective individual coping related to chronic illness.
(2) Social isolation of family unit related to altered state of health.
(3) Dysfunctional grief related to not accepting personal limitations.
(4) Risk of caregiver role strain related to overwhelming caregiving tasks and expectations.

10 Outcome criteria for successful counseling for the loss of a client's spouse would include the client's ability to:

(1) Avoid feelings about the spouse's death.
(2) Immediately memorialize the spouse.
(3) Attend grief support groups.
(4) Avoid sharing loss with significant others.

See pages 277–278 for Answers and Rationales.

I. Overview of Loss, Grieving, and Death

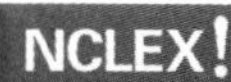

A. Definition of *loss*—the actual or potential situation in which something that is valued is changed, no longer available, or gone

1. Losses are experiences that affect not only the client and the client's family but also affect the nurse
2. Change in status of significant other
3. Any change that reduces the possibility of achieving implicit or explicit goals
4. Experience of deprivation or complete lack of something that was previously present

B. Types of loss

1. Actual: can be identified by others and can arise in response to or in anticipation of a situation (e.g., death of significant other)

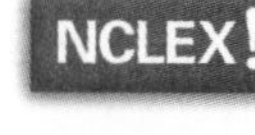

2. Perceived: is experienced by one person but cannot be verified by others (e.g., loss of self-esteem)
3. Anticipatory: is experienced before the loss actually occurs (e.g., terminal illness)

C. Time period of loss

1. Temporary: deprivation and later restoration of something that was previously present (e.g., missing child)
2. Permanent: irreversible deprivation (e.g., paralysis)

D. Circumstances of loss

1. Maturational: results from normal life transitions (e.g., parents' feeling sadness when their youngest child leaves for college)
2. Situational: loss occurs in response to a specific event

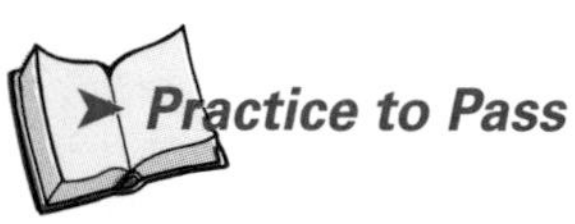

A client recently lost a partner of 20 years to acquired immunodeficiency syndrome (AIDS). What physiological and psychological responses by the client would you expect to observe?

E. Sources of loss

1. Aspect of self: loss of a valued part of oneself—a body part (e.g., amputation of an extremity), a physiologic function, or a psychological attribute
2. External objects: loss of inanimate objects (e.g., property) or loss of animate object (e.g., family pet)
3. Familiar environment: separation from an environment and people who provide security (e.g., placement in a nursing home)
4. Loved one: loss of a significant person or valued person (or pet) through illness, separation or death (e.g., death from AIDS)
5. Loss of life: loss of a significant person or loss of one's own life (e.g., terminal illness)

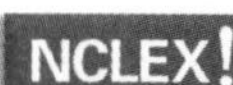

F. Physiological responses related to loss or grief

1. Crying and sobbing
2. Sighing respirations
3. Shortness of breath and palpitations

4. Fatigue, weakness, and exhaustion
5. Insomnia
6. Loss of appetite
7. Choking sensation
8. Tightness in chest
9. Gastrointestinal disturbances

NCLEX!

G. Psychological responses related to loss or grief

1. Intense loneliness and sadness
2. Depressed mood
3. Anxiety or panic episodes
4. Difficulty concentrating and focusing
5. Anger or rage directed toward self or others
6. Ambivalence and low self-esteem
7. Somatic complaints

H. Self-assessment and self-awareness

1. Is critical in order for the nurse to be sensitive and therapeutic with clients who have experienced loss

NCLEX!

2. Explore personal attitudes, feelings, and values related to loss and grief

I. Bereavement, mourning, and grief

NCLEX!

1. **Bereavement:** a change in status caused by losing a family member, friend, colleague, or other significant person through death
2. **Mourning:** the expression of the sorrow of loss and grief in a manner understood and approved by the culture

NCLEX!

3. **Grief:** a pervasive, individualized, and dynamic process that may result in physical, emotional, or spiritual distress because of loss or death of a loved one or cherished object

NCLEX!

   a. **Abbreviated grief:** mild anxiety and sorrow experienced for a brief period but genuinely felt

NCLEX!

   b. **Anticipatory grief:** anxiety and sorrow experienced prior to an expected loss or death

NCLEX!

   c. **Disenfranchised grief:** a response to a loss or death in which the individual is not regarded as having the right to grieve or is unable to acknowledge the loss to other persons (e.g., a gay partner unable to acknowledge the loss of his or her significant other)

NCLEX!

   d. **Dysfunctional grief:** unresolved or inhibited grief that does not lead to a successful conclusion

      1) **Unresolved grief:** prolonged or extended in length and severity of response (e.g., after a prolonged period, an individual continues to search for a lost person)

2) **Inhibited grief:** suppressed response that may be expressed in other ways, such as somatic complaints (e.g., physically symptomatic on the anniversary of a loss or during holidays)

3) **Delayed grief:** postponed response in which the bereaved person may have a reaction at the time of the loss, but it is not sufficient to the loss; a later loss may trigger a reaction that is out of proportion to the meaning of the current loss (e.g., loss of a pet triggers a suicidal reaction in a woman after not being able to grieve her husband's death 3 years ago)

J. Stages of grief: labels for stages must be used with caution because each individual processes grief in different ways and at different rates

NCLEX!

1. Stages should be used as descriptive of the grieving process rather than prescriptive of the grieving process (see Table 13-1)

NCLEX!

2. There have been many theories on the stages of grief; the central themes of these theories include:

a. Shock and disbelief (1 to 3 weeks)

1) Numbness

2) Denial

3) Passive

4) Unaware of others

b. Searching and protesting (3 weeks to 4 months)

1) Crying and yearning

Table 13-1

Engel's Stages of Grieving

Stage	Behavioral Response
Shock and disbelief	Refusal to accept loss Stunned feelings Intellectual acceptance but emotional denial
Developing awareness	Reality of loss begins to penetrate consciousness Anger may be directed at agency, nurses, or others
Restitution	Rituals of mourning (e.g., funeral)
Resolving the loss	Attempts to deal with painful void Still unable to accept new love object to replace lost person or object May accept more dependent relationship with support person Thinks over and talks about memories of the lost object
Idealization	Produces image of lost object that is almost devoid of undesirable features Represses all negative and hostile feelings toward lost object May feel guilty and remorseful about past inconsiderate or unkind acts to lost person Unconsciously internalizes admired qualities of lost object Reminders of lost object evoke fewer feelings of sadness Reinvests feelings in others
Outcome	Behavior influenced by several factors: importance of lost object as source of support, degree of dependence on relationship, degree of ambivalence toward lost object, number and nature of other relationships, and number of previous grief experiences (which tend to be cumulative)

Source: Engel, G. L. (1964). Grief and grieving. *American Journal of Nursing 64* (9), 93–98.

A client is expected to die from lung cancer within the next few months. The client's wife tells you, "I can't help with my husband's care right now. He keeps wanting to talk about his dying, and I just can't talk about that right now because it is too hard to lose him." You suspect the wife is experiencing what type of grief? Why?

2) Guilt
3) Intense and conflicting emotions, such as sadness and anger
4) Empty feeling
5) Identification and preoccupation with thoughts of loss or death
6) Dependent
7) Self-destructive behaviors

c. Disorientation (4 to 14 months)
1) Depression and despair
2) Apathy and loss of interest
3) Aimlessness
4) Disorganization
5) Insomnia
6) Inability to maintain work and family responsibilities
7) Confusion and slowed thinking
8) Social withdrawal

d. Reorganization and resolution (14 months throughout rest of life)
1) Acceptance of loss, letting go
2) Awareness of having grieved
3) Ability to talk about deceased or loss without intense pain
4) New or renewed social relationships
5) New or renewed interest
6) Process that may typically last up to 1 year

NCLEX!

3. Kübler-Ross's stages of death and dying: were originally intended to be used for individuals dying of terminal illness, but have been used to describe the grieving process of loss

a. Denial: disbelief or refusal to acknowledge that loss or death is happening

b. Anger: expression of overt hostility toward loss object, dying person, or others

c. Bargaining: attempts to negotiate to prolong one's life or to erase the loss

d. Depression: sense of sadness over loss or death

e. Acceptance: comes to terms with loss or death

4. Worden's four tasks of mourning: implies that persons who mourn can be actively involved in helping themselves and can be assisted and influenced by the nurse in resolving their grief

a. Task I: to accept the reality of the loss

b. Task II: to work through the pain of grief

c. Task III: to adjust to the environment in which the deceased or loss person/object is missing

d. Task IV: to emotionally relocate the deceased and move on with life

K. Factors influencing the grief response

1. Age (see Table 13-2)

NCLEX!

a. Childhood

1) Preschool children (aged 3 to 5) fear separation from parents and do not understand the finality of death

2) Children aged 5 to 6 see death as reversible

3) Children aged 6 to 9 begin to accept death as a destructive force and as a final event

4) Children at age 10 realize that death is inevitable

5) Adolescents intellectualize awareness of death, but tend to repress feelings about it

b. Early and middle adult

1) View loss and death as normal developmental tasks

2) Potential loss from impaired health or body function

3) Change in various role functions

Table 13-2

Development of the Concept of Death

Age	Beliefs/Attitudes
Infancy to 5 years	Does not understand concept of death Infant's sense of separation forms basis for later understanding of loss and death Believes death is reversible, a temporary departure, or sleep Emphasizes immobility and inactivity as attributes of death
5 to 9 years	Understands that death is final Believes own death can be avoided Associates death with aggression or violence Believes wishes or unrelated actions can be responsible for death
9 to 12 years	Understands death as the inevitable end of life Begins to understand own mortality, expressed as interest in afterlife or as fear of death
12 to 18 years	Fears a lingering death May fantasize that death can be defied, acting out defiance through reckless behaviors (e.g., dangerous driving, substance abuse) Seldom thinks about death, but views it in religious and philosophic terms May seem to reach "adult" perception of death but is emotionally unable to accept it May still hold concepts from previous developmental stages
18 to 45 years	Has attitude toward death influenced by religious and cultural beliefs
45 to 65 years	Accepts own mortality Encounters death of parents and some peers Experiences peaks of death anxiety Death anxiety diminishes with emotional well-being
65+ years	Fears prolonged illness Encounters death of family members and peers See death as having multiple meanings, (e.g., freedom from pain, reunion with already deceased family members)

Source: Kozier, B., Erb, G., Berman, A.J., & Burke, K. (2000). *Fundamentals of nursing: Concepts, process, and practice.* Upper Saddle River, NJ: Prentice-Hall, Inc., p. 981.

NCLEX!

c. Older adult

1) Loss of health, function, and/or independence

2) Potential change in living accommodations

3) Loss of longtime mate or significant other

4) Multiple losses (i.e., control, competence, and material possessions) and deaths of friends, family, and significant others

2. Significance of the loss

a. Value placed on the loss person, object, or function

b. Degree of change required because of loss

c. The person's belief and values

3. Culture

NCLEX!

a. Dictates customs and rituals used to express grief

1) In cultures where strong kinship ties are maintained, physical and emotional support and assistance are provided by family members

2) Spiritual beliefs and practices greatly influence both a person's reaction to loss and subsequent behavior

b. Describes the nature of life after death

NCLEX!

c. Explains the meaning of death

NCLEX!

d. Defines the relationship between the dead and the living

e. Designates the processes of bereavement

NCLEX!

f. Delineates the appropriate expression of feelings

1) Some cultures endure grief internally and privately, favoring a quiet and stoic expression of grief

2) Some cultures value social support and the outward expression of loss, such as, wailing, crying, and physical prostration

g. Determines patterns of behavior specific to age and gender

4. Gender

NCLEX!

a. Male or masculine grief

1) Expression of feelings are limited and toned down

2) Thinking precedes and often dominates feelings

3) Focus is on problem-solving rather than expression of feelings

4) Outward expression of feelings often involve anger and/or guilt

5) Internal adjustments to the loss are usually expressed through activity

6) Intense feelings may be experienced privately; there is a general reluctance to discuss these with others

7) Intense grief is usually expressed immediately after the loss, often during post-death rituals

Practice to Pass

A client recently lost his wife to breast cancer. He is withdrawn, stoic, and quiet during the funeral and while visiting with family and friends. He does not cry or openly share any feelings of sadness or loss. When asked how he is feeling he primarily responds with anger and states how he plans to survive the future without his wife. How would you interpret this behavior?

b. Female or feminine grief

1) Expression of feelings is more overt
2) May verbally express for longer period of time
3) More communicative about their loss
4) Usually exhibit a wider range of emotions and openly share their feelings with others
5) More often seek and accept support in one-to-one relationships or as members of support groups
6) Usually assume supportive roles for other survivors of loss through volunteering or other activities

5. Socioeconomic status

a. Socioeconomic status often affects the support system available at the time of loss

b. A loss of function or body part may cause a change in socioeconomic status due to loss of work or vocation

6. Support system

a. People closest to the grieving individual can often provide emotional, physical, and functional assistance

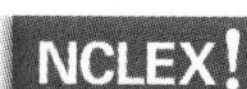

b. Because of being uncomfortable with loss or death, support people may withdraw from the grieving individual

c. Support may be available when the loss is first recognized, but as the support people return to their usual activities, the need for ongoing support is often unmet

7. Cause of loss or death

a. Views that society places on the cause of the loss or death

b. Loss or death caused by murder, suicide, or other tragic cause may be more difficult to accept and process

c. A loss or death that is beyond one's control (e.g., cancer) may be more acceptable than one that is preventable (e.g., drunk driving accident)

d. Loss of death occurring during respected activities (e.g., police officer in the line of duty) are considered honorable, whereas those occurring during illicit activities (e.g., accidental drug overdose) may be considered the individual's "just rewards"

L. Definitions and Signs of Death

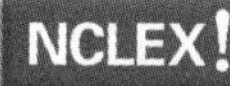

1. Death: cessation of physiologic processes that sustain life; a passing or parting; letting go of this life, or loss of life

a. Death represents the ultimate loss

b. Death is part of the continuum of life and as such is a universal and inevitable part of the human experience

c. Death is often viewed as a mystical event that may generate great fear and anxiety

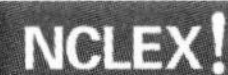

2. **Dying:** the dynamic and individualized process of death

NCLEX!

3. Clinical signs of death
   - **a.** Total lack of response to external stimuli
   - **b.** No muscular movement, especially breathing
   - **c.** No reflexes
   - **d.** Flat electroencephalogram

NCLEX!

4. In instances of artificial support, absence of electric currents from the brain (measured by an electroencephalogram) for at least 24 hours is an indication of death

NCLEX!

5. Cerebral death or higher brain death: occurs when the higher brain center, the cerebral cortex, is irreversibly destroyed

M. Byocak's developmental landmarks and tasks at the end of life

1. Sense of completion with worldly affairs: transfer of fiscal, legal, and formal social responsibilities
2. Sense of completion in relationships with community
   - **a.** Closure of multiple social relationships (employment, commerce, organizational, and congregational)
   - **b.** Components include: expressions of regret, expressions of forgiveness, acceptance of gratitude and appreciation
   - **c.** Leave taking; the saying of goodbye
3. Sense of meaning about one's individual life
   - **a.** Life review
   - **b.** Telling of "one's stories"
   - **c.** Transmission of knowledge and wisdom
4. Experience love of self
   - **a.** Self-acknowledgment
   - **b.** Self-forgiveness
5. Experience love of others: acceptance of worthiness
6. Sense of completion in relations with family and friends
   - **a.** Reconciliation, fullness of communication and closure in each of one's important relationships
   - **b.** Component tasks include expressions of regret, expressions of forgiveness and acceptance, expressions and acceptance of gratitude and appreciation, expressions of affection
   - **c.** Leave-taking; saying goodbye
7. Acceptance of the finality of life—of one's existence as an individual
   - **a.** Acknowledgment of the totality of personal loss represented by one's dying and experience of personal pain of existential loss

b. Expression of the depth of personal tragedy that dying represents

c. Decathexis (emotional withdrawal) from worldly affairs and cathexis (emotional connection) with an enduring construct

d. Acceptance of dependency

8. Sense of new self (personhood) beyond personal loss: developing self-awareness in the present

9. Sense of meaning about life in general

a. Achieving a sense of awe

b. Recognition of a transcendent realm

c. Developing and achieving a sense of comfort with chaos

10. Surrender to the transcendent, to the unknown—"letting go"; the ego accepts the volition to surrender

N. Legalities related to death and dying

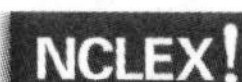

1. **Advance directive:** is a general term that refers to a client's written instructions about future medical care, in the event that the client becomes unable to speak or incapacitated; each state regulates the use of advance directives differently

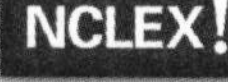

a. **Living will** (durable power of attorney for health care): provides specific instructions about what medical treatment the client chooses to omit or refuse (e.g., ventilator support) in the event that the client is unable to make those decisions

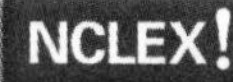

b. **Healthcare proxy:** is a document appointing someone else (e.g., a relative or trusted friend) to manage healthcare treatment decisions when the client is unable to do so

2. Organ donation: under the Uniform Anatomical Gift Act and the National Organ Transplant Act, people 18 years or older and of sound mind may make a gift of all or any part of their own body for the following purposes:

a. Medical or dental education

b. Research

c. Advancement of medical or dental science, therapy, or transplantation

3. **Euthanasia:** is the act of painlessly putting to death persons or animals suffering from incurable or distressing disease

a. Voluntary active euthanasia: occurs when the person being euthanized has agreed and volunteered for death

1) Example: a terminally ill client taking a medication to hasten the end of life

2) Current Oregon law permits voluntary active euthanasia with physician assistance under certain circumstances

b. Involuntary active euthanasia: occurs when the person being euthanized has not agreed or volunteered for death (e.g., the lethal injection of a death row inmate)

c. Voluntary passive euthanasia: occurs when treatment is intentionally withheld by voluntary consent of the individual who is dying (e.g., an individual who has requested through a living will not to be placed on life support for an end-stage condition, such as massive brain trauma)

d. Involuntary passive euthanasia: occurs when treatment is intentionally withheld without voluntary consent from the person who is dying (e.g., the decision not to treat pneumonia or an opportunistic infection in an immobilized and cognitively impaired long-term clients who have not made their wishes known through an advance directive)

NCLEX!

4. **Do-not-resuscitate order (DNR):** a physician's order of "no code" or "do not resuscitate" for clients who are in a stage of terminal, irreversible illness or expected death; the American Nurses Association (ANA) makes the following recommendations related to DNR orders:

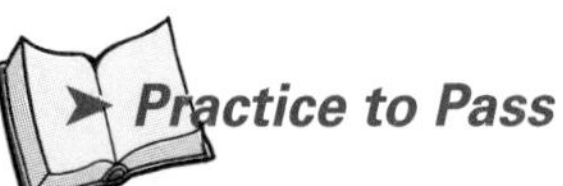

A client asks you to explain the difference between a living will and choosing a healthcare proxy. What would you include in client teaching?

a. The competent client's values and choices should always be given highest priority, even when these wishes conflict with those of the family or healthcare provider

b. When the client is incompetent, an advance directive or the surrogate decision-makers acting for the client should make healthcare treatment decisions

c. A DNR decision should always be the subject of explicit discussion between the client, family, any designated surrogate decision-maker acting on the client's behalf, and the healthcare team

d. DNR orders must be clearly documented, reviewed, and updated periodically to reflect changes in the client's condition

e. A DNR order is separate from other aspects of a client's care and does not imply that other types of care should be withdrawn (e.g., nursing care to ensure comfort or medical treatment for chronic but non-life-threatening illnesses)

f. If it is contrary to the nurse's personal belief to carry out a DNR order, the nurse should consult the nurse manager for a change in assignment

5. Comfort measures only order: a physician's order indicating that the goal of treatment is a comfortable, dignified death and that further life-sustaining measures are not indicated

O. Death-related religious and cultural practices

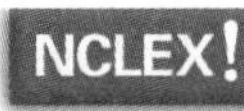

1. Serve primarily to assist individuals coping with the experiences of loss or death

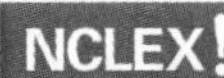

2. Knowledge of the client's religious and cultural heritage helps the nurse provide individualized care to clients and families, even though they may not participate in the rituals associated with loss or death

3. Dying in solitude is generally unacceptable in most cultures

4. Most cultural heritages support the individual's preference to a peaceful death at home rather than in the hospital

5. Some members of ethnic groups may request that health professional not reveal the prognosis of a terminal illness or impeding death to a dying client

6. Beliefs and attitudes about death, its cause, and the soul vary among cultures
7. Beliefs about preparation of the body, death-related rituals, autopsy, organ donation, cremation, and prolonging life are closely allied to the person's religious beliefs and cultural heritage

II. Assessment of Loss, Grieving, and Death

A. **Knowledge:** client and family understand the implication of the loss or death

1. **Closed awareness**—the client and family are unaware of impending loss or death
2. **Mutual pretense**—the client, family and healthcare provider know that the prognosis is terminal but do not talk about it and make an effort not to raise the subject
3. **Open awareness**—the client and individuals involved know about the impending loss or death and feel comfortable discussing it, even though it may be difficult

B. **Self-care abilities:** client's ability to care for self based on any physical or psychological limitations that may have been altered by the loss

C. **Current and previous coping strategies:** stage in the grieving or bereavement process and the use of previous and current coping skills in dealing with past loss or death

D. **Current manifestations of the grief response:** adaptive or maladaptive signs and symptoms including cultural and spiritually based behaviors

E. **Role expectations:** client's and family's perception and expectations of the need to return to work, social, or family roles

F. **Support people's availability and skills:** sensitivity to the client's emotional and physical needs; ability to provide an accepting environment

G. **Advance directive**

1. Does the client have basic information about advance care directives, including living wills and durable power of attorney?
2. Does the client wish to initiate an advance directive?
3. If the client has prepared an advance directive, did the client bring it to the healthcare agency or can the client locate the advance directive?
4. Has the client discussed end-of-life choices with the family or designated a surrogate, physician, or other healthcare team worker?

H. **Resources:** availability and familiarity with possible sources of assistance such as grief support groups, religious or spiritual services, counseling services, physical care providers, or hospice programs

III. Nursing Diagnoses/Analysis

A. **Bereavement, mourning, and grief:** Grieving; Anticipatory grief; Dysfunctional grief; Altered family processes; Altered nutrition: Less than body requirements; Altered role performance; Anxiety; Impaired adjustment; Ineffective family coping: Compromised; Family coping: Potential for growth; Risk for loneliness; Social isolation

B. Death or dying client: Fear; Hopelessness; Powerlessness; Risk for caregiver role strain; Altered family processes; Impaired adjustment; Self-esteem disturbance; Spiritual distress

IV. Planning and Implementation

A. Nursing care goals and interventions for loss and grief

1. Goals
   a. Understand personal feelings about and reaction to loss and grief
   b. Able to discuss response and reaction to loss and grief
   c. Resume baseline sleeping and eating patterns
   d. Resume daily activities and roles as they accept loss

NCLEX!

2. Interventions
   a. Establish rapport and build trust
   b. Facilitate grief work of client and family (see Box 13-1)
   c. Encourage clients to express feelings and assist them to identify their fears concerning the loss
   d. Accept negative feelings and use of defense mechanisms
   e. Provide client with opportunities to release tension, guilt
   f. Promote an adequate balance of rest, sleep, and activities
   g. Explain grieving and mourning processes and relate to client and family responses
   h. Discuss potentially difficult times such as holiday seasons or anniversary dates

Box 13-1

Facilitating Grief Work with Clients and Families

- Explore and respect the client's and family's racial, cultural, religious and personal values in their expression of grief.
- Explain the various common grief responses: denial, anger, depression, guilt and isolation, and describe ways that the client and family member can identify these.
- Teach the client and family what to expect in the grief process, such as that certain thoughts and feelings are normal (acceptable) and that labile emotions, feelings of sadness, guilt, anger, fear and loneliness will stabilize or lessen over time. Knowing what to expect may lessen the intensity of some reactions.
- Encourage the client to express and share grief with support people. Sharing feelings reinforces relationships and facilitates the grief process.
- Teach family members to encourage the client's expression of grief, and not to push the client to move on or enforce their own expectations of appropriate reactions. If the client is a child, encourage family members to be truthful and to allow the child to participate in the grieving activities of others.
- Encourage the client to resume normal activities on a schedule that promotes physical and psychological health. Some clients may try to return to normal activities too quickly. However, a prolonged delay in return may indicate dysfunctional grieving.

i. Assist grieving person to seek new meanings with both death or loss, as well as life

j. Encourage clients to implement religious beliefs and rituals surrounding death or loss

k. Mobilize the client's support systems

l. Refer client and family to self-help groups for survivors of loss, families for mentally ill persons, and individuals who are psychiatrically disabled

B. Nursing care goals and interventions for clients and families facing death

1. Goals

a. Assist the client in achieving his or her potential

b. Assist the client to maintain optimum comfort

c. Help family support the client and be with client as much as possible

d. Provide the client and family the opportunity to discuss what death means and to progress through stages of dying

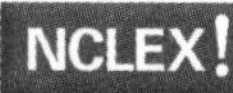

2. Interventions

a. Recognize that client and families have own way of dealing with death and dying

b. Use silence and personal presence along with techniques of therapeutic communication (see Chapter 2); these techniques enhance exploration of feelings and let clients know that the nurse acknowledges their feelings

c. Accept and support the client's and family's use of coping mechanisms

d. Accept denial and negative responses from clients and families

e. Encourage client to participate in decisions

f. Encourage client and family to discuss feelings related to death and dying

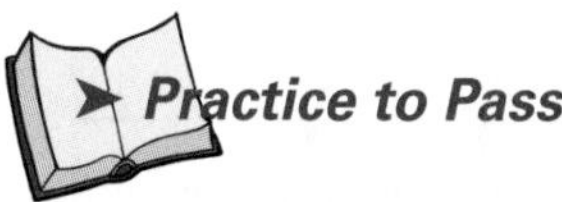

A client has just been diagnosed with a life-ending illness. What are your immediate assessments and goals?

g. Encourage family to communicate openly with client; acknowledge the family's grief

h. Support client and family as they work through the dying process

i. Assist client and family to adapt to changes in roles and lifestyles

j. Provide appropriate information regarding how to access community resources: clergy, support groups, counseling services

k. Support staff and seek support for self when dealing with dying client and grieving family

V. Evaluation/Outcomes

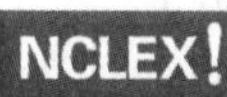

A. Outcomes of grief and loss

1. Client and family express feelings about grief and loss

2. Client and family describe the meaning of loss

3. Client and family progress through grieving and mourning process

4. Client and family are able to share loss with significant others
5. Client and family report decreased preoccupation with loss and resumed involvement in all possible usual activities
6. Client and family report adequate sleep and nutritional intake
7. Client and family verbalize positive expectations for the future
8. Client and family participate in decision-making regarding daily activities
9. Client and family recognize events that may result in additional stress on altered function
10. Client and family seek necessary support groups or other resources

NCLEX!

B. Outcomes of dying and death

1. Client takes opportunity to discuss feelings about dying and impeding death and eventually acknowledges inevitable outcome
2. Client is comfortable and participates in self-care for as long as possible
3. Client maintains personal control over present situation
4. Client accepts declining health status
5. Family discusses feelings about loss of loved one

Case Study

R. E., a 7-year-old male client, is expected to die from childhood leukemia. You are the nurse working in the home where the child has gone to prepare for death.

❶ Based on the child's age, how would you expect him to view his impending death?

❷ What assessment information would you expect to obtain from the child and family?

❸ What would be the important nursing diagnoses for this child and family?

❹ How would you determine the child and family have obtained goals?

❺ Once the child has died, describe bereavement, grief, and mourning by the family.

For suggested responses, see pages 310–311.

Posttest

1 In a child newly diagnosed with leukemia, which nursing care measure would the nurse identify as a teaching priority for the child and family?

(1) Comfort measures
(2) Distraction activities
(3) Anticipatory grieving
(4) Bereavement counseling

2 **In counseling a mother who has recently placed her newborn baby up for adoption, it is important for the nurse to have already dealt with feelings about adoption, grief, and loss. This self-awareness would:**

(1) Prevent the nurse from being personally affected by the client's choice in adoption.
(2) Prevent the nurse from sharing any personal feelings with the client.
(3) Assist the nurse in avoiding discussion of unpleasant feelings with the client.
(4) Assist the nurse in helping the client to express her grief fully.

3 **During a counseling session, a young client with schizophrenia verbalizes feelings of sadness and anger about having to drop out of college and not being able to keep a job. The most applicable nursing diagnosis would be:**

(1) Grief related to inability to achieve developmental milestones.
(2) Anxiety related to fear of unknown and fear of failure.
(3) Ineffective individual coping related to feelings of hopelessness and anger.
(4) Dysfunctional grief related to unrealistic expectations of abilities and lack of achievement.

4 **The nurse working with terminally ill clients understands that culture influences a client and family's reaction to grief, loss, and death by:**

(1) Ignoring inappropriate grieving behaviors.
(2) Tolerating any expression of grief or loss.
(3) Establishing symbolic rituals.
(4) Supporting all individual responses.

5 **Ever since her husband's death 4 years ago, a client experiences migraine headaches and severe nausea around the anniversary of his death each year. The nurse suspects the client is experiencing:**

(1) Delayed grief.
(2) Inhibited grief.
(3) Disenfranchised grief.
(4) Unresolved grief.

6 **A gay client who has just lost his significant other of 15 years to cancer is unable to attend his partner's funeral because the family told him he was not invited and the family does not acknowledge that their son was gay nor that he was living with another man for the past 15 years. The nurse suspects the client may experience:**

(1) Delayed grief.
(2) Inhibited grief.
(3) Disenfranchised grief.
(4) Unresolved grief.

7 **The nurse informs a 20-year-old client that her mother, father, and two older brothers were killed in an automobile accident. Based on an understanding of the stages of grief, the nurse would expect the client to exhibit behaviors that exhibit which of the following?**

(1) Acceptance
(2) Depression
(3) Bargaining
(4) Denial

8 **When questioned by a client about what an advance directive or living will is, the nurse should respond that it states:**

(1) What treatment should be provided or omitted if the client becomes incapacitated.
(2) The practitioners who are allowed to provide care at the end of life.
(3) The caregiver's role in providing care at the end of life.
(4) The inheritance requirements for those relatives who are living.

9 **A 3-year-old client whose grandfather just died is most likely to tell the nurse:**

(1) "Grandfather would not have died if I had wished a little harder."
(2) "Grandfather will be waiting for me when I die."
(3) "Grandfather will be back to take me to the ballgame next week."
(4) "Grandfather is gone, and now I have to be strong and not cry."

10 An outcome criterion for a client who is expected to die from lung cancer within 3 months would be to:

(1) Avoid negative feelings about the caregiver's burden and unrealistic expectations.
(2) Take opportunities to discuss feelings of impending death and acknowledge inevitable outcome.
(3) Verbalize understanding of need to remain pain free and maintain clear and coherent thinking.
(4) Allow caregivers to provide as much care as possible to reduce stress and to preserve energy.

See pages 278–279 for Answers and Rationales.

Answers and Rationales

Pretest

1 **Answer: 2** ***Rationale:*** A perceived loss is experienced by one person but cannot be verified by others (e.g., loss of self-esteem or body image). An actual loss can be identified by others and can arise in response to or in anticipation of a situation (e.g., death of significant other). An anticipatory loss is experienced before the loss actually occurs (e.g., terminal illness), and a permanent loss is an irreversible deprivation (e.g., paralysis).
Cognitive Level: Application
Nursing Process: Analysis; ***Test Plan:*** PSYC

2 **Answer: 1** ***Rationale:*** The capacity for self-awareness allows the nurse to reflect and make choices. Nurses who understand their own feelings and beliefs will be able to be therapeutic when clients need to address issues which are disturbing and difficult. The death of a child will personally affect the nurse, and it is critical for the nurse to share these feelings with others, including the parents. The nurse must be available both physically and emotionally for the parents in discussing unpleasant and difficult feelings.
Cognitive Level: Application
Nursing Process: Analysis; ***Test Plan:*** PSYC

3 **Answer: 1** ***Rationale:*** Although the loss of a child can be devastating, the ability of a parent to reintegrate involvement in usual activities is important to successfully resolving grief and loss. Options 2, 3, and 4 are normal responses to the death of a child.
Cognitive Level: Analysis
Nursing Process: Analysis; ***Test Plan:*** PSYC

4 **Answer: 4** ***Rationale:*** Dsyfunctional grief occurs because of unresolved or inhibited grief that does not lead to a successful conclusion. The client is exhibiting unresolved grief for a prolonged length of time and severity of response. She has been unable to return to her previous roles and function.
Cognitive Level: Analysis
Nursing Process: Analysis; ***Test Plan:*** PSYC

5 **Answer: 3** ***Rationale:*** Spiritual beliefs and practices greatly influence both a person's and family's reaction to death and subsequent behavior. Although options 1 and 2 are correct, option 3 is more correct because their spiritual and cultural beliefs dictate these behaviors. The family may or may not trust the healthcare system.
Cognitive Level: Analysis
Nursing Process: Analysis; ***Test Plan:*** PSYC

6 **Answer: 1** ***Rationale:*** Male or masculine expression of loss or death is commonly limited and toned down. Intense feelings are usually experienced privately with a general reluctance to discuss these with others. Option 2 would not be indicated at this time because the father is probably not experiencing dysfunctional grief. There is not enough data to support options 3 and 4.
Cognitive Level: Analysis
Nursing Process: Analysis; ***Test Plan:*** PSYC

7 **Answer: 2** ***Rationale:*** Preschool children (ages 3 to 5) do not understand the finality of death and children aged 5 to 6 see death as reversible. Magical thinking is usually common in younger children. The child is not experiencing delusions or making up a story to avoid feelings. A child who is 5 years old truly believes in the power of wishes.
Cognitive Level: Analysis
Nursing Process: Assessment; ***Test Plan:*** PSYC

8 **Answer: 2** ***Rationale:*** With mutual pretense, the client, family and/or healthcare providers know that the prognosis is terminal but agree not to talk about it and make an effort not to raise the subject. With closed awareness, the client and family are unaware of impending loss or death. With open awareness, the client and individuals involved know about the impending loss or death and feel comfortable discussing it, even though it may be difficult.
Cognitive Level: Application
Nursing Process: Analysis; ***Test Plan:*** PSYC

9 **Answer: 4** ***Rationale:*** As the care receiver becomes more chronically ill and the caregiving burden becomes more demanding, a great strain can be placed on the caregiver's emotional and physical health. There is not enough data to suggest any of the other nursing diagnoses.
Cognitive Level: Analysis
Nursing Process: Analysis; ***Test Plan:*** PSYC

10 **Answer: 3** ***Rationale:*** A major outcome of grief counseling is to assist the client in sharing his or her loss and to accept support from others. It is critical for the spouse to share the feelings of loss and grief with others. It is too early to memorialize the spouse; the client must grieve the loss of client first.
Cognitive Level: Application
Nursing Process: Evaluation; ***Test Plan:*** PSYC

Posttest

1 **Answer: 3** ***Rationale:*** The child and family will be overwhelmed with such a life-threatening illness; anticipating the loss of a child would be a priority for the family. The other listed measures are pertinent but would not be priority with a new diagnosis.
Cognitive Level: Analysis
Nursing Process: Analysis; ***Test Plan:*** PSYC

2 **Answer: 4** ***Rationale:*** Self-awareness is a key component of any nurse-client experience. The nurse must be able to examine personal feelings, actions, and reactions in order to better assist the client in fully expressing his or her own feelings and thoughts. A firm understanding and acceptance of self allows the nurse to acknowledge a client's differences and uniqueness. The remaining options focus on preventing the expression of feelings.
Cognitive Level: Application
Nursing Process: Analysis; ***Test Plan:*** PSYC

3 **Answer: 1** ***Rationale:*** Schizophrenia most often occurs in young adults who are in the prime of life and attempting to achieve a normal adulthood. The individual experiences many losses and the nurse should assist the client through the grieving process.
Cognitive Level: Application
Nursing Process: Analysis; ***Test Plan:*** PSYC

4 **Answer: 3** ***Rationale:*** Culture dictates acceptable customs and rituals used in the expression of grief, as well as, delineate the appropriate expression of feelings and behaviors.
Cognitive Level: Comprehension
Nursing Process: Analysis; ***Test Plan:*** PSYC

5 **Answer: 2** ***Rationale:*** Inhibited grief is a suppressed response to loss that may be expressed by somatic complaints, such as, physical symptoms around the anniversary of a loss or during holidays. Delayed grief is a postponed response in which the bereaved person may have a reaction at the time of the loss, but it is not sufficient to the loss. However, a later loss may trigger a reaction that is out of proportion to the meaning of the current loss. Disenfranchised grief is a response to a loss or death in which the individual is not regarded as having the right to grieve or is unable to acknowledge the loss to other persons. Unresolved grief is a response that is prolonged or extended in length and severity of response.
Cognitive Level: Analysis
Nursing Process: Analysis; ***Test Plan:*** PSYC

6 **Answer: 3** ***Rationale:*** Disenfranchised grief is a response to a loss or death in which the individual is not regarded as having the right to grieve or is unable to acknowledge the loss to other persons. Delayed grief is a postponed response in which the bereaved person may have a reaction at the time of the loss, but it is not sufficient to the loss. However, a later loss may trigger a reaction that is out of proportion to the meaning of the current loss. Inhibited grief is a suppressed response to loss that may be expressed by somatic complaints, such as physical symptoms around the anniversary of a loss or during holidays. Unresolved grief is a response that is prolonged or extended in length and severity of response.
Cognitive Level: Application
Nursing Process: Analysis; ***Test Plan:*** PSYC

7 **Answer: 4** ***Rationale:*** Although the stages of grief should be used with caution in labeling expected behaviors and feelings, many clients will experience the five stages of grief as denial or shock, anger, bargaining, depression, and acceptance.
Cognitive Level: Application
Nursing Process: Analysis; ***Test Plan:*** PSYC

8 **Answer: 1** ***Rationale:*** Advance directive is a general term that refers to a client's written instructions about future medical care, in the event that the client becomes unable to speak or is incapacitated. Specific instructions about what medical treatment the client chooses to omit or refuse (e.g., ventilator support) in the event that the client is unable to make those decisions is also included. The other options are not part of an advance directive.
Cognitive Level: Application
Nursing Process: Implementation; ***Test Plan:*** PSYC

9 **Answer: 3** ***Rationale:*** Preschool children believe death is reversible. They do not have a developed sense of death, and they are unable to understand the permanent impact of death and dying, while children between 5 and 9 years of age believe wishes or unrelated actions can be responsible for death.
Cognitive Level: Analysis
Nursing Process: Analysis; ***Test Plan:*** PSYC

10 **Answer: 2** ***Rationale:*** To evaluate the achievement of client goals, the nurse collects data in accordance with the desired outcomes established in the plan of care. The clients should be encouraged to freely discuss their feelings related to death and dying. The remaining responses do not adequately provide the client the opportunity to ventilate feelings or thoughts.
Cognitive Level: Analysis
Nursing Process: Planning; ***Test Plan:*** PSYC

References

American Nurses Association. (1991). *Position statement on nursing and the patient self-determination act.* Washington, DC: Author.

American Nurses Association. (1992). *Position statement on nursing care and do-not-resuscitate decisions.* Washington, DC: Author.

Brady, P. (1999). Grief and loss. In K. L. Fontaine & J. S. Fletcher (Eds.). *Mental health nursing* (4th ed.). Menlo Park, CA: Addison-Wesley. pp. 402–412.

Engel, G. L. (1964, September). Grief and grieving. *American Journal of Nursing 64,* 93–98. (Classic.)

Fortinash, K. M. & Holoday-Worret, P. A. (1999). *Psychiatric nursing care plans* (3rd ed.). St. Louis: Mosby, pp. 247–251.

George, J. B. & Frisch, L. E. (1998). Theory and neuroscience as basis for practice. In N. C. Frisch & L. E. Frisch (Eds.), *Psychiatric mental health nursing: Understanding the client as well as the condition.* Albany, NY: Delmar, p. 53.

Kastenbaum, R. J. (2001). *Death, society and human experience* (7th ed.). Boston: Allyn and Bacon.

Kozier, B., Erb, G., Berman, A. J., & Burke, K. (2000). *Fundamentals of nursing: Concepts, process, and practice* (6th ed.). Upper Saddle River, NJ: Prentice Hall, Inc., pp. 970–997.

Kubler-Ross, E. (1969). *On death and dying.* New York: Macmillan. (Classic.)

Olson, M. (1997). Death and grief. In B. Montgomery Dossey (Ed.), *Core curriculum for holistic nursing.* Gaithersburg, MD: Aspen Publishing, pp. 126–133.

Shives, L. R. (1998). *Basic concepts of psychiatric-mental health nursing* (4th ed.). Philadelphia: Lippincott, pp. 259–277.

Stuart, G. W. (1998). Therapeutic nurse-patient relationship. In G. W. Stuart & M. T. Laraia (Eds.), *Principles and practices of psychiatric nursing* (6th ed.). St. Louis: Mosby, pp. 18–22.

Townsend, M. C. (2001). *Nursing diagnoses in psychiatric nursing: Care plans and psychotropic medications* (5th ed.). Philadelphia: F. A. Davis.

CHAPTER 14

Psychological Adaptation to Medical Illness

Sara L. Campbell, DNS, RN

CHAPTER OUTLINE

OBJECTIVES

- Identify four emotional responses to medical illness.
- Identify common clinical symptoms of psychotic disorders due to medical illness.
- Differentiate intervention strategies for clients experiencing critical acute illness and chronic illness.
- Discuss the psychological effects of acquired immunodeficiency syndrome (AIDS) and other life-ending illnesses.

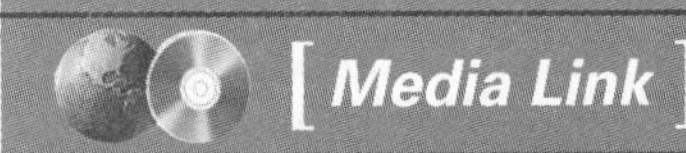

Use the CD-ROM enclosed with this text, or log onto the address given to access the free, interactive Companion Website created for this series. The CD-ROM and Companion Website accompanying this book offer additional practice opportunities and information—NCLEX Review, Case Studies, Glossary, In Depth with NCLEX, and more.

www.prenhall.com/hogan

Review at a Glance

adaptive coping *an effective or appropriate response to a stressful event*

control *a feeling that an event can be managed*

coping *cognitive, physical, or emotional attempts to manage stress*

crisis *a state in which coping skills are no longer effective and disequilibrium occurs*

internal locus of control *a feeling that events can be controlled by the self*

maladaptive coping *an ineffective or inappropriate response to a stressful event*

precipitating stressors *a person's perception of something that results in feelings of anxiety*

Pretest

1 The client is two days postoperative from undergoing emergency surgery as the result of a severe automobile accident. Based on this type of illness, the nurse should plan to assist the client with what psychological adaptation?

(1) Controlling hallucinations
(2) Assisting with spiritual distress
(3) Perceived degree of autonomy and control
(4) Preventing suicidal ideation

2 The nurse assesses a client carefully who has which of the following medical diseases that often masquerades as a mental disorder?

(1) Hypertension
(2) Tumors
(3) Osteoporosis
(4) Asthma

3 The client has been diagnosed with a cardiovascular disease. The contributing behaviors to which personality type should be discussed when teaching the client about disease management?

(1) Borderline personality
(2) Antisocial personality
(3) Type A
(4) Type B

4 The client has the diagnosis of acquired immunodeficiency syndrome (AIDS). The nurse observes that the client is demonstrating psychotic symptoms that include memory difficulties, declining self-care of physical appearance, and angry, hostile behaviors that are different from those previously displayed by the client. The nurse should plan care based on the likely occurrence of what condition?

(1) Delirium
(2) Depression
(3) Hopelessness
(4) Dementia

5 When planning care for the client diagnosed with a life-changing medical illness, the nurse should assess for what common emotional response?

(1) Anger
(2) Anorexia
(3) Apathy
(4) Euphoria

6 In working with an adolescent diagnosed with a chronic medical illness, the nurse can anticipate the client needing assistance with issues related to what area?

(1) Family relationships
(2) Schoolwork
(3) Daily job functioning
(4) Sexuality

7 The client has been diagnosed with an acute medical illness. The nurse recognizes that the client's response to the illness initially will be least dependent on what factors?

(1) Precipitating stressors
(2) Number of friends of the client
(3) Level of economic status
(4) Cultural background

8 Psychological factors impact the occurrence of what types of medical illnesses?

(1) Fractures
(2) Gastrointestinal disorders
(3) Urinary infection
(4) Benign brain tumors

9 What is an expected outcome related to increasing the level of social support for the terminally ill client?

(1) Increased number of friends
(2) Increased independence
(3) Expression of emotions
(4) Expression of hope

10 The client diagnosed with a chronic medical illness arranged for a wheelchair ramp to be built onto his home to allow him easier access. This action demonstrates use of what kind coping behaviors?

(1) Adaptive
(2) Maladaptive
(3) Stress response
(4) Hopeful

See pages 293–294 for Answers and Rationales.

I. Overview of Psychological Aspects Related to Medical Illness

A. Factors influencing response to medical illness: the client's developmental/lifespan level, personality type/behaviors, coping behaviors, precipitating stressors, support systems, and nature of illness

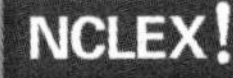

1. Developmental/lifespan issues: refers to the developmental stage of a client at the time of a medical illness diagnosis; influences the client's response to the illness; in addition, the medical illness can further affect client mastery of a developmental/lifespan level, which further affects how the client responds to the illness

a. Early/middle adulthood

1) Medical illnesses that occur when clients are in the early/middle adulthood developmental/lifespan phase can interfere with intimacy, sexuality, and career goals

2) An adolescent with an illness of chronicity is at high risk, and this may result in severe emotional stress, depression (see Chapter 4), anxiety (see Chapter 5), and possible suicidal ideation

b. Late adulthood: medical illnesses that occur when clients are in the late adulthood developmental/lifespan phase can interfere with self-care and daily functioning, which may result in severe emotional stress

2. Personality traits: refer to a client's predictable pattern of response to events; based on a client's personality behaviors, the nurse can predict how a client will respond to a medical illness diagnosis, which then assists the nurse with planning care

a. Type A personality trait behaviors: increase the likelihood that medical illness will occur and contribute to unhealthy responses to medical illness; these traits include rapid speech, irritability, rapid movements, time consciousness, difficulty relaxing, internalization of feelings, excessive dependence on approval of others, and low self-esteem

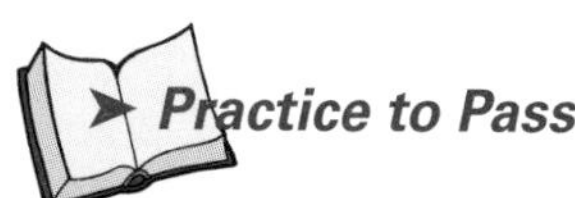

The parents of an adolescent recently diagnosed with a medical illness are concerned with their child's depressed response to the diagnosis. How should the nurse respond?

b. Type B personality trait behaviors: contribute to healthy responses to medical illness, and include easygoing manner, more "laid-back" in behaviors, relaxed and goal-directed behaviors

c. The behaviors that place clients at greater likelihood for occurrence of medical illness include pessimism, repression, limited/guarded social interactions, hostility, and despair

d. Behaviors that place clients at lesser likelihood of medical illness occurrence include behaviors that are self-healing, energetic, questioning, humorous, inspirational, and that demonstrate good interpersonal skills

3. Coping behaviors: a client's response to a medical illness diagnosis is affected by the coping behaviors that the client is able to utilize; **coping** (cognitive, physical, or emotional attempts to manage stress) implies that the client is attempting to lower tension in order to manage the situation effectively; both adaptive and maladaptive coping behaviors are typically manifested

NCLEX!

a. **Adaptive coping** behaviors: if a client can utilize adaptive coping behaviors, the client is capable of mobilizing internal/external resources and is able to sustain general homeostasis

NCLEX!

b. **Maladaptive coping** behaviors: if a client utilizes maladaptive coping behaviors, disorganization occurs because resources cannot be mobilized; ineffective and destructive behaviors appear; and general homeostasis is not preserved

NCLEX!

4. **Precipitating stressors**

a. Are defined as events occurring prior to a medical illness that initiated a stress response of physiological and psychological alterations

b. Precipitating stressors can influence a client's response to medical illness because the client may already be in an emotionally compromised state prior to the medical illness diagnosis

5. Support systems: the presence or absence of strong support systems influences a client's response to medical illness; strong family, friend, and community support systems can result in positive or negative responses

6. Nature of illness: a client's response to medical illness can depend on whether the illness is of an acute (or short-lasting) type, chronic (long-lasting) type or terminal, a life-ending type

a. Acute illness: sudden onset, may be caused by an accident, or other fast onset type of illness

1) This often results in crisis for client and family

2) **Crisis** refers to an event in which the client's regular coping mechanisms are inadequate

3) The client may demonstrate a short attention span and a tendency to be unproductive and impulsive

b. Chronic illness: the client must cope with illness that may be long-standing and debilitating in nature; this often results in ongoing stress for client and family; the client often feels frustrated, hopeless, and fatigued

c. Terminal illness: a terminal illness diagnosis may place the client and family in a crisis mode

1) This type of illness continues to be extremely disruptive to client and family functioning

2) The client often exhibits signs of anger, hopelessness/helplessness, and despair

II. Associated Common Psychological Symptoms

A. **Certain psychological symptoms are common** to clients diagnosed with a medical illness

B. **These include anger, depression, anxiety, helplessness, and hopelessness**

NCLEX!

C. **Anger**

1. Clients with a medical illness diagnosis typically demonstrate behaviors that are indicative of anger
2. These behaviors reflect feelings of helplessness and frustration about the illness and the effects the illness has on daily functioning
3. Behaviors likely to be exhibited include demanding types of action, loud verbalization, slamming of items, and social withdrawal

D. **Depression**

1. Clients with a medical illness diagnosis typically demonstrate symptoms of depression related to the disruption of daily functioning
2. Signs associated with depression include feelings of helplessness/hopelessness, flat affect, poor eye contact, disrupted eating/sleeping patterns, absence of motivation and compliance, and a decreased energy level (see Chapter 4)

NCLEX!

E. **Anxiety**

1. Clients with a medical illness diagnosis typically demonstrate feelings and behaviors of anxiety
2. This reflects feelings of real or imagined threat to body image
3. Anxiety results in autonomic nervous system stimulation with increased heart rate, increased respirations, increased visual acuity, diaphoresis, shortness of breath, and restlessness

F. **Helplessness/hopelessness**

1. Clients with medical diagnoses typically demonstrate feelings of helplessness/hopelessness
2. Helplessness relates to feelings of powerlessness associated with being unable to change what is happening, while hopelessness relates to feelings of despondency and loss of optimism
3. This is reflected in feelings of loss of **control** (feeling that an event can be managed) and individuality and increased dependency on others

III. Medical Conditions Contributing to Psychological Symptoms

A. **Critical/acute illness:** may occur without warning and immediately affect a client's daily functioning; clients typically experience feelings of loss of control, anxiety, helplessness, and anger

1. Cardiovascular illnesses
   a. Have been linked to the occurrence of stress
   b. Include myocardial infarction, cerebrovascular accident, and hypertension
   c. Stress levels can influence the course and/or the outcomes of the medical illness
2. Trauma
   a. May be the result of an accident or crime
   b. Behavioral and physiological responses occur and are demonstrated in client social isolation, agitation, nightmares, and numbness
   c. The client typically struggles to control episodes of anxiety related to the traumatic event
3. Surgery as the result of a critical or an acute medical condition may be disfiguring or incapacitating; surgical procedures can result in alterations of client daily functioning and changes in the client's perception of self-image
4. Pain can accompany many acute illnesses; the client's response is based on a need to protect oneself from harm

B. **Chronic illness:** produces effects that are long-term and implies that the client will need to cope with the illness and its effects for a longer time; these illnesses can be unpredictable in nature and will require use of adaptive coping behaviors in an ongoing manner; lower socioeconomic status increases the likelihood of multiple ongoing health problems that are influenced by reduced access to health care and financial resources to adhere to treatment plans

1. Pulmonary diseases
   a. Include disorders such as chronic obstructive pulmonary disease and asthma
   b. Higher stress levels lead to increased secretions and airway spasms and will result in increased episodes of breathing difficulties
2. Gastrointestinal (GI) diseases
   a. Irritable bowel syndrome, peptic ulcer, and ulcerative colitis are stress-related illnesses
   b. Involved are the GI tract and the autonomic nervous system; increased acid and increased parasympathetic stimulation of the lower bowel occurs and exacerbates symptoms when stress levels increase
3. Medical illnesses that result in chronic pain can have a profound effect on clients and their adaptive and maladaptive coping behaviors; clients respond to pain in a psychological and physiological manner that requires them to continually attempt to adapt

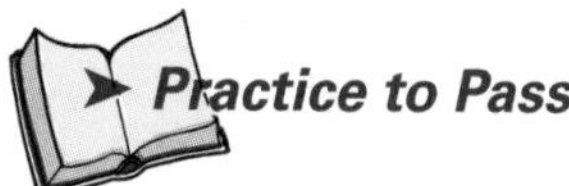

Family members of a client hospitalized with asthma become upset when the treatment team talks about psychological factors of asthma. They feel asthma is "just" a medical illness. How should the nurse respond?

C. Life-ending illnesses

1. HIV/AIDS: human immunodeficiency virus (HIV) and acquired immunodeficiency syndrome (AIDS) result simultaneously in a compromised immune system and occurrence of a psychiatric disorder; this further compromises the health and well-being of the person diagnosed with HIV/AIDS

NCLEX!

   a. Assessment of clients diagnosed with HIV disease is crucial because of the occurrence of psychiatric symptoms/illness, and the enormous losses that the client and family endure

   b. Psychosocial factors influencing occurrence of psychiatric symptoms/illness include fear that the diagnosis will be exposed to others, concern related to the stigma of the diagnosis, intimacy and sexual disruptions, and employment/insurance issues

   c. There are overlapping symptoms of HIV and psychiatric illness, especially with symptoms of depression and anxiety

      1) Fatigue, hopelessness/helplessness, weight loss, aching muscles, and diarrhea are some of the symptoms associated with AIDS that are also indicative of depression and anxiety

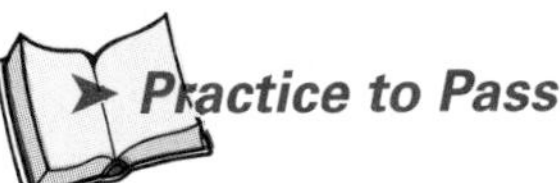

A friend of a client dying with HIV/AIDS states concern that everyone will think the client is "crazy" because of the memory problems and bizarre behaviors. How should the nurse respond?

      2) Other psychiatric symptoms specifically related to HIV/AIDS diagnosis include irritability, paranoia, psychosis, substance abuse, and suicidal ideation

   d. Cognitive changes related to HIV/AIDS diagnoses include dementia and delirium

      1) Dementia is a chronic irreversible brain disorder with symptoms of memory difficulties, impaired judgment, personality changes, and decline in physical appearance

      2) Delirium is an acute reversible brain disorder characterized by inability to be attentive, cloudy consciousness, apathy, and bizarre behaviors

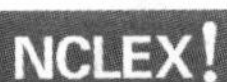

   e. Interventions for clients with the HIV/AIDS should include those that relate to AIDS dementia/delirium, changes in body image/self-esteem, imminent death, support of family/significant others, and management of pain

2. Other life-ending illnesses

   a. The dying client experiences feelings of helplessness and hopelessness

   b. In addition, feelings of depression, anger, and hostility are experienced

   c. The client's response to a life-ending diagnosis will be affected by coping skills, developmental/lifespan level, spiritual, cultural, biological, and psychosocial factors (see Chapter 13)

NCLEX!

   d. Interventions for clients with a life-ending illness should include use of empathy and compassion; a focus on aspects of the client's life that were positive; spirituality assessment and reinforcement; support of family and significant others; and allowing client dignity, client control, and use of pain management

IV. Associated Psychiatric Symptoms

A. **Psychosis** is the inability of a client to understand and know reality or cope with demands of daily living

B. **Psychotic symptoms** that may be demonstrated in clients with selected medical illness diagnoses include evidence of delusions and hallucinations, thought process disruption, and difficulty in caring for oneself (see Chapter 9)

1. Delusions may be persistent and recurrent, and are beliefs that are false but cannot be altered by reason or evidence

2. Hallucinations may be persistent and recurrent, and are defined as an occurrence of a sight, sound, smell, taste, or touch when there is no external stimulus to the corresponding sensory organ

V. Assessment

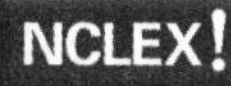

A. **The nurse uses various resources** to collect psychological, biological, and social data

B. **Subjective and objective symptoms,** family/significant other reports, and diagnostic reports are considered in the assessment phase

NCLEX!

C. **Psychological assessment**

1. Elicits clients' emotional reaction to the medical illness diagnosis, coping abilities, and support resources

NCLEX!

2. A stress appraisal should be done with identification of the source of stress, number of stressors, and duration of stressors

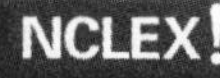

3. Depression symptom assessment should be completed with notation of time of initial symptoms, duration of symptoms, and physical appearance

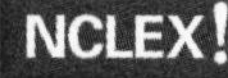

4. Identification of coping behaviors is part of the psychological assessment and includes assessment of adaptive and maladaptive behaviors that reflect a client's ability to identify problems and analyze feelings

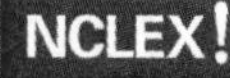

5. Assessment of substance abuse/dependence is crucial in the assessment phase because it can contribute to symptoms of depression, anxiety, hopelessness, helplessness, and eating/sleeping disruptions

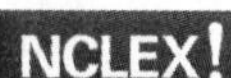

6. The assessment phase should also include identifying the emotional stage of the medical illness

a. Clients often progressively move through stages of illness and interventions should be planned according to the emotional stage

b. These stages include:

1) Denial of the medical illness and associated limitations

2) Anger at loss of control and associated limitations

3) Bargaining, with a plea for another chance and a seeking of new answers/treatments

4) Depression when grieving occurs due to loss or anticipated loss

5) Acceptance/adaptation when conflicts are resolved and the client participates in care

NCLEX!

D. Biologic assessment

1. This type of assessment is done to understand how stress might alter a client's internal body functioning
2. Biological changes can assist the nurse with determining the severity of an illness
3. Assessment of recent/past health conditions that may contribute to current level of physical and psychological functioning should be done; recent and chronic illnesses alter the client's immune system and raise susceptibility to additional healthcare problems
4. A complete physical exam should be conducted to reveal any physical conditions contributing to psychological symptoms; some medical illnesses will cause the client to exhibit psychological symptoms that may be misdiagnosed as a mental health disorder
5. A thorough neurological status exam should be conducted to reveal current neurological state and any changes; findings will provide a baseline level of functioning and may alert the nurse to medical problems
6. Laboratory results should be carefully explored as these can provide insight into the occurrence of psychological symptoms
7. The nurse should assess the client's current abilities with physical functioning/activities/exercise to identify baseline information from which the plan of care can be developed
8. Sleep patterns should be investigated with sleep disruptions being noted, such as inability to fall asleep, stay asleep for the night, or desire to sleep all of the time; sleep disruptions may be indicative of either physiological or psychological problems
9. Nutritional pattern assessment should be done, noting disruptions such as lack of appetite, failure to enjoy previously enjoyable food, and overeating; eating disruptions can be indicative of either physiological or psychological stress
10. Pharmacological assessment should be done, noting medications that the client is currently taking that could account for level of physical/psychological functioning

NCLEX!

E. Social assessment

1. A social assessment should be included as part of the total client assessment
2. Social assessment explores family history, client lifestyle, life-changing events, and presence of social support systems (appraisal of networks that are supportive or not, negative or positive)
3. Recent life-changing events that may have an impact on adaptation to current illness should be explored with the client
4. The client's lifestyle patterns should be discussed as well as any potential impact of lifestyle choices on development/progression of the disease
5. The client's cultural practices should be noted for unique aspects that may indicate specific responses or need for special interventions
6. Assess family communication patterns, level of cohesion, flexibility, functioning, and general support

A client has been admitted to the hospital with various physical symptoms. The nurse should be sure to assess what major areas of the person's life?

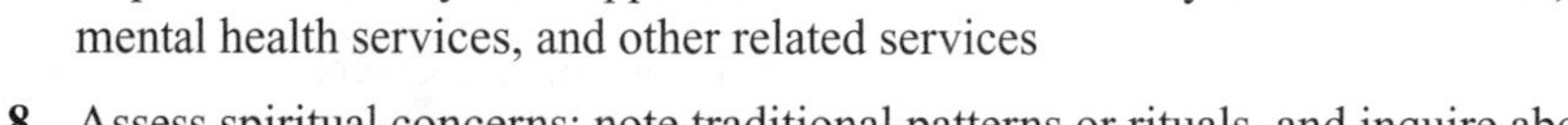

7. Explore community and support resources for availability of home services, mental health services, and other related services
8. Assess spiritual concerns; note traditional patterns or rituals, and inquire about other forms of spirituality that may be important to the client
9. Do an occupational assessment: determine if the client can continue in current occupation or whether it will be disrupted, and whether or not there will be an opportunity to continue it in the future
10. Determine economical status, specifically whether there are finances to support current and future expenses

VI. Nursing Diagnoses/Analysis

A. **Nursing diagnoses** are used to describe health problems and needs that nursing interventions can address

B. **Problems may be either actual or potential in nature**

C. **Commonly used nursing diagnoses in the care of clients** requiring psychological adaptation to medical illness include:

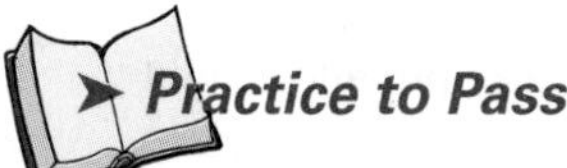
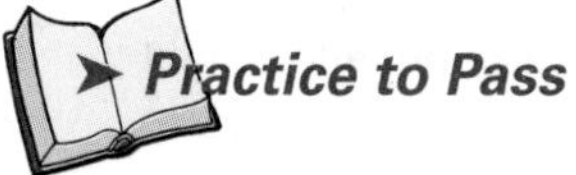

A client is feeling depressed about how the right leg appears following a traumatic automobile accident and multiple surgeries to correct problems. What nursing diagnoses should the nurse consider?

1. Ineffective denial related to changes in physical and psychosocial abilities following a chronic or acute medical illness diagnosis
2. Body image disturbance related to occurrence of a medical illness
3. Impaired adjustment related to function changes needed following medical illness diagnosis
4. Ineffective individual coping related to occurrence and effects of a medical illness diagnosis
5. Self-care deficit related to function changes associated with a medical illness diagnosis
6. Alterations in self-image and self-esteem related to function changes associated with a medical illness diagnosis
7. Anxiety related to occurrence of a medical illness diagnosis

VII. Empowering Strategies

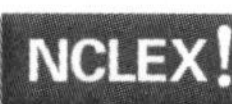

A. Interventions

1. The nurse collaborates with the client and family members to develop a plan of care for the client in which client response can be monitored
2. Interventions serve as the foundation for all client care and are subject to change as the condition of the client changes
3. Specific interventions that exemplify empowering strategies include the following
   a. Increase client control; provide opportunities for client decision-making regarding care
   b. Engage in therapeutic interactions—empathetic listening
   c. Recommend psychotherapy when deemed appropriate to assist client with adaptation and support
   d. Assist with stress management—teach relaxation methods, imagery, biofeedback, exercise

e. Reinforce current positive, adaptive coping behaviors

f. Promote comfort and healing

g. Utilize spiritual resources—provide opportunities for client to engage in spiritual traditions/rituals; offer resources related to complementary medicine if desired

B. Differential interventions for critical/acute versus chronic illnesses

1. Critical/acute illnesses typically result in abrupt interruption of a client's usual daily activities; this can precipitate a crisis stage if client perceives events as a threat to safety, self-esteem, or self-image

a. Seek immediate ways to increase client's control

b. Engage in therapeutic interactions with client and family; encourage verbalization of feelings

c. Assist with immediate anxiety reduction through use of relaxation techniques

d. Use firm, direct limit-setting to assist client with staying focused

2. Chronic illnesses typically require ongoing adaptation as long-term effects are unpredictable; chronic illnesses often deplete energy levels, support systems, coping reserves, economic abilities, and may lead to suicidal ideation

a. Increase self-care responsibilities as appropriate to preserve/facilitate functioning/self-esteem/image

b. Reward positive adaptive coping behaviors

c. Reinforce existing support network linkages and assist client with creating new linkages; identify support groups, self-help groups, and special interest groups

VIII. Evaluation/Outcomes

A. Preservation of healthy physiological function

B. Disease process reduction/cessation: client learns about the illness and ways to decrease the disease process, such as diet, exercise, and stress reduction activities

C. Development/reinforcement/strengthening of adaptive coping behaviors: this includes ability to express feelings related to the medical illness diagnosis and effects of the illness; it also includes productive interdependence of client with ongoing support systems, such as family and friends

D. Participation in treatment/rehabilitation process

E. Optimal level of functioning

F. Independence in self-care

G. Development of functional support systems

H. Decreased anxiety

I. Evidence of an *internal locus of control:* clients who believe that they have ability and responsibility in their lives to decrease the likelihood of illness or effects of illness have an internal locus of control and are less likely to experience symptoms of distress

Case Study

A 20-year-old female client has been diagnosed with HIV/AIDS. The client is feeling depressed and hopeless about the future. You are the nurse working with this client.

❶ What are the symptoms indicative of depression?

❷ What other assessments do you need to make?

❸ What are possible nursing diagnoses?

❹ What interventions should you consider?

❺ If the client asks you why she should feel anything but hopeless about the future, how would you respond?

For suggested responses, see page 311.

Posttest

1 A client with a recent leg amputation as a result of a car accident is ready for discharge. The nurse has been talking with the client about signs and symptoms of depression. The nurse feels that the client has a good understanding of depression related to the accident when the client states:

(1) "I realize that I might feel a little down after this accident, but I know that if I'm not sleeping or eating well or if I feel like things do not matter anymore, that I should seek help."
(2) "I realize that accidents happen to good people too. I just need to be tougher and not let this accident get me down. I should look at the positive side—at least I'm still alive."
(3) "I need to get medicine for depression, just in case."
(4) "If I stay busy, I won't get depressed."

2 A client diagnosed with ulcerative colitis is preparing for discharge from the hospital. In evaluating the coping strategies learned during the hospitalization, the nurse notes that the client understands the relationship between the disease and stress. The nurse bases this conclusion on what statement made by the client?

(1) "I will be OK if I just take my medicine."
(2) "I am glad I am learning how to cope with stressors in my life."
(3) "Now that this has been diagnosed, I really don't have to worry about stress anymore."
(4) "It's my family's fault that I feel stressed about things."

3 The client who has a diagnosis of acquired immunodeficiency syndrome (AIDS) has a nursing diagnosis of Alteration in self-esteem. The nurse should incorporate which of the following behaviors when working with this client?

(1) Avoid looking directly at the client.
(2) Maintain a formal relationship with the client.
(3) Keep contact with the client at a minimum.
(4) Listen attentively.

4 The nurse is developing a stress management seminar for clients recently discharged from a cardiac care unit. Which of the following concepts should be included in the seminar?

(1) Learning to develop a large network of friends
(2) Developing additional social activities
(3) Personality types and how these impact cardiac illness
(4) Use of confrontation as a beneficial way to decrease tension

5 The client who has a chronic medical illness diagnosis that results in physical disability should be carefully assessed for what possible severe response to the illness?

(1) Suicidal ideation
(2) Depression
(3) Anxiety
(4) Helplessness

6 **The nurse understands that the client in pain is experiencing an event that is physiological and psychological in nature. The nurse bases pain management strategies on knowledge that the psychological component comes from the need to:**

(1) Express feelings.
(2) Protect oneself from harm.
(3) Feel sorry for self.
(4) Keep feelings inside.

7 **What would be an effective intervention for a client with a medical illness diagnosis who is struggling with loss of independence?**

(1) Help the client with all activities
(2) Ignore the client during activity time
(3) Wait until the client requests help before providing assistance
(4) Allow the client to join the treatment team

8 **The nurse knows that once the client with a medical diagnosis is assessed and has been found to have psychological symptoms, the next step is to develop a:**

(1) Process.
(2) Intervention.
(3) Nursing diagnosis.
(4) Plan of evaluation.

9 **The client and family who have learned healthy coping skills for adjusting to the physical limitations of a medical illness will exhibit which of the following?**

(1) Unproductive interdependence
(2) Productive dependence
(3) Productive interdependence
(4) Unproductive dependence

10 **A client with a medical illness diagnosis is found to be at a low socioeconomic level of income. The nurse anticipates that this client is more likely to experience which of the following?**

(1) Increased grief
(2) Increased pain
(3) Loss of control
(4) Higher number of other illnesses

See pages 294–295 for Answers and Rationales.

Answers and Rationales

Pretest

1 **Answer: 3** ***Rationale:*** Accidents are classified as an acute/critical illness that result in the client assessing own degree of autonomy and level of control related to care. Option 1 does not relate to accidents. Option 2 may relate to some persons, but is not primary for all clients. Option 4 does not relate to accidents.
Cognitive Level: Application
Nursing Process: Analysis; ***Test Plan:*** PSYC

2 **Answer: 2** ***Rationale:*** There are specific medical problems that can appear as a mental disorder without further investigation. Tumors of the frontal, occipital, parietal, and temporal lobes often produce symptoms that are mistaken for a mental disorder. Options 1, 3, and 4 do not typically masquerade as mental disorders.
Cognitive Level: Application
Nursing Process: Assessment; ***Test Plan:*** PHYS

3 **Answer: 3** ***Rationale:*** Options 1 and 2 refer to personality disorders, which have not been found to be directly related to cardiovascular illness. Option 4 refers to a personality type in which persons are more relaxed and less time-oriented. Option 3, Type A personality behaviors, consist of anger, hostility, a sense of urgency, becoming easily frustrated, and having workaholic type behaviors. Research has indicated that persons with Type A personalities are more likely to be diagnosed with a cardiovascular disease and to have more difficulty controlling the disease once it has been diagnosed.
Cognitive Level: Application
Nursing Process: Planning; ***Test Plan:*** HPM

4 **Answer: 4** ***Rationale:*** Option 1 does not refer to a common occurrence of symptoms related to the AIDS diagnosis. Options 2 and 3 refer to symptoms/feelings that might occur in conjunction with the illness. Option 4, dementia, can be understood by the related symptoms. The nurse should understand that the occurrence of symptoms indicates progression of the AIDS illness and that care should be planned accordingly.
Cognitive Level: Application
Nursing Process: Planning; ***Test Plan:*** PSYC

5 **Answer: 1** ***Rationale:*** Option 1, anger, is included in the stages of grief as clients grieve for what has been lost. Although clients may experience multiple emotional feelings in response to diagnosis of a life-changing medical illness, anger is one of the most common emotional responses because of the sudden and often dramatic change in lifestyle. Options 2 and 3 might occur but are not considered primary responses. Option 4 is inappropriate and typically does not occur.
Cognitive Level: Application
Nursing Process: Assessment; ***Test Plan:*** PSYC

6 **Answer: 4** ***Rationale:*** Chronic medical illnesses might affect options 1, 2, and 3 but are not considered to be related to developmental level of the client. Option 4 is related to the developmental level of the adolescent client. Medical illnesses that occur during adolescence typically interfere with sexuality because of the stage of life development of the client.
Cognitive Level: Analysis
Nursing Process: Planning; ***Test Plan:*** HPM

7 **Answer: 3** ***Rationale:*** The level of economic status will not initially affect one's response to illness. Precipitating stressors (option 1) initially indicate how the client will respond to an acute medical illness diagnosis because they relate to the level of coping that a person brings to any given situation such as illness. Culture (option 4) influences how a person perceives a stressful event, as does social support (option 2).
Cognitive Level: Analysis
Nursing Process: Assessment; ***Test Plan:*** HPM

8 **Answer: 2** ***Rationale:*** Gastrointestinal disorders are influenced by psychological factors. Appetite changes, dietary intake alterations, digestion, and elimination patterns occur in conjunction with emotional stress. Options 1, 3, and 4 are not the result of psychological factors.
Cognitive Level: Comprehension
Nursing Process: Analysis; ***Test Plan:*** HPM

9 **Answer: 3** ***Rationale:*** The client's engagement with social supports would hopefully result in increased ability to express emotions with others. Option 1 does not necessarily indicate a strong level of social support. Options 2 and 4 are not related to social support.
Cognitive Level: Analysis
Nursing Process: Evaluation; ***Test Plan:*** PSYC

10 **Answer: 1** ***Rationale:*** Option 1, adaptive, indicates that the client is able to mobilize internal/external resources to cope with the chronic illness and its effects. Option 2 relates to a response that is negative in nature. Options 3 and 4 are not related.
Cognitive Level: Application
Nursing Process: Evaluation; ***Test Plan:*** PSYC

Posttest

1 **Answer: 1** ***Rationale:*** Option 1 indicates that the client understands the disruption of the accident and that feeling down might be expected, but the client is able to differentiate between mild and more severe depressive symptoms. Options 2 and 4 indicate that the client thinks he/she can have control over depressive symptoms following the accident and that if the "right things" are done, depression will not occur. Option 3 indicates that the client views medicine as a necessity.
Cognitive Level: Analysis
Nursing Process: Evaluation; ***Test Plan:*** PSYC

2 **Answer: 2** ***Rationale:*** The client has verbalized that there is a relationship between the disease and stress and has learned how to deal with the stress. Options 1 and 3 indicate no understanding of the relationship and option 4 indicates blaming.
Cognitive Level: Application
Nursing Process: Evaluation; ***Test Plan:*** HPM

3 **Answer: 4** ***Rationale:*** Option 4 indicates interest and concern about the client and facilitates open communication. Options 1, 2, and 3 indicate that the nurse wants distance from the client.
Cognitive Level: Application
Nursing Process: Implementation; ***Test Plan:*** PSYC

4 **Answer: 3** ***Rationale:*** Option 3 indicates knowledge related to how personality types impact cardiac illness. Options 1 and 2 do not have anything to do with understanding stress and cardiac disease. Option 4 is not a beneficial way to decrease tension.
Cognitive Level: Application
Nursing Process: Assessment; ***Test Plan:*** HPM

5 **Answer: 1** ***Rationale:*** Although options 2, 3, and 4 should be assessed, option 1 is indicative of the most severe response to illness that results in physical disability.
Cognitive Level: Application
Nursing Process: Assessment; ***Test Plan:*** SECE

6 **Answer: 2** ***Rationale:*** Option 2 is the normal response that a person engages in when threatened in any way, such as with pain. Options 3 and 4 are inap-

propriate responses of coping with pain. Option 1 is not an option related to psychological nature of pain.
Cognitive Level: Analysis
Nursing Process: Analysis; ***Test Plan:*** PHYS

7 **Answer: 4** ***Rationale:*** Option 4 allows the client to be a part of his/her own care and supports interdependence. Option 1 does not promote feelings of independence; option 2 could lead to client isolation; and option 3 places undue pressure on the client to feel that he/she should be doing things by him/herself.
Cognitive Level: Analysis
Nursing Process: Implementation; ***Test Plan:*** PSYC

8 **Answer: 3** ***Rationale:*** The next logical step in the nursing process is the nursing diagnosis that flows from the assessment. Options 1, 2, and 4 are part of the care plan and flow from the nursing diagnosis.
Cognitive Level: Comprehension
Nursing Process: Analysis; ***Test Plan:*** PSYC

9 **Answer: 3** ***Rationale:*** The goal for the client is to have him/her adjust to any physical limitations by understanding own capabilities and being able to ask for assistance when necessary. This creates interdependence. Options 1, 2, and 4 are not signs of healthy coping with physical limitations.
Cognitive Level: Analysis
Nursing Process: Assessment; ***Test Plan:*** SECE

10 **Answer: 4** ***Rationale:*** Research indicates that a lower socioeconomic level does lead to a higher number of illnesses in these clients. Options 1, 2, and 3 are not related to socioeconomic level.
Cognitive Level: Analysis
Nursing Process: Planning; ***Test Plan:*** HPM

References

Fontaine, K. L. & Fletcher, J. S. (1999). *Mental health nursing* (4th ed.). Menlo Park, CA: Addison Wesley Longman, pp. 70–113, 401–410, 516–591.

Fortinash, K. M. & Holoday-Worret, P. A. (2000). *Psychiatric mental health nursing* (3rd ed.). St. Louis: Mosby, pp. 696–725.

Stuart, G. W. & Laraia, M. T. (2001). *Principles and practice of psychiatric nursing* (7th ed.). St. Louis: Mosby, pp. 227–245, 299–314, 460–481, 783–787.

Townsend, M. C. (2000). *Psychiatric mental health nursing: Concepts of care* (3rd ed.). Philadelphia: F. A. Davis, pp. 167–232, 428–440, 711–734.

Appendix

➤ Practice to Pass Suggested Answers

Chapter 1

Page 4: *Solution*—There is neither a universally accepted definition of "normal" or "abnormal" nor clear parameters of mental health versus mental illness. Mental health and mental illness can be viewed as end points on a continuum, with movement back and forth throughout life. One out of four individuals will suffer from mental illness in their lifetime. Everyone is susceptible to mental illness. The continuum could be used to demonstrate to the group how cultural, interpersonal, and individual factors contribute to mental health and illness.

Page 8: *Solution*—The client is most likely using the defense mechanism of denial. Denial is an unconscious attempt to screen or to ignore unacceptable realities by refusing to acknowledge them. Denial allows individuals to reduce their anxiety and not have to acknowledge unacceptable feelings, thoughts, or behaviors.

Page 10: *Solution*—Erikson's stage of growth and development experienced by a 72-year-old is "integrity versus despair." Individuals who experience "integrity" accept life as it has been by acknowledging both the good and bad aspects of one's life and maintaining a positive self-concept. This client is not currently achieving Erikson's developmental milestone because he is experiencing "despair." He finds life meaningless. He has no hope for the future and feels that he and others would be better off without him. The nurse could assist the client in conducting a life review, which may help this client in finding meaning to his life. Life review is a process of systematically evaluating one's successes and failures in life to resolve conflicts and to find meaning.

Page 12: *Solution*—The brain is the site of all integrative functions that govern our behavior, feelings, and thoughts. Neurotransmission is the electrochemical process in the brain that allows nerve signals to pass from one cell to another at the synapse. The synapse is a microscopic gap between where two neuron cells meet. Neurotransmitters act, as the word implies, to transmit signals across the synapse from one neuron to another. Serotonin is the neurotransmitter involved with depression. Decreases in serotonin levels can lead to depression. Antidepressant medications are the primary drugs that affect serotonin levels.

Page 19: *Solution*—

- Risk for other-directed violence related to confusion, memory loss, and intruding into others personal space.
- Chronic confusion related to memory loss and disorientation to place, time, and situation.
- Risk for injury related to wandering behaviors and wandering into unfamiliar areas.

Chapter 2

Page 35: *Solution*—

- Situational crisis is any event that poses a threat or challenge to an individual person.
- Maturational crisis is a stage in a person's life where adjustment and adaptation to new responsibilities and life patterns are necessary.
- Cultural crisis is a situation where a person experiences culture shock in the process of adapting/adjusting to a new culture or returning to one's own culture after being assimilated into another.
- Community crisis is a crisis of a proportion to affect an entire community of people. Natural disasters, armed conflicts, and significant social ills are community crises.

Page 35: *Solution*—

- The individual's perception of the crisis situation will dictate how the client will react to the situation.
- Past experience or lack of experience in coping with stress will impact how the client will react to the crisis situation.
- Established coping strategies will assist the client in dealing more effectively with current crisis situation.
- Availability of support persons gives the client the resources needed to deal with the crisis and to return to normal.

Page 35: *Solution*—

- Marked feelings of tenseness and anxiousness without feelings of fatigue, sadness, and depression
- Elevated motor-sensory behavior
- Elevated systolic blood pressure
- Elevated pulse
- Elevated respiration
- High score for verbal anxiety

Page 40: *Solution*—

- Depression
- Increased alcohol drinking
- Previous suicide attempts
- Buying a gun
- Stockpiling pills
- Giving away money or possessions
- Loss of interest in favorite activities
- Making or changing a will
- Making funeral plans
- Suspicious behavior
- Recent for death of spouse, child, or close friend
- Death of pet
- Major move
- Diagnosis of a terminal illness
- Retirement

Page 41: *Solution*—

- Removing sharp objects, such as knives, scissors, and mirrors, from the client's possession and access.
- Removing toxic substances, such as drugs and alcohol, and ensuring that unit medications are locked.
- Removing clothing that could be used for self-harm, such as neck ties, belts, shoe strings, stockings, and the like.
- Placing the client under close supervision, including one-to-one supervision with a staff member.

Chapter 3

Page 54: *Solution*—In some cases, antidepressants are prescribed for children with ADHD, especially venlafaxine (Effexor) and fluvoxamine (Luvox). More commonly, central nervous system (CNS) stimulants are prescribed. These medications increase the ability to focus attention by blocking out irrelevant thoughts and impulses. CNS stimulants lead to significant improvement in 70 to 75 percent of cases. The advantage of methylphenidate (Ritalin) and dextroamphetamine (Dexedrine) is that effectiveness is almost immediate, while the same effect with pemoline (Cyclert) may take up to 8 weeks.

Page 54: *Solution*—Common side effects include pallor, a pinched facial expression, dark hollows under the eyes, anorexia, insomnia, headache, and dryness of the mouth. Toxic effects may include overstimulation and sedation.

Page 55: *Solution*—

- Depressed mood, irritable, aggressive
- Academic difficulties
- Eating and sleeping disturbances
- Severe self-criticism and guilt
- Suicidal ideation and plans

Page 55: *Solution*—

- Intense mood swings
- Academic difficulties
- Argumentative and/or assaultive
- Risk-taking or antisocial behavior
- Hypersomnia
- Very low self-esteem

Page 58: *Solution*—Any of the following nursing diagnoses may apply:

- Altered nutrition: less than body requirements related to reduced intake; purging
- Anxiety related to fears of gaining weight and losing control
- Impaired thought process related to dichotomous thinking, overgeneralization, personalization, obsessions, and superstitious thinking
- Body image disturbance related to delusional perception of body in anorexia
- Powerlessness related to having no control over bulimic patterns

Chapter 4

Page 68: *Solution*—"You tried to hurt yourself and you are on suicide precautions. That means that someone must be with you at all times, 24 hours per day, until you are no longer a danger to yourself." Communicate to the client the understanding that it may be embarrassing, but the client's safety is the most important concern.

Page 70: *Solution*—Major depressive disorder is 1.5 to 3 times more common among first-degree biological relatives of persons with this disorder than among the general population. Clients have a right to feel angry about having depression, but it is important to reinforce that parents can't choose the traits they pass on to their offspring.

Page 71: *Solution*—Those who are depressed do not have the energy to talk or participate in an assessment for any longer than 15- to 20-minute segments. The client may be slow to respond as well, so the nurse needs to be patient with the client and allow sufficient time for client responses. The client who is diagnosed with a bipolar disorder is not able to concentrate for any longer than this, nor may the client be able to focus long enough to sit still for even this amount of time. The nurse also needs to know that this client may not always give accurate information.

Page 77: *Solution*—Five short-term goals for this client could include any of the following:

- Be free from self-inflicted harm.
- Engage in reality-based interactions.
- Demonstrate appropriate use of boundary setting with staff and other clients.
- Be oriented to person, place, and time.
- Express feelings directly with congruent verbal and nonverbal messages.
- Express anger or hostility outwardly in a safe manner.
- Participate in formulation of discharge plan.

Five long-term goals for this client could include any of the following:

- Be free of psychotic symptoms.
- Demonstrate functional levels of psychomotor activity.
- Demonstrate compliance and congruence with medication knowledge and regime (if prescribed).
- Demonstrate an increased level of coping with anxiety, stress, and/or frustration.
- Demonstrate appropriate coping if a loss or change occurs.
- Identify discharge plan and components.
- Verbally contract and begin to demonstrate compliance with plan of care components.

Page 85: *Solution*—The plan should include the following points:

- There is no clear evidence as to why the therapy works. There are indications that early morning light causes circadian rhythm shifts.
- Therapy involves a large time commitment.
- Usually clients spend 30 minutes to several hours each day in the light source depending on the light strength (2,500 lux is usually administered).
- Antidepressant effects can be full, partial, or not at all.
- If effective, results will usually be seen after 2 to 4 days and therapy is complete after 2 weeks.
- Maintenance consists of sitting in front of the lights for approximately 30 minutes each day.
- The therapy is usually necessary during the fall and winter months when the client is affected by the disorder.

Chapter 5

Page 103: *Solution*—It would be useful to explain to the client that while there is some evidence of a genetic predisposition to anxiety, many theorists believe anxiety is learned or acquired. It would also be helpful to explain to the client that new ways of coping with anxiety, regardless of its cause, can be learned.

Page 104: *Solution*—You should explain to the client that anxiety can occur in anybody at any time, and it is important to consider anxiety when designing a nursing care plan for the client. You might also explain that physical illness can increase anxiety, and anxiety can lead to physical illness. In addition, there is some evidence that admission to a hospital may increase a client's level of stress. Nurses need to be aware of how the admission process is affecting the client.

Page 109: *Solution*—Not all over-the-counter medications are safe for everyone. Benadryl can interact with other prescribed and nonprescribed medications, as well as alcohol. Benadryl can suppress the central nervous system and can be habit-forming. Because Benadryl interferes with REM sleep, the quality of the client's sleep may decrease over time leading the client to periodically increase the dosage to maintain the desired effect. Conveying information related to actions that facilitate sleep would also be helpful.

Page 111: *Solution*—Because agoraphobic clients frequently are fearful of leaving their homes and being trapped in situations they cannot escape, the first action would be assess the client's motivation and ability to participate in this group. It may be necessary for a helping person to accompany the client to the first few meetings to provide reassurance to the client and to promote safety. Teaching a relaxation exercise the client can use before and during the meeting might also be helpful. Assisting the client to contact the group leader before attending the first meeting might reduce some anticipatory anxiety.

Page 112: *Solution*—It is important to allow the client to discuss this fear openly and honestly and to take this concern seriously. Neglecting this important issue will increase the client's level of anxiety. The client should be reassured that this fear will be taken into consideration when planning nursing care. Whenever possible, medications should be given orally. During procedures where blood is involved, allow the client to avert his eyes. Do not ridicule this behavior. Teaching relaxation techniques might be useful. If the fear seriously limits the client's ability to obtain health care, some consideration might be given to involving the client in developing a systematic desensitization program.

Chapter 6

Page 126: *Solution*—The body responds to stress with a general increase in muscle tension that is felt in different parts of the body by different people. While some people have neck or shoulder pain, this client feels the muscle tension in the head and low back. The muscles tighten automatically, which lessens the blood flow to them. Not only do the tissues get decreased oxygen from the blood, but waste products like lactic acid do not get removed from the muscles. Lactic acid and other waste products are irritants to the muscle, and further increase the muscle tension. That is probably what causes the pain.

Page 127: *Solution*—The client *does* experience the symptoms, regardless of physical findings, so resuming activities must come gradually as the symptoms become less pronounced. Of great importance is the role of the symptoms in the client's and the family members' lives. Changing roles, even for the positive, require significant readjustment, particularly if there was gain from the sick role.

Page 128: *Solution*—First, emphasize that the purpose of reinforcing verbal expressions of the stresses of daily life or other events is to help the client express feelings through speaking, rather than through physical symptoms. It is not to punish. Second, remind family members that habits are difficult to break for all concerned, so they should not expect to do this perfectly every time. Next, suggest that when the client complains of physical symptoms to listen politely, but not make comments that encourage further elaboration. Rather, spend time really listening to the person when they are talking about *other* things in general, or their own stresses and conflicts. Often families have "turned off" listening at all—since hearing about physical problems most of the time, or having life revolve around illnesses, eventually becomes frustrating. The family has an important role to play in treatment, as does the client.

Page 131: *Solution*—Medications are only one part of the treatment plan, and they will be more effective if the client is involved in other aspects of pain management including exercise, physical therapy, and stress management. Often clients will need to face the fact that medication can only help to some extent, and learning to manage pain in other ways is essential. When using medications, the client must, in partnership with the provider, agree on how to best use the medication in terms of dose and frequency. The client must clearly understand the concept of tolerance and withdrawal in the use of habit-forming medications.

Chapter 7

Page 140: *Solution*—Explain to the client that stress or conflicts can cause anxiety. When that anxiety becomes too great, the mind can do many things, automatically, to protect the client. One of those things is dissociation. Dissociation is like being split off from reality or "spacing out." Although it is protective, dissociation can also impair how the client lives because she can lose full awareness of what is occurring.

Page 140: *Solution*—

- "As a child or as an adult, have you ever been physically hurt or abused by anyone?"
- "As a child or as an adult, have you ever been emotionally hurt or abused by anyone?"
- "As a child or as an adult, have you ever been sexually touched by anyone against your will? Abused sexually by anyone?"

Page 142: *Solution*—"Because visual imagery is created by internal stimuli, when you try to reduce stress, there is a tendency to dissociate, or "space out," especially if you already have a pattern of dissociating. If you feel dissociative, focus on external stimuli—what you can see, hear, and feel physically—which will "ground" you to reality, to the present by distracting you and interfering with the dissociative process. If you want to use stress-management techniques when you are not feeling dissociative, you could try progressive muscle relaxation or deep-breathing accompanied by counting inside your head. Stress-management techniques that are "physical" in nature are more grounding than those that are more mental or internal."

Page 142: *Solution*—Antianxiety agents are extremely effective in reducing anxiety, but are physiologically addictive, with the client developing tolerance (and withdrawal symptoms when the drug is removed). The agents are also psychologically addictive, and clients can come to believe they cannot cope without medication. Thus, antianxiety agents are best used to decrease anxiety to a lower level where the client can learn nonpharmacological techniques to control anxiety.

Page 142: *Solution*—Clients often dissociate or split off their affect off from an experience so that even horrific events are recounted with minimal emotional expression. This ability to dissociate affect from the traumatic event serves to numb. When a survivor of trauma remembers those events with appropriate affect, the nurse can expect anger, great fear, or sadness to be expressed freely.

Chapter 8

Page 155: *Solution*—Personality disorders are diagnosed when personality patterns or traits are inflexible, enduring, pervasive, maladaptive, and cause significant functional impairment or subjective distress.

Page 157: *Solution*—Personality patterns are ingrained and frequently ego-syntonic; thus, clients may lack motivation to change. Help individuals see how their behavior affects their lives may motivate them to change. Expecting radical, long-term change is unrealistic. Interventions should reflect short-term goals and focus on small steps to improve functioning or decrease distress.

Page 158: *Solution*—Individuals diagnosed with antisocial personality disorder frequently use manipulation to control others and their environment. Intervening in this behavior pattern by setting limits that deter the client from manipulating others is a small step toward effecting behavioral change. In addition, clients diagnosed with antisocial personality disorder frequently display diminished impulse control. Setting limits helps clients maintain impulse control in order to protect themselves and others from injury.

Page 158: *Solution*—Individuals diagnosed with borderline personality disorder tend to engage in dichotomous thinking or splitting—they tend to see themselves and others as all good or all bad. The tendency to idealize or devalue the self and others results in unstable interpersonal relationships. In addition, and more importantly, it is frequently reflected in rage directed at the self (self-mutilation) or at others (injury to others). Encouraging these clients to see that there is good and bad in all of us is a small step in decreasing the tendency to dichotomous thinking to protect client safety, decrease subjective distress and improve functioning.

Page 159: *Solution*—It is designed to support client safety by decreasing the risk of suicide or self-mutilation through the use of anti-harm contracts, close monitoring by both staff and client, identifying triggers and patterns related to self-destructive behavior, and identifying alternative coping strategies.

Page 159: *Solution*—To be effective, limits must be clearly stated, necessary, and enforceable. Clearly stating limits and seeking clarification from clients of their understanding of the limits decreases their ability to manipulate based on "not understanding what was expected." Establishing necessary limits establishes staff members as business-like authority figures rather than as being punitive or judgmental and diminishes a client's tendency to engage in a power struggle. Limits must be enforceable or they encourage rather than discourage the tendency to manipulate.

Page 162: *Solution*—

1. Individuals diagnosed with paranoid personality disorder do not try to establish social relationships because they distrust and are suspicious of others. They expect to be harmed or exploited by others.
2. Individuals diagnosed with schizoid personality disorder do not try to establish social relationships because they are emotionally aloof and have no interest in or desire to develop relationships.
3. Individuals diagnosed with schizotypal personality disorder do not try to establish social relationships because they are uncomfortable around people. Conversely, their odd/eccentric behavior causes other people to tend to avoid them.

Page 163: *Solution*—

1. Individuals diagnosed with antisocial personality disorder tend to establish relationships with others in order to manipulate others for their personal gain. They perceive themselves as more clever than other people.
2. Individuals diagnosed with borderline personality disorder seek out relationships with others as they fear abandonment. Their relationships are unstable since they tend to idealize others until they are threatened by a real or imagined fear of abandonment. They quickly then may devalue those others.
3. Individuals with histrionic personality disorder seek out relationships with others because they are uncomfortable unless they are the center of attention. They display attention-seeking behavior (dramatic, seductive) when interacting with others. Interpersonal relationships tend to be superficial.
4. Individuals with narcissistic personality disorder exploit others to achieve their personal goals. They lack empathy, seek constant admiration and display a sense of entitlement. They see themselves as more important/special than others.

Page 164: *Solution*—

1. Individuals diagnosed with avoidant personality disorder desire relationships but are reluctant to enter into them due to a fear or rejection and embarrassment. They view themselves as inadequate and inferior and are shy and inhibited.
2. Individuals diagnosed with dependent personality disorder seek out relationships because they are anxious when alone due to a fear of being unable to do things for themselves. They lack self-confidence and fear abandonment.
3. Individuals diagnosed with obsessive-compulsive personality disorder tend to be emotionally constricted. In addition, their devotion to work and productivity negatively affects their relationships with others.

Page 165: *Solution*—The personality patterns associated with the various personality disorders reflect differences in individuals' attitudes toward interpersonal relationships. Their attitudes toward others reflect their feelings toward themselves. In addition, their attitudes determine their response to nursing care.

Chapter 9

Page 175: *Solution*—Having knowledge about a genetic predisposition to schizophrenia can be helpful to family members and clients. The power of this knowledge can assist individuals in identifying early signs and symptoms of the illness for early intervention and prevention of acute, crisis states of schizophrenia. This knowledge may also be helpful for reproductive counseling services. Research indicates, however, that genetic factors alone do not cause the development of schizophrenia. Other factors, such as the environment and psychological effects from maladaptive relationships, seem to play an important role in the development of schizophrenia.

Page 177: *Solution*—When clients are experiencing psychosis, they are not in touch with reality. They are disoriented and safety is in jeopardy. The safety of the client, others around them, and yourself is priority. The environment must be secure and free of potentially dangerous elements. There should be low levels of stimuli and increased vigilance of the client. The client will most likely need to be medicated to treat the psychosis and decrease agitation. Only after safety issues are addressed could other interventions be carried forth. Reality orientation techniques are important interventions to bring the client back in touch with the real world. Providing emotional support to the client and the families may help decrease anxieties and fears. There may also be a need to assist the client with activities of daily living (ADLs) during the period of active psychosis.

Page 178: *Solution*—Clients with medication non-adherence problems may be appropriate candidates for antipsychotic depot injections. These depot injections only need to be administered every 4 to 6 weeks depending on the clients' therapeutic reactions to the medication. Before the depot injection is given, an oral form of the medication must be administered to that client to assess for any adverse reactions to that medication. If an adverse reaction to the oral medication does occur, then the depot form of that medication should not be administered.

Page 179: *Solution*—A simple tool used to screen for tardive dyskinesia (TD) is the Abnormal and Involuntary Movement Scale (AIMS). This scale assesses for abnormal, involuntary movements of the tongue, face, trunk, and extremities of the body. The client is observed in several body positions. Severity of the symptoms of abnormal, involuntary movements is rated on a scale of 0 to 4. Zero is the score given for no signs of abnormal, involuntary movements. A score of one to four is given for increasingly severe signs of abnormal, involuntary movements. A client that receives any score other than zero needs to be referred for further evaluation of possible TD. The AIMS should be administered to the client every 3 to 6 months while receiving antipsychotic medications.

Page 180: *Solution*—One of the most important interventions that may prevent relapse is education. Educating family members or significant others about early signs of behaviors indicating relapse is a priority. Early intervention will help decrease the number and severity of relapses. Client and family education regarding the need for medication adherence, management of side effects, need to report any adverse reactions, and possible drug interactions is imperative. Other important interventions include referrals to appropriate community support systems, improved housing conditions, financial assistance programs, and access to medical and psychiatric clinics for followup care.

Chapter 10

Page 193: *Solution*—Possible causes of confusion in clients with a fractured hip (or other trauma) include:

1. Substance-induced delirium from ingestion of alcohol or pain medications such as narcotics, muscle relaxants, or benzodiazepines.
2. Psychosocial stress related to pain or the unfamiliar acute hospital setting.
3. Poor cerebral blood flow caused by complications from the fracture such as fat emboli, pulmonary emboli, blood loss, shock, and tachycardia.
4. General medical conditions occurring concomitantly in older adults such as atherosclerosis, arrythymias, vitamin deficiency, diabetes mellitus, COPD, and liver and kidney disease.
5. Diseases that predispose clients to falls and fractures, such as dementia of the Alzheimer's type, Parkinson's disease, chronic alcoholism, and vascular dementia.

Page 193: *Solution*—

1. Most important to obtain would be the client's vital signs, especially temperature (infection) and blood pressure (indication of cerebral blood flow).
2. Questions regarding the onset of confusion, illicit drug use, allergies, medication history, medical history, and previous episodes of confusion should then be asked to determine possible underlying causes.

Page 196: *Solution*—

1. Eliminate distracting background noise or shadows. Leave light on in bathroom.
2. Provide safe area where client can move about freely. Remove obstacles, throw rugs, and hazardous objects.
3. Place bed in low position, lower one side rail to prevent client from crawling over the foot of the bed to get up.
4. Avoid the use of physical restraints as they cause clients to become terrified and combative. Use only as a last resort when client is in imminent danger.
5. Evaluate medications for paradoxical effects. Limit caffeine use at night. Initiate toileting program, assist client to bathroom on regular basis, especially at night.

Page 199: *Solution*—

1. Stiff neck and difficulty swallowing may indicate an acute muscle dystonia due to potent antipsychotic medications used to control agitation such as chlorpromazine (Thorazine) or haloperidol (Haldol). Tremors and abnormal involuntary movements are other extrapyramidal effects associated with these medications.
2. Do not administer another dose of the sedative. Ask a staff member to stay with the client and observe for signs of choking, especially when eating. These symptoms should be reported immediately to the physician so that an anticholinergic or antihistamine can be ordered. Older adults are especially prone to developing tardive dyskinesia. This condition is aggravated by anticholinergics; therefore, the physician may order diphenhydramine (Benadryl) to control the extrapyramidal symptoms.
3. Reassure the client and family (if present) that the muscle stiffness and difficulty swallowing are temporary and will lessen with proper medication.

Page 201: *Solution*—

1. Respond to her concerns in a nonjudgmental, open manner. Use therapeutic techniques to encourage the wife to explore her feelings. (e.g., "This must be very hard for you. What other feelings do you have?")
2. Make arrangements for her to meet with a counselor (e.g., nurse clinician, social worker) to identify feelings and define a plan to regain a sense of control and facilitate grief work.
3. Encourage her input and maintain her involvement in her husband's care to help reduce feelings of guilt. Suggest she assist routinely in feeding her husband or other tasks without overwhelming or creating a sense of obligation.
4. Provide information regarding appropriate support groups in the community.
5. Encourage the wife to stay with the client and help arrange outings or home visits for holidays and special occasions.

Chapter 11

Page 215: *Solution*—Ask your client what he is specifically concerned about. Based on his response, you can encourage him to call the local chemical dependence treatment facility and discuss his concerns with a trained professional. If the son has alcohol-dependence issues, you could refer your client to Al-Anon to learn more about how alcohol has affected the family dynamics and how to begin healing.

Page 220: *Solution*—You need assessment data that focuses on the use of mood-altering chemicals. This includes a physical assessment/systems review, personal family assessment, chemical use assessment, medication assessment, OTC or nutritional supplement assessment, social history assessment, and laboratory value assessment.

Page 221: *Solution*—You are concerned the client may be experiencing tolerance. Tolerance is identified by a need for markedly increased amounts of a substance to achieve intoxication or desired effect, or markedly diminished effect with continued use of the same amount of the substance. This could mean that the client would need a higher dose of pain medication for pain relief and that the client might have an addiction problem. You may need to discuss your concern with the physician that the client may need an increased medication dose and also educate the client about signs and symptoms of substance abuse.

Page 225: *Solution*—The concern is that the client may be drinking or experiencing a reaction to an ingredient in the cleaning solution. You ask her to come to the office and bring the cleaning solution in its original container. If the intoxilyzer reading is negative, but you still have reason to believe the client was drinking, the physician may order a urine or blood drug abuse survey. If there is no indication that the client has been drinking, then exposure to alcohol occurred from contact with the cleaning solution or another product. In that case, preventing exposure to the product will minimize the likelihood of a reaction.

Page 227: *Solution*—The client needs education on the dynamics of chemical dependence including signs, symptoms, and defense mechanisms. You recognize that she is in the pre-contemplation or contemplation stage of change. You will take a laid-back approach using reflective listening and validation. You will help her discuss both the positive and negative aspects of alcohol use.

Chapter 12

Page 224: *Solution*—Child: Physical signs of sexual abuse include frequent urination or dysuria; venereal disease or gonorrhea of throat; pain or difficulty walking or sitting; foreign matter in bladder, rectum, urethra, or vagina; sleep problems such as insomnia or nightmares; bruises in genital or rectal area; rashes or itching in genital area, rectum, or vagina; scars in labia or rectal fissures.

Behavioral signs include overly sexualized behavior, seductive or advanced sexual knowledge, fear of a particular person or place, promiscuity or prostitution, compulsive masturbation or precocious sexual play, sexually abusing another child, unexplained gifts or money from questionable sources, drop in school performance, sudden onset of enuresis or encopresis, excess anxiety, compulsive bathing, running away from home, suicide attempts and self-destructive behaviors such as head banging.

Parents: Relationship with child, stressful situations in life, history of childhood sexual abuse in either parent, social isolation, unrealistic expectations of child, maladaptive coping mechanisms, problems with impulse control or low self esteem, substance abuse in either parent. Traits of the family: father—domineering, impulsive or physically abusive; mother—assive and submissive, battered. Structure of the family system: closed with rigid rules and rigid external boundaries. Enmeshment: internal boundaries poorly defined and characterized by excessive dependence on family members for physical and psychological needs, role reversal.

Page 246: *Solution*—Child: Provide for protection of the child by reporting abuse following facility's policies; treat child's injuries; reassure child that abuse was not his or her fault and that the child will be protected.

Parents: Approach with nonpunitive manner. Do teaching on reporting process, normal growth and development, anger management, stress management, parenting skills, communication skills. Teach appropriate disciplinary methods, the availability of and need for treatment for substance abuse if indicated. Provide resources available to them such as Parent's Anonymous, support groups, parenting classes, or employment counseling if indicated.

Page 248: *Solution*—Assess for imminent danger of situation: escalation in violence with increase in severity or frequency of attacks, weapons in the home, increased in use of substances, threats of homicide, or suicide by abuser.

Develop a safety plan: Ask neighbors to phone police if violence begins. Establish a code with family and friends to signify violence. Plan an escape route if the abuser blocks main exit. Determine a place to go and how to get there. Keep an escape bag available in a safe place with extra clothing for victim and children, children's favorite toys, and cash. Keep hidden and available extra copies of important papers such as driver's licenses, birth certificates, marriage license, insurance papers, social security numbers, bank account numbers, and important phone numbers.

Provide information about resources available: community resources, crisis line numbers, women's shelters or safe houses, legal assistance.

Page 250: *Solution*—Client: Has the client experienced verbal assaults, threats or intimidation, restriction of social contacts, violation of personal rights, unreasonable confinement, forced isolation or denial of privacy, abandonment, or threats of abandonment? Is there evidence of denial of needed food, clothing, or medical care or misuse or misappropriation of client's funds? Is the client financially dependent on the caregiver? Is client mentally ill or abusing substances?

Client's physical status: malnutrition and/or dehydration, untreated medical conditions, poor hygiene, lack of dental care, bruises, broken bones, healing fractures, unusual pattern of bruises or lacerations such as rope burns on ankles or wrists.

Caregiver: Relationship with the client, personal problems, a lack of support systems, increased level of stress in caring for elder, a history of family violence, unresolved previous conflicts and power struggles, evidence the behavior may be in retaliation for past behavior of elder, attitude toward the client, evidence of mental illness or substance abuse. Are there signs of aggression within the relationship?

Page 254: *Solution*—

- Reassure clients that rape is not their fault and survival was the most important outcome.
- Advise about potential for pregnancy and sexually transmitted disease.
- Provide information about community services such as survivors groups, shelters for battered women, and legal service.
- If sexual assault is by a partner, provide options: staying with abuser, removing abuser through arrest, obtaining protective orders to keep abuser away, or leaving abuser.
- Assist with development of a safety plan if the victim is returning to the environment with the abuser.

Chapter 13

Page 262: *Solution*—Clients dealing with loss and the families of these clients often experience many physiological and psychological responses. Physiological responses may include crying and sobbing, fatigue, weakness and exhaustion, insomnia, and loss of appetite. Psychological responses may include intense loneliness and sadness, depressed mood, anxiety or panic episodes, difficulty concentrating and focusing, anger or rage directed toward self or others, ambivalence, and low self-esteem, as well as somatic complaints.

Page 265: *Solution*—You suspect the wife is experiencing anticipatory grief. Anticipatory grief is the process of disengaging or "letting go" that occurs before the actual loss or death has occurred. Significant others and family members may withdraw emotionally from the dying client in order to disengage or begin the "letting go" process for themselves. They may find it too difficult to provide physical as well as emotional support because they will be confronted with the reality of death.

Page 268: *Solution*—Males and females often express grief differently. Traditional approaches to bereavement counseling are designed to facilitate feminine grief. Most counselors emphasize showing empathy; some encourage, even insist, that the griever reminisce about the loss, experiencing and then expressing painful feelings. Masculine grievers find the focus on feelings unhelpful and may resent being urged to express them. Male or masculine grief is usually limited and toned down; thinking precedes and often dominates feelings; focus is on problem-solving rather than expression of feelings; outward expression of feelings often involve anger and/or guilt; and intense feelings may be experienced privately.

Page 271: *Solution*—An advance directive is a general term that refers to a client's written instructions about future medical care, in the event that the client becomes unable to speak or incapacitated. The client can choose between developing a living will or identifying a healthcare proxy or both. A living will or durable power of attorney for health care is a set of specifically written instructions about what medical treatment the client chooses to omit or refuse (e.g., ventilator support) in the event that the client is unable to make those decisions. A healthcare proxy is a document appointing someone else (e.g., a relative or trusted friend) to manage health care treatment decisions when the client is unable to do so.

Page 274: *Solution*—The nurse would assess the client's and family's current knowledge and understanding of the implication of the illness and impeding death, the client's ability to provide self-care, the client's and family's current and past coping strategies, current manifestations of grief, role expectations and role changes, availability of support people, client's knowledge and documentation of advance directives, as well as need for community resources. At the end of life, the nurse intervenes in ways that bring comfort to clients and families, even when hope for cure is gone. Promoting an environment that supports and fosters the completion of the essential tasks of bringing closure to life and relationships is the primary goal of nursing.

Chapter 14

Page 284: *Solution*—"It sounds like you are very concerned. However, it is typical that people feel somewhat depressed about a diagnosis that may disrupt one's usual level of functioning. Adolescents often feel upset as they are also struggling with issues related to self-image and self-esteem."

Page 286: *Solution*—"The occurrence of medical illnesses can be influenced by stress. Higher stress levels can result in an increased number of asthmatic episodes."

Page 287: *Solution*—"I can see that you are very concerned. It is important to understand that there are cognitive changes with the progression of HIV/AIDS that are not within the control of your friend. He needs continued support and care."

Page 290: *Solution*—Important assessments include psychological, biological, social, subjective/objective symptoms, family/significant other reports, and diagnostic reports.

Page 290: *Solution*—Priority nursing diagnoses include Body image disturbance and Alteration in self-image and self-esteem related to functional changes associated with medical illness diagnosis.

➤ Case Study Suggested Answers

Chapter 1

1. The nurse demonstrated two attentive skills toward the client that communicate respect for individuals. First, the nurse approached the client and sat down close to her. She complimented the client on her appearance and asked the client how she was doing. Second, the nurse offered herself by sharing with the client that she had an hour that she could use to spend with the client.

2. When the nurse approached the client and asked her how she was doing, the client leaned away, maintained a rigid posture, avoided eye contact, and only nodded her head in response. The nurse reacted by leaning back and crossing her arms over her chest to create what she thought would be a less threatening posture. However, leaning away from the client and crossing her arms over her chest communicated distance and unavailability to the client. In addition, the nurse communicated to the client that she would spend an hour with her; however, when the client would not respond, the nurse assumed the client did not want to talk and left after only 25 minutes. This was inconsistent communication. This would foster mistrust and lack of confidence in the client's feelings toward the nurse.

3. A depressed client often is quiet and noncommunicative. Clients experiencing depression often have difficulty identifying their own feelings and thoughts. The client could have been using the time to collect her own thoughts in order to communicate her feelings and thoughts more clearly to the nurse. The client may have been testing the nurse's trustworthiness by seeing if the nurse would do what she said she would do by spending the hour with the client, whether the client spoke or not.

4. Instead of initially reacting to the client by leaning back and crossing her arms over her chest, the nurse could have better communicated by leaning forward and having an open posture. Leaning forward and having an open posture communicates willingness to be present with the client. Once the nurse offered an hour of her time for the client, she should have stayed the entire hour even though the client did not want to share. This would have promoted trustworthiness. The nurse could have communicated that it was okay for the client to be silent and that the nurse would sit with her in silence for the hour or until the client was ready to share. Silence is an effective therapeutic technique.

5. The nurse assumed the client did not want to share. Instead of confirming with the client her assumption, she acted incorrectly on the client's silence. The nurse may have been uncomfortable with silence and felt the need to leave the situation. Nurses must understand the importance of silence as a therapeutic technique and respect a client's need to not share while remaining in the presence of the client.

Chapter 2

1. Risk factors for this client include:
   - Age over 50 years
   - Males are higher risk than females
   - Whites are at higher risk than non-whites (Native Americans or African Americans)
   - Single, divorced, or widowed
   - Retirement or loss of job
   - Mental illness diagnosis: major depression
   - Recent losses: moving from his home and loss of family pet
2. Priority nursing diagnoses include:
   - Risk for self-directed violence related to feelings of loss and hopelessness
   - Ineffective individual coping related to situational crisis (suicide attempt) and relocation
   - Hopelessness related to perception of worthlessness
3. Nursing interventions include:
   - Establish a therapeutic relationship
   - Ensure the safety of the client by communicating the potential for suicide
   - Stay with the client
   - Listen to the client's concerns
   - Give the client a message of hope
4. This client will:
   - Experience no physical harm to self
   - Set realistic goals for self and future
   - Express some optimism and hope for the future
5. The nurse should take the following precautions:
   - Initiate suicide precautions
   - Begin to establish trust
   - Establish in each 24-hour period a verbal contract to not harm self
   - Offer positive encouragement for the client remaining free of injury
   - Ensure a safe environment: remove sharp objects, toxic substances, and clothing that could be used for self-harm, and place client on close supervision

Chapter 3

1. Information about the behaviors that the boy displayed as an infant and as a small child would help make an accurate assessment. For instance, consider his ability to concentrate, ease of distractibility, overt acts of hostility, the manner in which he deals with frustration, and specific learning problems.
2. Severe and persistent antisocial behaviors would differentiate conduct disorder from ADHD. Behaviors include physical aggression and cruelty to people and animals, anger, and no indication of guilt or remorse for actions.

3. The boy has the ability to communicate with others and is not severely socially impaired. He exhibits no ritualistic behaviors or unusual motor behaviors that are associated with autistic disorders.

4. CNS stimulants increase the child's ability to focus attention by blocking out irrelevant thoughts and impulses. Some stimulants are effective immediately (Ritalin and Dexedrine) and they lead to significant improvement in 70 to 75 percent of ADHD cases.

5. There are several interventions that could be helpful for this client. Socialization enhancement will increase his ability to negotiate stressful interpersonal situations with his siblings, parents, and classmates. It will also help him develop a more positive self-perception. Self-esteem enhancement allows a shift in focus from negative behaviors to positive behaviors, making the client feel better about himself.

Chapter 4

1. Initial questions should include topics related to suicidality, reason for being brought/coming to the unit, and recent significant stressors (within the last few months) that may have contributed to this manic state/relapse. It is also important for the nurse to assess the presence of hallucinations, flight of ideas, or delusions. The following are examples of appropriate questions:
   - "How did you get to the hospital today?"
   - "Have you ever been hospitalized before? Where? When? For how long?"
   - "Do you feel you want to hurt yourself right now?" If yes, inquire about a plan.
   - "Has anything happened in the last few months that you think could be significant to your being here today?"
   - "Are you hearing voices or seeing things that are unusual?"
   - Can you tell me what you usually do on a typical Tuesday from the time you get up in the morning until you go to bed at night?"

2. Based on the intake assessment data, this client will need to have a physical examination, safe environment, and frequent checks by healthcare workers until the staff is sure the client is no longer a safety risk to self or others.

3. This client will probably be prescribed lithium carbonate (Lithium) PO. If the assessment data indicates, he may also be given a benzodiazepine or an antipsychotic if necessary until the effects of the Lithium can be seen (2 to 4 weeks). Then, these medications can be slowly withdrawn.

4. The nurse will recognize the cues indicating fatigue/need for sleep and will:
   - Decrease environmental stimuli in room and common areas.
   - Restrict intake of caffeine (coffee, tea, cocoa, cola, etc.).
   - Offer small snack/warm milk at bedtime or when awake during the night.

Chapter 5

1. Based on what is known about this client, either social isolation or impaired social interactions would probably be the most appropriate nursing diagnosis.
2. Additional information related to the client's level of self-esteem, quality and quantity of social support, and effective coping strategies used for similar problems would be essential. Specific examples of the client's perceptions of stressors in social situations that lead to anxiety, and examples of interactions with other people that have been both positive and negative, would also enhance understanding of the client.
3. Several steps may prove useful to achieve this outcome. Such steps might include:
   - Establishing a trusting one-to-one therapeutic relationship with the client.
   - Encouraging the client to verbalize feelings about interactions with others.
   - Teaching and role-playing interpersonal skills.
   - Introducing the client to other people on the unit.
   - Assisting the client to identify people on the unit with whom she might like to interact.
   - Involving the client in an activity she enjoys, and ask one other person to join in the activity.
   - Gradually including more people in the activity.
   - If the client's anxiety increases beyond the moderate level while engaged in an activity with others, allowing the client to leave the activity and discussing the incident with her.
   - Providing positive reinforcement when the client interacts with others.
4. Because the client complains of muscle tension, the best relaxation technique would be some form of progressive muscle relaxation.
5. The first step would be to ask the client to clarify what feeling "more comfortable" means by asking for specific examples of what the client would like to accomplish. Changes in behaviors and feeling could then be compared to baseline data. The staff could keep a record of the frequency and duration of the client's interactions with others and compare finding over time. Direct observation and evaluation of the quality of interactions with others would provide useful information. Asking the client to use a diary to record relevant information could provide a useful self-assessment tool. Using a standardized assessment tool to measure the client's level of anxiety before and after interactions could provide more objective data for the evaluation process.

Chapter 6

1. Pain symptoms are "real" and the nurse should not dismiss them as "only in the client's head." In order to not reinforce the pain symptoms, however, the nurse must assess the pain before and after G. A. receives analgesics with a concerned, but matter-of-fact attitude. Because G. A.'s pain symptoms may be his predominant way of expressing himself and be-

cause he is unlikely to be aware of the relationship between mind and body, the nurse should also encourage him to talk, to express verbally his concerns or difficulties in his life. If the pain is significant, talk *after* the medication has taken effect. If easily distracted during the assessment, the nurse may encourage verbalization at that time.

2. Chronic pain often results in hopelessness, helplessness, irritability, and other symptoms of depression.
3. The nurse should acknowledge G. A.'s pain and the use of medications, but help him to understand the role of other therapies such as group therapy that may help him decrease his stress (hence, muscle tension and pain): "When you are hurting, it's hard to think about going to group or thinking that talking will help. Talking about what is going on in your life can help reduce stress, because pain is worsened when stress causes an increase in muscle tension."
4. Somatoform disorders, of which pain disorder is a part, often originate when clients are unable to verbally express problems, conflicts, or dependency needs. Pain disorder is not caused by consciously wanting to avoid work, nor is it "pretending" to have pain. Rather, the pain symptoms "speak" for G. A.
5. The nurse could teach G. A. about the stress-tension-pain cycle, thus setting up the groundwork for relaxation training techniques. Autogenic training, progressive muscle relaxation, and visualization are all effective relaxation training techniques. In addition, the teaching plan could include the effective use of medication (noting the effect of alcohol on pain medications), distraction, and physical activity.

Chapter 7

1. Given the diagnoses of both depression and dissociative identity disorder, several safety issues should be anticipated. First, physical safety may be an issue if the client is suicidal; hence, initial and continued assessment for suicidal ideation is indicated. Physical safety may also be jeopardized by self-mutilation. Although rarely lethal, self-mutilation can be serious with deep burns or cuts that require extensive treatment if severe. Different alters (personalities) may also be more self-destructive than others, and talking about difficult memories in therapy may produce sufficient affective instability and pain that the client feels self-destructive. The emotional safety of the client is also an issue. Having experienced a childhood of abuse, the client does not readily trust or feel safe.
2. Dissociative disorders are rare and fascinating, but they are painful in origin and painful to endure. Talking with the nursing assistants about dissociative identity disorder and its origins, including the dehumanization of the child, may help them see the client not as a curiosity, but as a human being struggling to cope. In addition, introducing the nursing assistants (individually) to the client will reduce the exotic nature of the disorder and create an opportunity for a therapeutic relationship with all staff.
3. "Mapping" (sketching) the personality system, noting age, gender, and other characteristics, including which alters share consciousness and memories, can decrease confusion. The client's alter personalities may be helpful in creating the map, depending upon the level of acceptance of the diagnosis and the cooperation of various personalities. The host personality is initially unaware of the alters. Additionally, when unsure with whom you are speaking, the nurse can ask, "With whom am I speaking?" or "Who is here now?" when the client is nonverbal.
4. All family members are affected by the behavior and mood of the client with dissociative identity disorder. Family therapy can be helpful in a number of ways. First, teaching the family about the disorder names and identifies the phenomenon so that imagination and fears do not fill the information gap. Second, children are keen observers and are quite aware of the client's affective and behavioral "switches," and they need to learn to deal with, and not manipulate child alters, in particular. Third, family members can learn how to help the client avoid dissociating and how to handle hostile personalities. Finally, the family therapist can work with the family's own interactional patterns so that the family is a healthy place for all members as healing takes place.
5. It is not uncommon for even professional staff to doubt the validity of the disorder itself, or to make the error in logic that an effect (getting "attention" during hospitalization and therapy) is the intention. The possession of material resources or even good family support will not prevent the pain of dissociative identity disorder, nor will it prevent *any* mental disorder. Both family and material resources can make the healing process less difficult, but not easy. The nurse may be uneducated, manifesting counter-transference, or have issues regarding power in relationships (seeing and concerned with client "manipulation").

Chapter 8

1. Priority nursing diagnoses include:
    - High risk for violence, self-directed (self-mutilation) related to intense emotional pain including rage and a sense of emptiness coupled with poor impulse control.
    - Impaired social interaction related to overidealization and devaluation of the self and others.
    - Personal identify disturbance related to feelings of emptiness.
2. The priority goal is maintenance of client safety—client will not harm herself. Secondary goals include to begin to recognize the tendency to dichotomous thinking—idealizing and devaluing others in response to a fear of abandonment, and to begin to recognize the effect of a feeling of emptiness on functioning and mood.
3. It is especially important to promote client collaboration in the maintenance of her own safety. Her collaboration in the development of the other goals will depend in part on her level of insight into the effect of her behavior on her functional impairment and subjective distress.

4. Nursing interventions include:
   - To maintain client safety, the implementation of an anti-harm contract, staff and client self-monitoring, and identifying behavioral triggers and alternative coping strategies are all important.
   - As a step in diminishing the tendency toward dichotomous thinking, the nurse can help the client recognize when it is occurring.
   - As a step in enhancing client's sense of self, encouraging her to identify her own strengths is important.
5. The nursing interventions should be evaluated in relationship to the goals—the most important goal being maintenance of client safety.

Chapter 9

1. Clients with a diagnosis of schizophrenia, paranoid type typically present with auditory hallucinations and delusional thought processes. Delusions are usually of a persecutory type. This client may appear hostile and angry. Disorganized speech patterns, behaviors, and flat or inappropriate affect are not present to any significant degree.
2. This client's priority of care is safety of self and others. During an acute phase, safety is a critical issue. As a result of this client's paranoid delusional system, potential for violence is high. Environmental safety factors should include a milieu free of potential harmful objects/sharps and special client observation protocols/vigilance.
3. Several nursing diagnoses may be appropriate for this client's plan of care. The nursing diagnoses that are *most likely* to be included consist of:
   - Risk for violence directed at self or others
   - Altered thought processes
   - Social isolation
   - Sensory or perceptual alterations
   - Impaired home maintenance management
4. Paranoid schizophrenic clients have difficulty establishing trust as a result of their suspicious delusions. Several interventions may be helpful to begin fostering trust with this client. The nurse must be consistent and honest with the client. Communication must be clear and concise. Promises should never be made to the client. The nurse should avoid challenging the content of the client's delusions. Objectivity must be maintained, and the nurse should listen actively to the client's verbalizations. Maintaining the client's personal space and using touch carefully is important. The nurse may offer the client food and beverages in closed, sealed containers. The client's care should be provided by staff members consistently assigned to him/her.
5. This client has had multiple hospital admissions because of a history of poor medication adherence with antipsychotic medications. To prevent this problem from repeatedly occurring in the future, the nurse may explore several interventions. First of all, the reason for the poor medication adherence must be determined. It may be that the client is having adverse reactions or side effects from psychotropic medications. If this is the reason, an option may be to change to another antipsychotic medication with a different mechanism of action. Anticholinergic medications may be helpful. Other reasons for poor medication adherence may be a lack of support systems at home. Support systems are very important for prevention of exacerbation in chronic illnesses such as schizophrenia. Community resources must be explored before this client is discharged from the hospital. Administration of antipsychotic medications in the form of depot injections should be explored for overcoming nonadherence issues.

Chapter 10

1. The initial assessments to make include:
   - Baseline vital signs, which are necessary to ascertain signs of infection, cardiac arrythmia, or vascular problems.
   - Mini-Mental State Examination, which is important to determine an objective measure of cognitive impairment for future comparison.
   - Head-to-toe physical assessment, concentrating on abnormal findings to determine a possible physiological cause for the confusion.
   - Further pertinent information; if any family members are present, ask them to provide further information regarding preferred routines, food likes and dislikes, and family information that would be helpful when communicating with G. B.
2. The three nursing diagnoses that are appropriate in the care of G. B. are:
   - Risk for injury or trauma related to episodes of confusion.
   - Sleep pattern disturbances related to sundown syndrome.
   - Anxiety related to fear of cognitive deficits and unfamiliar surroundings.
3. The outcome/evaluation criteria that might be appropriate for G.B. include:
   - The client will be free of injury as evidenced by absence of falls, burns, or bruises.
   - The client will sleep 5 to 7 hours per night and remain calm and quiet in the evening.
   - The client will verbalize decreased anxiety and intact orientation to person, place, and time, especially in late afternoon and early evening hours.
4. Four nursing interventions aimed at promoting safety and security for G. B. and her family could include:
   - Eliminate distracting background noise or shadows. Leave light on in bathroom.
   - Place bed in low position; lower one side rail to prevent client from crawling over the foot of the bed to get up.
   - Provide a simple, structured environment with consistent personnel to minimize confusion and provide a sense of security and stability in the client's environment.
   - Allow client to have familiar objects around her to maintain reality orientation and enhance self-worth and dignity.

5. Your response to G. B.'s daughter might include:
   - Encouraging the daughter to reflect the underlying feeling of concern (e.g., "You miss Daddy. It must be lonely here without him.")
   - Encouraging the daughter to discuss topics that are meaningful to her mother, such as past events occurring in the family; bring and discuss photos of her children and grandchildren.
   - Explaining that reality orientation and validation therapy that is geared toward the person and place rather than to the time is more effective in decreasing confusion.

Chapter 11

1. Important additional information includes:
   - Blackout or lost consciousness. Blacking out or passing out can be related to one's use of alcohol or other substances.
   - Changes in bowel movement. Persons using alcohol and/or drugs frequently can experience changes in bowel movement. Changes range from diarrhea related to drinking to constipation related to using pain medications frequently. Withdrawal from narcotics can cause diarrhea.
   - Weight loss or weight gain. Persons using alcohol or drugs regularly may experience weight loss/gain and/or poor nutritional balance.
   - Experiencing stressful situations. Stress can precipitate an increase in drinking; stress can also result from drinking or using drugs regularly.
   - Sleep problems. Persons using alcohol and/or other drugs experience all sorts of sleep problems. One may start using alcohol to promote sleep, but once someone develops tolerance, sleep is more difficult.
   - Chronic pain. Persons experiencing chronic pain may use drugs and/or alcohol to self-medicate.
   - Concern over substance use. If friends and relatives worry about substance use, it is generally because there is something to be concerned about.
   - Cutting down on alcohol consumption (or drug use, prescription medications, gambling, or addictive behavior). If a person feels that he or she must cut down, it is usually because there are problems.
   - Infections: systemic, viral, sepsis or localized infection. IV drug abuse and alcohol abuse can cause these medical problems: hepatitis, HIV, TB, endocarditis, kidney abscesses, unexplained urosepsis, syphilis, and infection/abscess at local injection sites.
   - Anorexia, nausea, vomiting, hematemesis. Cirrhosis can be caused by alcohol abuse or narcotic abuse.
   - Cardiac rhythm disturbances. Persons who regularly abuse cocaine suffer from electrocardiographic abnormalities.
   - Dyspnea, wheezing, tachypnea, wheezing cyanosis. Cocaine abusers suffer from abnormal pulmonary function tests.
   - Flank pain radiating to groin, hematuria, urinary frequency. Alcohol abuse can cause pathologic renal conditions.
2. The nursing assessment should focus on the following body systems:
   - Gastrointestinal
   - Liver
   - Cardiac
   - Respiratory
   - Neurologic
   - Endocrine
   - Reproductive
   - Nutritional status
3. The following lab values would be helpful:
   - Gamma glutamyl transferase (GGT)
   - Aspartate aminotranferase (SGOT/SGPT)
   - Alkaline phosphatase (AK)
   - Lactate dehydrogenase (LD)
   - Mean corpuscular volume (MCV)
   - Urine toxicology and blood screen for drugs of abuse is also an essential component of the substance use evaluation.
4. Obtain the following information:
   - Type of substance used
   - Type of compulsive behavior
   - Pattern/frequency
   - Amount
   - Age at onset
   - Age of regular use
   - Changes in use patterns
   - Periods of abstinence in history
   - Previous withdrawal symptoms
   - Date of last substance use/compulsive behavior
   - Ask about each substance or behavior separately
5. Focus is on safety:
   - Maintain safe environment.
   - Orient to time, place, and person.
   - Maintain adequate nutrition and fluid balance.
   - Monitor for beginning of withdrawal signs and symptoms.
   - Create a low-stimulation environment.
   - Monitor vital signs and withdrawal symptoms: nausea/vomiting, tremor, paroxysmal sweats, anxiety, agitation, tactile disturbances, auditory disturbances, visual disturbances, headache or fullness in head, disorientation and sensorium
   - While female clients may have been initially screened for pregnancy, they should be screened later in the episode of care be sure that any medication use potentially harmful to the fetus is minimized. Alcohol is the most harmful drug of all and the most harmful to the fetus of any drug at all.
   - Monitor for delirium tremens, psychotic symptoms, and suicide/seizure risk.
   - Administer the withdrawal medication: anticonvulsants; benzodiazepines, sedative vitamins, or other medications

as ordered thiamine help to prevent confusion and other mental status changes.

- Maintain adequate nutrition and fluid intake.
- Maintain normal comfort measures.
- Monitor for covert substance use during detox period.
- Provide emotional support and reassurance to client and family.
- Provide reality orientations and address hallucinations in a therapeutic manner.
- Advise client of the depressive uneasy feelings and the fatigue that is usually experienced during withdrawal.
- Begin to educate the client about the disease of addiction and the initial treatment goal of abstinence.

Chapter 12

1. Important information to gather includes:
   - Do the details about the cause of injuries match the actual injuries?
   - When did the injury take place; was there a delay in seeking treatment?
   - Relationship to the child; family structure; patterns and methods of discipline; unreasonable expectations of the child; problems with pregnancy, labor, or delivery with this child; substance abuse in the family; history of family violence; mother being battered.
   - Availability and use of support systems; social isolation.

2. *Current injuries*: Unusual pattern such as bite marks, burns in shape of objects, or glove-like burns from immersion in hot liquids; bruises in various stages of healing, especially on head and neck; bald spots that would indicate hair pulled out; old fractures, scars, welts, lacerations, or internal injuries.

3. Behavioral extremes such as rage, aggression, or passivity; fear of parents or caregiver; apprehension when other children cry; verbal reports of abuse; hyperactivity; distractibility or hypervigilance; disorganized thinking; self-injurious or suicidal behavior; running away from home or illegal behaviors; school performance; poor relationships with peers; inappropriately dressed for weather; regressed behaviors such as enuresis, encopresis, and thumb-sucking.

4. The child's safety and well-being would be the priority. Report the suspected abuse following facility policies and procedures; reassure the child that he or she is not to blame; treat the child's immediate injuries.

5. Mother needs to be approached nonjudgmentally and taught normal child growth and development to reduce unrealistic expectations of the child that are often present with child abuse. If the mother is not the abuser, she should be taught how to keep the child safe. Teach parenting skills, anger management, stress management, communication skills, and what resources are available to the family.

Chapter 13

1. Adults often believe—or want to believe—that children do not understand death and should be protected from all death-related situations or discussions. The facts are quite different. Children are naturally curious about loss, dying, and death. Furthermore, no child is too young to experience the anxiety associated with separation experiences. Children between the ages of 5 and 9 years understand that death is final; however, they believe their own deaths can be avoided. Many of these children will fear the dying and death process because they may associate death with aggression or violence. They may view death as a person who comes and takes them away from their family. In addition, these children may experience guilt or shame because they believe past wishes or unrelated actions are responsible for their death.
2. Assessment of children and family members in the grieving or mourning process includes an accurate perception of the loss from their viewpoint. The nurse begins by identifying the loss and the family's perception of the impact of their loss. The nurse should use the opportunity for the child to express his concerns through conversation, play, drawing, and writing. The nurse should seek to understand the nature of the family's attachment to the lost child, assess past experience with loss, and determine the impact those have on the family's present experience. It is important for the nurse to assess cultural rituals and rules about mourning to understand the unique experience of grieving individuals.
3. Important nursing diagnoses for the child and family who are experiencing impeding death include Fear, Hopelessness, Powerlessness, Risk for caregiver role strain, Altered family processes, Impaired adjustment, Self-esteem disturbance, and Spiritual distress. Possible nursing diagnoses for survivors of a family member who has died include Anticipatory grieving; Dysfunctional grieving; Social isolation; Altered role performance; Risk for altered parenting; Ineffective family coping: compromised; and Family coping: potential for growth.
4. Living with loss is a normal but very stressful part of life. When coping with loss through grieving or mourning, people may respond in adaptive or maladaptive ways. Some never lose their sense of despair. The loss of a child is one of life's most difficult losses. When evaluating the family's movement toward goals, the nurse should evaluate the family's personal understanding of their feelings about and reaction to loss and grief, the family's ability to discuss their response and reaction to loss and grief, whether family members have resumed baseline sleeping and eating patterns, and have resumed daily activities and roles as they accept their loss.
5. Once the child has died, the family will experience bereavement of their loss. Bereavement is a change in status caused by losing a family member, friend, colleague, or other significant person through death. The family will experience a

shifting mix of feelings, including disbelief, anxiety, anger, sadness and confusion. This condition is known as grief. The family will express their bereavement and loss to others in ways that are culturally patterned. This is known as mourning.

Chapter 14

1. Symptoms of depression include feelings of hopelessness/helplessness, flat affect, poor eye contact, disrupted patterns of eating or sleeping, absence of motivation/compliance, and decreased energy level.
2. Important assessments include spirituality, cultural, biological, psychosocial assessments; also assess developmental level and coping skills.
3. Nursing diagnoses include Ineffective individual coping related to occurrence and effect of medical illness; Alteration in self-esteem and self-image related to function changes associated with medical illness diagnosis.
4. Nursing interventions include empathy, compassion, spirituality reinforcement, support, dignity, control, and pain management.
5. "It sounds like it is difficult to find meaning in your life."

Credits

Chapter 1

Fig. 1-1 Art, Source: *Mental Health Nursing,* by K. L. Fontaine, J. S. Fletcher, Edition 4, 1999, Addison-Wesley, Menlo Park, CA; Page 5, Fig. 1-1; Precision Graphics.

Fig. 1-2 Art, Source: *Mental Health Nursing,* by K. L. Fontaine, J. S. Fletcher, Edition 4, 1999, Addison-Wesley, Menlo Park, CA; Page 91, Fig. 5-1; Precision Graphics.

Fig. 1-3 Art, Source: *Mental Health Nursing,* by K. L. Fontaine, J. S. Fletcher, Edition 4, 1999, Addison-Wesley, Menlo Park, CA; Page 62, Fig. 3-1; Precision Graphics.

Chapter 4

Fig. 4-1 Art, Source: *Mental Health Nursing,* by K. L. Fontaine, J. S. Fletcher, Edition 4, 1999, Addison-Wesley, Menlo Park, CA; Page 236, Fig. 11-1; Precision Graphics.

Chapter 6

Fig. 6-1 Art, © Prentice Hall Health, Upper Saddle River, New Jersey; Precision Graphics.

Fig. 6-2 Art, © Prentice Hall Health, Upper Saddle River, New Jersey; Precision Graphics.

Chapter 7

Fig. 7-1 Art, © Prentice Hall Health, Upper Saddle River, New Jersey; Precision Graphics.

Fig. 7-2 Art, © Prentice Hall Health, Upper Saddle River, New Jersey; Precision Graphics.

Chapter 10

Fig. 10-1 Art, From *Medical Surgical Nursing: Critical Thinking in Client Care,* by Priscilla LeMone, Karen M. Burke, Edition 2, © 2000 by Prentice-Hall, Inc., Upper Saddle River, New Jersey; Page 1818, Fig. 42-1; Artist: Kristin N. Mount.

Index

Page numbers followed by *f* indicate figure; those followed by *t* indicate table; those followed by *b* indicate box.

D

T

U

V